BMA

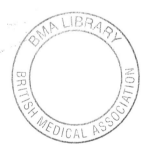

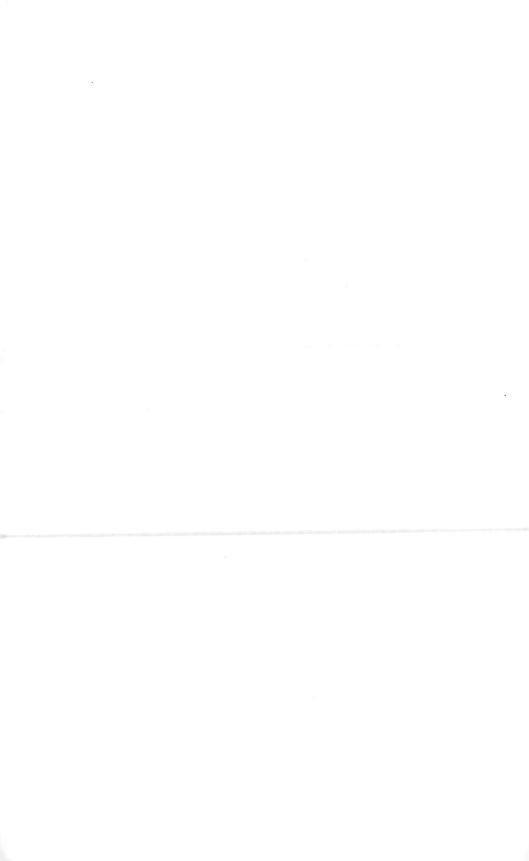

PERSONALISED MEDICINE, INDIVIDUAL CHOICE AND THE COMMON GOOD

Hippocrates famously advised doctors, 'it is far more important to know *what person the disease has* than *what disease the person has*'. Yet 2,500 years later, 'personalised medicine', based on individual genetic profiling and the achievements of genomic research, claims to be revolutionary. In this book, experts from a wide range of disciplines critically examine this claim. They expand the discussion of personalised medicine beyond its usual scope to include many other highly topical issues, including:

- human nuclear genome transfer ('three-parent IVF')
- stem cell-derived gametes
- private umbilical cord blood banking
- international trade in human organs
- biobanks such as the US Precision Medicine Initiative
- direct-to-consumer genetic testing
- health and fitness self-monitoring

Although these technologies often prioritise individual choice, the original ideal of genomic research saw the human genome as 'the common heritage of humanity'. The authors question whether personalised medicine actually threatens this conception of the common good.

BRITTA VAN BEERS is an associate professor at VU University Amsterdam. As a legal philosopher she explores the notions of personhood and corporality within the regulation of biomedical technologies, such as assisted reproductive technologies, markets in human body materials and biomedical tourism. In 2011 she received the Praemium Erasmianum Research Prize for her PhD dissertation on the legal relationship between persons and their bodies in the era of medical biotechnology (2009). Recent publications include the co-edited volumes *Humanity in International Law and Biolaw* (Cambridge University Press, 2014) and *Symbolic Legislation and Developments in Biolaw* (2016).

SIGRID STERCKX is a founding member of the Bioethics Institute Ghent. Her current research projects focus on ethical and legal aspects of: human tissue research and biobanking; patenting in biomedicine and genomics; organ transplantation; medical end-of-life practices; neuroethics; and global justice. She has published more than 150 articles, book chapters and books on these issues, including the co-authored book *Exclusions from Patentability* (Cambridge University Press, 2012) and the co-edited volume *Continuous Sedation at the End of Life: Ethical, Clinical and Legal Perspectives* (Cambridge University Press, 2013). Sigrid also serves on various advisory committees, including the Ethics Committee of Ghent University Hospital.

DONNA DICKENSON is the author of one of the first books to take a balanced critical stance on personalised medicine, *Me Medicine vs We Medicine: Reclaiming Biotechnology for the Common Good* (2013). She is Emeritus Professor of Medical Ethics and Humanities at the University of London and a research associate at the HeLEX Centre at the University of Oxford. Previously she taught at Imperial College School of Medicine, London. For many years she served on the Ethics Committee of the UK Royal College of Obstetricians and Gynaecologists. She has written or edited twenty-five books, as well as over one hundred articles and chapters. In 2006 she became the first woman to win the international Spinoza Lens Award for her contribution to public debate on current ethical issues about the impact of biotechnology on our society.

CAMBRIDGE BIOETHICS AND LAW

This series of books was founded by Cambridge University Press with Alexander McCall Smith as its first editor in 2003. It focuses on the law's complex and troubled relationship with medicine across both the developed and the developing world. Since the early 1990s, we have seen, in many countries, increasing resort to the courts by dissatisfied patients and a growing use of the courts to attempt to resolve intractable ethical dilemmas. At the same time, legislatures across the world have struggled to address the questions posed by both the successes and the failures of modern medicine, while international organisations such as the WHO and UNESCO now regularly address issues of medical law.

It follows that we would expect ethical and policy questions to be integral to the analysis of the legal issues discussed in this series. The series responds to the high profile of medical law in universities and in legal and medical practice, as well as in public and political affairs. We seek to reflect the evidence that many major health-related policy debates in the UK, Europe and the international community involve a strong medical law dimension. With that in mind, we seek to address how legal analysis might have a trans-jurisdictional and international relevance. Organ retention, embryonic stem cell research, physician-assisted suicide and the allocation of resources to fund health care are but a few examples among many. The emphasis of this series is thus on matters of public concern and/or practical significance. We look for books that could make a difference to the development of medical law and enhance the role of medico-legal debate in policy circles. That is not to say that we lack interest in the important theoretical dimensions of the subject, but we aim to ensure that theoretical debate is grounded in the realities of how the law does and should interact with medicine and health care.

Series Editors

Professor Graeme Laurie, *University of Edinburgh*
Professor Richard Ashcroft, *Queen Mary University of London*

PERSONALISED MEDICINE, INDIVIDUAL CHOICE AND THE COMMON GOOD

Edited by

BRITTA VAN BEERS
VU University Amsterdam

SIGRID STERCKX
Ghent University

DONNA DICKENSON
Birkbeck College, University of London

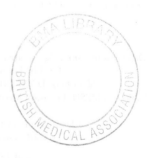

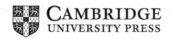

CAMBRIDGE
UNIVERSITY PRESS

CAMBRIDGE
UNIVERSITY PRESS

University Printing House, Cambridge CB2 8BS, United Kingdom

One Liberty Plaza, 20th Floor, New York, NY 10006, USA

477 Williamstown Road, Port Melbourne, VIC 3207, Australia

314–321, 3rd Floor, Plot 3, Splendor Forum, Jasola District Centre,
New Delhi – 110025, India

79 Anson Road, #06–04/06, Singapore 079906

Cambridge University Press is part of the University of Cambridge.

It furthers the University's mission by disseminating knowledge in the pursuit of
education, learning, and research at the highest international levels of excellence.

www.cambridge.org
Information on this title: www.cambridge.org/9781108473910
DOI: 10.1017/9781108590600

First published 2018

Printed and bound in Great Britain by Clays Ltd, Elcograf S.p.A.

A catalogue record for this publication is available from the British Library.

Library of Congress Cataloging-in-Publication Data
Names: Beers, Britta Chongkol van, 1977– editor. | Sterckx, Sigrid, editor. | Dickenson,
Donna, editor.
Title: Personalized medicine, individual choice and the common good / edited by Britta van
Beers, Sigrid Sterckx, Donna Dickenson.
Description: Cambridge, United Kingdom; New York, NY: Cambridge University Press,
2018. | Includes bibliographical references and index.
Identifiers: LCCN 2018022368 | ISBN 9781108473910 (hardback)
Subjects: | MESH: Precision Medicine | Personhood | Genome – ethics | Ethics, Clinical |
Philosophy, Medical
Classification: LCC R733 | NLM WB 102 | DDC 610–dc23
LC record available at https://lccn.loc.gov/2018022368

ISBN 978-1-108-47391-0 Hardback

CONTENTS

CONTRIBUTORS

KRISTOF VAN ASSCHE is a research professor in health law and kinship studies at the University of Antwerp, Belgium. His research and numerous publications focus on the legal aspects of organ trafficking, surrogacy and experimental assisted reproductive technologies. He is a member of the Declaration of Istanbul Custodian Group, a member of the Ethics Committee of The Transplantation Society, and a member of the working group established by the Belgian government to implement the Council of Europe Convention against Trafficking in Human Organs.

FRANÇOISE BAYLIS is Professor and Canada Research Chair in Bioethics and Philosophy at Dalhousie University. She is an elected fellow of the Royal Society of Canada and the Canadian Academy of Health Sciences. At the centre of her research lie questions of justice, especially intergenerational justice as it applies to our responsibilities to future generations when we undertake research programmes that may alter the nature of humans.

BRITTA VAN BEERS is an associate professor in the Department of Legal Theory at the VU University Amsterdam. A recurring theme in her work is the legal relationship between persons and their bodies in various biomedical contexts, such as assisted reproductive technologies, markets in human body materials and biomedical tourism. Recent publications include the co-edited volumes, *Humanity in International Law and Biolaw* (Cambridge University Press, 2014) and *Symbolic Legislation and Developments in Biolaw* (2016).

ALANA CATTAPAN is an assistant professor at the Johnson Shoyama Graduate School of Public Policy at the University of Saskatchewan. A long-time feminist researcher and activist, she studies women's participation in policymaking, identifying links between the state, the commercialisation of the body, biotechnologies and reproductive labour. She is currently co-editing a volume on surrogacy in Canada and conducting research on the concept of 'women of childbearing age' in public health policy and biomedical research.

JULIAN COCKBAIN is a consultant European patent attorney based in Ghent, Belgium, and Oxford, UK. He has written numerous articles on patent-related matters and co-authored the book *Exclusions from Patentability: How Far has the European Patent Office Eroded Boundaries?* (Cambridge University Press, 2012) with Sigrid Sterckx. He is also frequently invited to lecture on patent law and innovation policies.

CHRISTIAN DETWEILER is a design lecturer and researcher at The Hague University of Applied Sciences. His current research focuses on normativity in personal informatics technologies and its implications for design. Christian was previously a PhD candidate at Delft University of Technology, where he worked on his dissertation project, *Accounting for Values in Design*.

DONNA DICKENSON is Emeritus Professor of Medical Ethics and Humanities at the University of London. Her writings comprise over seventy academic articles and twenty-five books, including her study of personalised medicine, *Me Medicine vs. We Medicine: Reclaiming Biotechnology for the Common Good* (2013).

SANDI DHEENSA is a research associate at the Cardiff School of Social Sciences, Cardiff University. A common theme throughout her career so far has been the ethical and social challenges that evolving technologies pose, especially in the genomics field.

JYOTSNA AGNIHOTRI GUPTA is an assistant professor in gender and diversity (emerita) and a senior research associate at the University of Humanist Studies in Utrecht, The Netherlands. She is the author of *New Reproductive Technologies, Women's Health and Autonomy: Freedom or Dependency?* (2000), and of numerous published articles. Her research has concentrated on reproductive technologies and reproductive health issues from a gender and diversity perspective.

KLAUS HOEYER is Professor of Medical Science and Technology Studies at the University of Copenhagen. His research interests include ethics as policy work and the social organisation of health data, biobanks and transplant services. He has published in a variety of journals and is the author of *Exchanging Human Bodily Material: Rethinking Bodies and Markets* (2013).

STUART HOGARTH is a lecturer in sociology of science and technology in the Department of Social Science at the University of Cambridge. His research focuses on the political economy of diagnostic innovation. His work combines empirical research on the development, assessment and adoption of diagnostic technologies with normative analysis of public policy and commercial strategy. He has produced reports on intellectual property rights and regulatory frameworks in personalised medicine for the European Commission, Health Canada and the Human Genetics Commission.

MARLI HUIJER is a professor of philosophy at Erasmus University Rotterdam. In early 2015 she was named Thinker Laureate of The Netherlands. Her books include *Rhythm: In Search of a Recurring Time* (in Dutch, 2011) and *Discipline: Survival in Surfeit* (in Dutch, 2013).

HEIDI MERTES is a professor of ethics at Ghent University, a founding member of the Bioethics Institute Ghent (BIG) and a researcher at the Research Foundation – Flanders. Her main area of interest is bioethics, more specifically the topics of embryo research, stem cell research, reproductive medicine, fertility preservation and prenatal genomics. She has published numerous articles on these issues.

ROBIN PIERCE is an associate professor at the Tilburg Institute for Law, Technology and Society (TILT) of Tilburg Law School. She obtained her PhD from Harvard University in Health Policy, with a focus on comparative genetic privacy. She also holds a Juris Doctor from Boalt Hall School of Law at the University of California at Berkeley. Her research and numerous publications explore policy, legal and ethical issues of translational research in the life sciences, most recently involving synthetic biology, neuroscience and nanomedicine.

SIGRID STERCKX is a professor of ethics and political and social philosophy at the Department of Philosophy and Moral Sciences of

Ghent University. Her current research projects focus on: global justice (with particular attention to climate change); human tissue research and biobanking; patenting in biomedicine and genomics; organ transplantation; neuroethics; and end-of-life decisions. She has published more than 150 books, book chapters and articles in international academic journals on these issues, including the co-edited volume *Continuous Sedation at the End of Life: Ethical, Clinical and Legal Perspectives* (Cambridge University Press, 2013). Sigrid is a member of the Belgian Advisory Committee on Bioethics, which advises the Federal Government.

HUB ZWART is a professor of philosophy at the Faculty of Science of the Radboud University Nijmegen. In 2004, he established the Centre for Society and Genomics (CSG) in this department, and acted as CSG's scientific director. In 2005, he established the Institute for Science, Innovation and Society (ISIS). He is also Editor-in-Chief of the journal *Life Sciences, Society and Policy*. He has published ten books and seventy-five articles.

1

Introduction

DONNA DICKENSON, BRITTA VAN BEERS AND SIGRID
STERCKX

1.1 What Is Personalised Medicine?

Hippocrates famously advised physicians that it is more important to know *what person the disease has* than *what disease the person has.* So it might well be thought that all good medical practice is personalised, and that there is nothing new about that. But the phenomenon that has been widely presented as a paradigm shift in medicine – and which is our concern in this volume – is both more specific and more general.

In the specific sense, *personalised* or *precision medicine* builds on the achievements of genomic science, aiming to offer doctors and patients more sophisticated tools of molecular profiling to identify and treat genetic variants implicated in disease risk and treatment. Pharmacogenetics, probably the most advanced arm of personalised medicine, aims to minimise adverse drug reactions and produce better responses by tailoring pharmaceutical regimes in cancer care and other branches of medicine to the patient's individual genome. For example, the application of whole-genome sequencing to the care of a patient with early onset breast and ovarian cancer but no significant family history revealed unsuspected genetic defects, enabling clinicians to change her treatment plan from bone marrow transplantation to successful targeted chemotherapy.[1] Outside oncology, treatment for the liver disease hepatitis has been successfully personalised to avoid the worst side effects for patients whose genetic variation makes them more responsive to a lower drug dosage.[2] The discovery of a 'Goldilocks' gene affecting patients' inflammatory

---

[1] Daniel C. Link et al., 'Identification of a novel PT3 cancer susceptibility mutation through whole-genome sequencing of a patient with therapy-related AMl' (2011) 305 *Journal of the American Medical Association* 1568–76.
[2] Amy Maxmen, 'Pharmacogenetics: playing the odds' (2011) 474 *Nature* S9–S10.

response to tuberculosis could be crucial, particularly in the Third World, in determining who will contract the disease and who would benefit from steroids.[3]

Such is the sense captured in the following description:

> Precision medicine is an approach to disease treatment and prevention that seeks to maximize effectiveness by taking into account variability in genes, environment and lifestyle. Precision medicine seeks to redefine our understanding of disease onset and progression, treatment response, and health outcomes through the more precise measurement of molecular, environmental, and behavioral factors that contribute to health and disease. This understanding will lead to more accurate diagnoses, more rational disease prevention strategies, better treatment selection, and the development of novel therapies. Coincident with advancing the science of medicine is a changing culture of medical practice and medical research that engages individuals as active partners—not just as patients or research subjects.[4]

This is the goal underpinning the announcement made by President Obama in January 2015 of a $215 million Precision Medicine Initiative (PMI), coupled with plans to recruit a million participants into the accompanying 'PMI-Cohort' programme. As a junior senator, Obama had already championed the bill that was to become the Genomics and Personalized Medicine Act 2007, remarking: 'We are in a new era of the life sciences, but in no area of research is the promise greater than in personalized medicine.' In these initiatives the language of *individualisation* was powerfully dominant, despite the 'rhetorical reform' implicit in the change of nomenclature from 'personalised' to 'precision' between the 2007 statute and the 2015 initiative.[5] In the words of the White House statement accompanying the PMI announcement:

> Until now most medical treatments have been designed for the 'average patient'. As a result of this 'one-size-fits-all' approach, treatments can

---

[3] Linda Wijlaars, '"Goldilocks" gene response to TB suggests best treatment' (6 February 2012) *Bionews*.

[4] Precision Medicine Initiative (PMI) Working Group Report to the Advisory Committee to the Director, NIH, *The Precision Medicine Initiative Cohort Program – Building a Research Foundation for 21st Century Medicine* (2015), September 17, p. 1. See also Maya Sabatello and Paul S. Appelbaum, 'The precision medicine nation' (2017) 47(4) *Hastings Center Report* 19–29.

[5] Eric Juengst, Michelle L. McGowan, Jennifer R. Fishman et al., 'From "personalized" to "precision" medicine: the ethical and social implications of rhetorical reform in genomic medicine' (2016) 46 *Hastings Center Report* 21–33.

be very successful for some patients but not for others. Precision Medicine, on the other hand, is an innovative approach that takes into account individual differences in people's genes, environments, and lifestyles.[6]

1.2   The Personalisation of Medicine and the Common Good

However, this emphasis on individualisation – 'Me Medicine', as one of us has termed it[7] – is controversial, despite Hippocrates' dictum. To begin with, it is extremely unlikely that completely individualised treatments are ever going to be feasible. Many commentators and clinicians acknowledge that the best aspiration is to deliver diagnoses and treatments stratified into patient groups by genomic science:

> I don't think that we can ever, ever become truly personal and truly individualized ... [T]he way I look at personalized medicine is whereby we can stratify patient groups respective of ancestry, ethnicity, into individuals who are more likely to respond using novel technologies ... So I see a way of being able to subphenotype individuals in the way they're going to respond to drugs, and that's what I see as personalized medicine. So I don't see it as individual.[8]

The term 'stratified' medicine, however, lacks the powerful appeal of 'personalised' medicine, with its promises of greater *individual choice* and patient empowerment. These claims have been made most explicitly by the direct-to-consumer (DTC) genetic testing sector, in which firms offer customers whole- or partial-genome sequencing analyses of their risks for particular diseases. As one firm put it, 'We use the latest science and technology to give you a view into your DNA, revealing your genetic predisposition for important health conditions and empowering you with knowledge to help you take control of your health future.'[9] Direct-to-consumer genetic testing is the self-proclaimed vanguard of the personalised medicine movement, with leading proponents advocating a proactive approach

---

[6] Quoted in J. Patrick Woolley, Michelle L. McGowan, Harriet J. A. Teare et al., 'Citizen science or scientific citizenship? Disentangling the uses of public engagement rhetoric in national research initiatives' (2016) 17(33) *BMC Medical Ethics*, pp. 7–8.

[7] Donna Dickenson, *Me Medicine vs We Medicine: Reclaiming Biotechnology for the Common Good* (New York, NY: Columbia University Press, 2013).

[8] A senior editor of a genomics journal, interviewed in Juengst et al., 'From "personalized" to "precision" medicine', p. 23.

[9] Navigenics advertising, quoted in Dickenson, *Me Medicine vs We Medicine*, p. 32.

to individual health that stresses the importance and validity of DTC tests in taking control of one's own health.[10]

But are these promises of empowerment illusory? 'The weakness of "personalized genomic medicine", as a promissory label for what genomics might bring to health care, is that it promises more than genomics can actually deliver – both in terms of increased patient empowerment and in terms of the individualization of care.'[11] Perhaps personalised medicine might even *diminish* patient choice by denying patients treatments which they would like to have but to which they are unlikely to respond. Or it might leave that decision more firmly in the hands of physicians and genetic counsellors, operating on the pharmacogenetic ethos of 'the right treatment for the right patient at the right time'. But the inevitable corollary is 'the wrong treatment for the wrong patient at the wrong time', conceivably meaning 'no treatment' for patients whose genomic profiles make them less likely to respond.[12]

Rationing decisions such as these are only the start of the ethical and social issues arising from personalised medicine. Interpreted broadly, personalised medicine can encompass a whole gamut of new biotechnologies, united mainly by their common emphasis on patient choice and empowerment. As a prominent example, 'enhancement technologies', such as neurocognitive stimulation techniques, brain–computer interfaces, drugs to improve mental functioning, and, most controversially, germline genetic modification, can be seen as a form of personalised medicine. They are typically predicated on the individualistic ethos of 'being the best Me I can possibly be'.[13]

Yet the original ideals behind the rise of genomic medicine were communitarian, not individualistic: they symbolise 'We' rather than 'Me' Medicine. This 'We' may refer to a variety of concerns: our genetic relatedness, ideals of solidarity and distributive justice, or global public goods such as the genetic commons. The ideal of the genome as the common heritage of humanity permeates the international scientific community's 1996 'Bermuda statement', which declares: 'All human genome sequence information from a publicly funded project should be freely available in the public

[10] E.g. Francis Collins, *The Language of Life: DNA and the Revolution in Personalized Medicine* (New York, NY: Harper Collins, 2010).
[11] Juengst et al., 'From "personalized" to "precision" medicine', p. 30.
[12] Dickenson, *Me Medicine vs We Medicine*, p. 72.
[13] Dickenson, *Me Medicine vs We Medicine*, p. 113.

domain.'[14] Likewise, article 1 of the 1997 UNESCO Universal Declaration on the Human Genome and Human Rights stipulates: 'In a symbolic sense, the human genome is the common heritage of humanity.'

Does personalised medicine undermine and threaten this conception of the 'common good'? If more resources are dedicated to precision medicine, for example, will less attention be paid to public health?[15] That could be counterproductive in overall population terms, bearing in mind that it was public health initiatives such as improved sanitation and screening that radically improved lifespan figures in the twentieth-century Western world by lessening the incidence of contagious disease.

This phenomenon is not 'merely' historic; nor is it limited to infectious disease. 'Most of the recent successes in cancer care have resulted from the traditional public health measures of screening, early detection and smoking reduction as well as some immunologic therapies.'[16] Even two of the most prominent 'poster children' for genomic medicine, the BRCA1/2 genes implicated in some breast and ovarian cancers and the discovery of specific cystic fibrosis mutations responsive to recently developed drugs, have arguably had less effect than 'We Medicine'. 'Although well-deserved recognition has accompanied these genetic discoveries, neither has been a significant factor in the substantial reduction in mortality from the two target diseases during the past 25 years. The commitment to screening technology and adherence to best practices has proven far more important to the lives of affected patients.'[17] More broadly, it has been argued that a solidarity-based 'We Medicine perspective' could allow us to formulate better policies in areas ranging from palliative care to organ donation.[18]

[14] HUGO (Human Genome Organization), *Summary of Principles Agreed at the International Strategy Meeting on Human Genome Sequencing ('Bermuda Statement')* (London: Wellcome Trust, 1996).
[15] W. Burke et al., 'Extending the range of public health genomics: what should be the agenda for public health in an era of genome-based and "personalized" medicine?' (2010) 12 *Genetics in Medicine* 785–91.
[16] Michael J. Joyner and Nigel Paneth, 'Seven questions for personalized medicine' (2015) 314(10) *JAMA* 999–1000, p. 999.
[17] Ibid.
[18] Barbara Prainsack, 'The "We" in the "Me": solidarity and health care in the era of personalized medicine' (2018) 43(1) *Science, Technology and Human Values* 21–44.

1.3   Digital Health and Personalised Medicine

All these developments regarding personalised medicine need to be seen in connection with the digital health (or e-health) revolution. In 2017 the digital health industry was already worth US$25 billion globally.[19] Digital health includes diverse technologies, e.g. automated algorithm-based decisional support systems, mobile health apps (m-health) monitoring health-related behaviours, remote consultations (or 'telemedicine') and Electronic Health Records (EHRs). Staggeringly, 153,000 m-health apps have been released since 2015, bringing the worldwide total to 320,000.[20] For most of these technologies, robust governance is lacking.[21]

These technologies also result in an increasing 'pile' of Big Data. Increasingly, as in other contexts (not only businesses but also election campaigns, for example), in healthcare, too, attempts are made to link disparate data sets at the individual person level. New kinds of data collection, linkage and analysis are expected to profoundly transform clinical medicine, public health and epidemiology.

In her hugely impressive article in *The Lancet* on 'The art of medicine', Inmaculada de Melo-Martin analyses the impact on current-day medicine of the Cartesian concept of the human body as a machine. Although this model has resulted in unquestionable benefits from the biomedical sciences, she adds this caveat:

> [I]t also underlies the belief that the goal of medicine is to somehow eliminate human vulnerability. Because contemporary biomedical sciences ask questions oriented to that end, it is not surprising that their responses tend to sustain medical practices that are directed to produce cures. Of course, we cannot emphasise enough the importance of curing human diseases. But excessive emphasis on this goal runs the risk of disregarding those things that cannot be cured, such as disabilities and chronic illnesses. This goal also underscores the emphasis on individual solutions to problems that might best be addressed by attending to social and economic aspects, and hence the common lack of attention given to public health solutions.[22]

[19] 'Does mobile health matter?' (2017) 390 *The Lancet* 2216. doi:10.1016/S0140-6736(17)32899-4.

[20] IQVIA, 'The growing value of digital health in the United Kingdom: evidence and impact on human health and the healthcare system' (7 November 2017). www.iqvia.com/institute/reports/the-growing-value-of-digital-health (Accessed 11 February 2018).

[21] Rishi Duggal, Ingrid Brindle and Jessamy Bagenal, 'Editorial: Digital healthcare: regulating the revolution' (2018) *British Medical Journal* 360:k6. doi:10.1136/bmj.k6.

[22] Immaculada de Melo-Martin, 'The art of medicine – Vulnerability and ethics: considering our Cartesian hangover' (2009) 373 *The Lancet* 1244–45.

Promises of ever more cures where none were previously available can be found throughout the 'personalised medicine' rhetoric, to an increasingly embarrassing extent, as explained powerfully by Stanford epidemiologist John Ioannidis:

> I have had great excitement about the prospects of omics, big data, personalized medicine, precision medicine, and all. Much of my effort has been to put together these efforts with rigorous statistical methods and EBM (Evidence-Based Medicine) tools. But I am tired of seeing the same overrated promises recast again and again. For example, several years ago I gave an invited lecture at a leading institution on the danger of making inflated promises in personalized medicine. Right after my talk, everybody rushed to hear the launch of a new campaign, where the leader of the institution singled out this unique historic moment: that institution would single-handedly eliminate most major types of cancer within a few years. Several years have passed, and none of these cancer types have disappeared. I recently tried to find the name of that campaign online but realized that this institution has launched many similar campaigns. Which among many was the unique historic moment that I happened to be at? Multiply this by thousands of institutions, and there are already millions of unique historic moments where cancer was eliminated. The same applies to neurologic diseases and more. I do not understand why academic leaders and politicians need to make such self-embarrassing announcements now and then.[23]

1.4 Me Medicine vs We Medicine

To examine these wide-ranging and global questions, this volume brings together an international array of scholars from various disciplines, including law, bioethics, anthropology and sociology, to exchange ideas on the tensions between Me Medicine and We Medicine.

One of the recurring questions in the contributions to this book is what *Me* and *We* exactly mean in this context. As various authors argue, personalised medicine gives rise to new conceptions of the self and the communal. What kind of concept of the person is implied by the notion of personalised medicine: a geneticised self, quantified self, potential self, fictional self, consumer self? And what is the nature of community and the common good implicit in We Medicine: collective morality, social solidarity or rather new types of commons, such as 'genome-commons' (e.g. the human genome as common heritage of mankind), 'bio-

---

[23] John Ioannidis, 'Evidence-based medicine has been hijacked: a report to David Sackett' (2016) 73 *Journal of Clinical Epidemiology* 82–6.

commons' (e.g. sharing DNA samples) and 'data-commons' (e.g. promotion of early data disclosure and release)?[24]

Moreover, many of the chapters offer reflection on the causes of the spectacular rise of the rhetoric of personalised medicine. One of us has argued[25] that four possible explanations can be distinguished, with some emerging from further analysis as more plausible than others. These four explanations also resurface in most of the chapters and can be characterised as follows.

A first possibility is that the personalisation of healthcare is rooted in a more general sense of threat and contamination in society. For example, the fear of contamination can be recognised in the growing lack of confidence in public health resources. Second, the popularity of products and services in the field of Me Medicine, such as DTC tests, could be understood against the background of a broader trend towards narcissism and a fixation on the self. Third, it seems likely that corporate interests also fuel the fascination for personalised medicine. The highly lucrative and still expanding market in products and services based on personalised medicine suggests a correlation between the emergence of personalised medicine on the one hand, and the rise of neoliberal politics and the privatisation of most domains of life on the other. Last, the rhetoric surrounding personalised medicine alludes to a celebration of personal choice, personal empowerment and personal autonomy. From this perspective, the belief in personalised medicine as the new panacea is intimately connected to modern society's belief in the 'sacredness of personal choice and individualism'.[26]

These four hypotheses have engaged the attention of many of our contributors, allowing a more sophisticated and multi-disciplinary analysis of the phenomenon of personalised medicine to be united under a shared framework. In the next section we summarise each of their contributions separately.

1.5 Overview

In their chapter, 'Personalised Medicine and the Politics of Human Nuclear Genome Transfer', philosopher and bioethicist Françoise

---

[24] Bartha M. Knoppers and Vural Özdemir, 'The concept of humanity and biogenetics' in Britta van Beers, Luigi Corrias and Wouter Werner (eds.), *Humanity across International Law and Biolaw* (Cambridge: Cambridge University Press, 2014).

[25] Dickenson, *Me Medicine vs We Medicine*, pp. 10–29.

[26] Dickenson, *Me Medicine vs We Medicine*, p. 24.

Baylis and feminist political scientist Alana Cattapan offer an important contribution to the debate on the governance of human nuclear genome transfer, commonly (but incorrectly) known as 'mitochondrial replacement'. This emerging reproductive technology aims to provide women who are genetic carriers of certain mitochodrial diseases with the possibility of reproducing without passing on their mitochondrial DNA to their offspring. The result would be the creation of 'three-parent babies', with genetic material from two women and one man. In their thought-provoking analysis Baylis and Cattapan argue that the rise of human nuclear genome transfer should be understood as part of the current movement towards the personalisation of healthcare; as such, they claim, it deserves a critical examination. They subsequently argue against the implementation of this technology by fruitfully engaging with Dickenson's aforementioned four possible explanations for the rise of personalised medicine. According to Baylis and Cattapan, Dickenson's first explanation resurfaces in the context of human nuclear genome in the shape of a fear of genetic contamination of one's familial DNA, against which this technology would offer protection. They then engage with Dickenson's second hypothesis – narcissism and bowling alone – by highlighting how an important part of this technology's appeal rests on a short-sighted prioritisation of genetic relatedness above all other interests. As to Dickenson's third explanation, Baylis and Cattapan describe how the fertility industry's huge commercial interests are steering the development and marketing of this reproductive technology. Finally, they argue that 'the sacredness of personal choice' has also clearly affected the reception of human nuclear genome transfer. The rhetoric surrounding this technology emphasises the right to have genetically related children who are free of mitochondrial disease, and obfuscates the risks that are at stake, such as the intergenerational effects of altering the genome.

Extending the scope of personalised medicine beyond genomic science into an unexpected and novel area, bioethicist Heidi Mertes applies the concept to 'Stem Cell-Derived Gametes and Uterus Transplants'. Although both of these experimental techniques are far from being mainstream, they implicitly rely for their justification on the conventional view of 'reproductive autonomy' as a personal right. The sacredness of personal choice and the importance attached to genetic parenthood chime with this view. Likewise, the hypothesis that 'Me Medicine' derives its popularity from a fear of threat and contamination also seems to be supported by fear of third-party involvement in the formation of a family, Mertes suggests. However, she concludes that 'it is far from obvious that the desire for genetic or gestational parenthood can trump considerations for the welfare of the future child and for the safety of the other parties involved (in the case of uterus transplantation), or that it can justify resource allocation to these new reproductive technologies.' She ends her analysis by exploring what measures a less individualistic approach to infertility might entail: one rooted in the 'We Medicine' concept of the common good.

Reproductive ethics is also the concern of Jyotsna Agnihotri Gupta, a sociologist who works on reproductive and genetic technologies from a gender perspective, in her original and important study combining media analysis, interviews and participant observation: 'Personalising Future Health Risk through "Biological Insurance": Proliferation of Private Umbilical Cord Blood Banking in India'. Private cord blood banking epitomises 'Me Medicine' in its ostensible concentration on the individual's future well-being, rather than the collective's health, which is better served by public banks. In India, however, public banks are few and far between, whereas private banking is very much on the rise. Gupta provides extensive detail on the Indian private cord blood industry – potentially the largest supplier in the world – along with interview results from patients and doctors alike. Locating the private cord blood phenomenon not only within the 'Me Medicine' framework but also in the literature on risk theory, Gupta documents the construction of a new kind of patient: the 'at-risk' individual who needs a form of personalised medicine from birth: the moment when cord blood is taken.

A different dimension of the tensions between We Medicine and Me Medicine is explored in the chapter, 'Combating the Trade in Organs: Why We Should Preserve the Communal Nature of Organ Transplantation' by Kristof Van Assche. Van Assche, who is a legal expert on organ donation and transplantation, offers a powerful and highly critical examination of recent proposals to introduce elements of free market economics into systems of organ donation. Even if organ selling is still banned in most legal systems, 'as altruistic kidney donation symbolizes We Medicine at its noblest',[27] the call for a regulated market in organs is becoming louder in reaction to the continuing shortage in organs. Van Assche's ardent defence of the existing altruistic system rests on two lines of argumentation. His first argument is that a regulated organ market is likely to lead to the exact opposite of what proponents

---

[27] Dickenson, *Me Medicine vs We Medicine*, p. 72.

hope to achieve. As a result of the inability to control all market transactions, such a system cannot prevent organ patients from accessing black markets for organs, either in their own country or abroad. Moreover, a regulated market may crowd out altruistic organ donation. Finally, he stresses the problematic account of autonomy that underlies proposals to allow individuals to sell their organs. In the second part of his chapter, Van Assche expands his critical analysis of regulated markets in organs by connecting the issue with the debate on the commodification of the human body and by engaging with different theories of property. He argues that both utilitarian and Lockean theories of property fail to properly justify property rights in organs. Conversely, according to Van Assche, only personhood theories of property are able to recognise the grave immaterial harms at stake in organ vending.

In her chapter on one of the greatest global challenges in the twenty-first century, Alzheimer's disease – an untreatable disease whose prevalence and financial and social consequences are reaching epidemic proportions – legal scholar Robin Pierce addresses the We/Me Medicine aspects of research and development of diagnostic tests and therapeutic treatments. It may well be that Alzheimer's disease is in fact an umbrella term covering a range of separate diseases, some of which have a genetic cause while others do not. Until the cause of and possible treatments for the disease are discovered, research and development clearly falls into the We Medicine category, even though some of the diagnostic tests being developed are so complicated and expensive that their widespread deployment could currently only be considered to belong to the realms of research and Me Medicine. However, as Pierce powerfully explains, there is a danger that any cures which are developed would be applicable to and affordable by only a small minority. Thus, the development of such cures by commercial entities risks being Me Medicine only. Indeed, 'When There Is No Cure: Challenges for Collective Approaches to Alzheimer's Disease' shows that public pressure may be necessary to ensure that cures are developed for more than just a 'favoured few': without deliberate consideration throughout the R&D and translational process, collective approaches to the Alzheimer's crisis may lose ground to commercially more profitable individualised approaches.

In his chapter, 'Lost and Found: Relocating the Individual in the Age of Intensified Data Sourcing in European Healthcare', Klaus Hoeyer, who specialises in anthropology and medical science and technology studies, investigates the implications of 'data sourcing'. To an increasing extent, health data are created, collected, curated, stored and used for diverse purposes. Denmark is the primary example described in this chapter because the Danish government prescribes a form of solidarity that Hoeyer associates with We Medicine: people deliver data in the process of receiving, or in exchange for, publicly financed healthcare; and the data can be used for research that promotes the common good. Thanks to the use of personal identity numbers in all encounters with public services, Danish health data can be combined with data on socio-economic and educational status from employers and tax authorities. Denmark takes a more radical approach to the facilitation of research than the other Nordic countries: since 2014, Danish citizens can no longer opt out from being contacted by researchers wanting further information from them. Hoeyer considers the rights and wrongs of establishing such comprehensive national public health and social information databases, based on what boils down to 'conscription' of personal data. Moreover, these data registries are increasingly used by the government to attract international investment in the Danish pharmaceutical industry. Hoeyer argues that the Danish registries hold great promise for the development of new therapeutic treatments and the improvement of current ones, for example, by allowing the identification of unknown side-effects of drugs. Although identifying some Me Medicine aspects in the Danish approach, he concludes that its We Medicine associated benefits outweigh the drawbacks. Nonetheless, a key task is to ensure that the collective goods do not become redirected into private pockets and that collectives help each other to counter individual risks.

In their chapter, 'Presuming the Promotion of the Common Good by Large-Scale Health Research: The Cases of care.data 2.0 and the 100,000 Genomes Project in the UK', philosopher and bioethicist Sigrid Sterckx, social scientist Sandi Dheensa and patent attorney Julian Cockbain offer an analysis of recent efforts by the UK government to expand the possibilities for collecting health-related data from UK citizens. The first part of their chapter consists of an examination of the political statements, official reports and legal documents used by the government to introduce both care.data and the 100,000 Genomes Project. In the second part, they build on this analysis to identify several ethically highly problematic aspects of these recent initiatives, such as their under-lying consent model. One of the most striking findings of the authors' ethical analysis is that the UK government tries to promote its policy by appealing to what are essentially We Medicine values. However, as the authors argue, upon closer inspection it emerges that behind this thin layer of obfuscatory language hides a Me Medicine approach to health data, rooted in what, essentially, is a neoliberal political agenda.

In their chapter, 'My Genome, My Right', sociologist Stuart Hogarth, patent attorney Julian Cockbain and bioethicist Sigrid Sterckx consider the claim that people have the right to *access* their genomic data, e.g. using direct-to-consumer genetic testing companies such as 23andMe, and that that right extends to the use (and publication) of such data in any desired way. In effect, the claim is to an *ownership* right that corresponds to the central libertarian claim to self-ownership of the body and all body material. The authors, however, argue that the libertarians conflate a right to ownership of material, a rivalrous good, with a right to *own* information, a non-rivalrous good to which others may also legitimately claim control rights since genetic information is shared with relatives, at least. Accordingly, while the authors propose a human right to access personal genetic information, subject to regulatory control to ensure counselling where appropriate, they argue that, to protect the rights of others, not least to privacy, the person has no right to publish their 'own' genetic data. The 'Me Medicine' of personal control is trumped by the 'We Medicine' of privacy.

'"The Best Me I Can Possibly Be": Legal Subjectivity, Self-Authorship and Wrongful Life Actions in an Age of "Genomic Torts"', written by legal scholar and philosopher Britta van Beers, demonstrates the necessity of a legal perspective on personalised medicine. This chapter demonstrates how the 'person' in personalised medicine is connected with the legal understanding of a 'person' as a bearer of legal rights and responsibilities. However, this emphasis is changing. In her analysis of new types of legal claims that affect the law's understanding of the 'person', van Beers focuses on the emerging area of 'genomic torts'. Who, if anyone, is liable to compensate the children or their parents if children are conceived and born with disabling conditions that could have been detected or predicted before birth, or sometimes even before conception? Should responsibility lie with the physician who fails to offer appropriate tests, the parents who, knowingly or not, allow pregnancy to go to term, or society in general? Recently, two forms of legal action have come into focus: wrongful birth (an action against the physicians by the parents) and wrongful life (an action against the parents by the children). Britta van Beers investigates two different interpretations of a wrongful life claim (a right not to be born or a right to be born in a different body) and explains why both are problematic. Interestingly, she also discusses the potential effects that recent developments in gene-editing, such as the

CRISPR-Cas9 technique, may have on wrongful life actions. Moreover, gene-editing and preimplantation diagnostics run the risk of enhancing parental antenatal and pre-conception obligations and of transforming the responsibility for ensuring the welfare of the handicapped child from being a societal responsibility into a personal one. The analysis undertaken by van Beers clearly shows why wrongful birth and wrongful life claims are emblematic of a Me Medicine approach to regulation, i.e. an approach that views the legal issues involved in reproductive medicine as disputes between *individuals* about *personal* rights and entitlements, and why we should be concerned about the radically individualistic model of self-authorship that underlies this approach.

In their innovative chapter, 'I Run, You Run, We Run: A Philosophical Approach to Health and Fitness Apps', philosopher Marli Huijer and design researcher and philosopher Christian Detweiler focus on self-tracking technologies as a new kind of Me Medicine. Also known as *Quantified Self* or *Personal Informatics*, these popular applications ostensibly reflect the individualistic enhancement ideal of 'becoming the best Me I can possibly be'.[28] However, Huijer and Detweiler question whether these technologies do actually empower individuals. A Foucauldian analysis, they argue, might instead suggest that 'there is concern that personal informatics technologies submit their users to disciplinary forces that seduce or force the individual to take responsibility for their own health' as a means of governing the self, a form of voluntary self-surveillance. By expanding the scope of what counts as personalised medicine and sceptically questioning its rhetoric of individual choice and empowerment, the authors offer an unexpected counter-analysis to the prevalent optimistic discourse on precision medicine.

Similar concerns are further developed from a psychoanalytical perspective by philosopher of science Hub Zwart in his chapter, 'The Molecularised Me: Psychoanalysing Personalised Medicine and Self-Tracking'. The emergence of wearable tracking devices can be seen as a 'second revolution', bringing together paradigm shifts in computer technology and genomic sequencing. A 'quantified self' has emerged: what Zwart calls 'a digital version of the superego'. Self-knowledge in this new context links to but transcends narcissism: as Zwart puts it, 'Self-tracking devices purport to provide access to our molecularised unconscious.' Supposedly, these developments transform us all into proactive and empowered bio-citizens, reducing physicians to mere assistants or

---

[28] Dickenson, *Me Medicine vs We Medicine*, p. 113.

managers and promoting the ideal of citizen health science. But do they actually represent a new form of surveillance like Jeremy Bentham's panopticon? – what Zwart calls 'a ubiquitous electronic panopticon, a molecularised version of the super-ego, the voice of conscience of the terabyte age'. Like Huijer and Detweiler, Zwart is concerned that this enhancement-orientated form of Me Medicine actually forces a powerful new form of discipline on its users, rather than increasing their autonomy.

Each chapter in this book in its own way offers a critical exam- ination of the grand claims made by the 'evangelists' of personalised medicine. Does personalised medicine truly bring about a revolution in medicine by offering tailor-made medical treatment? Can this new approach indeed do justice to patients' biogenetic uniqueness and as such empower them to make better-informed choices about their health? Which values and interests are championed by Me Medicine's promissory discourse, and which are neglected? And how can the sudden rise and wide appeal of personalised medicine be explained?

As both the disciplinary richness of the chapters and the wide variety of themes with which they engage indicate, the increasing dominance of Me Medicine approaches over We Medicine approaches is also inti- mately connected to other developments, such as the hegemony in bioethics and biolaw of the principle of autonomy,[29] the dominance of rights discourse at the cost of attention for more collective interests,[30] the commodification of the human body[31] and human reproduction,[32] and

---

[29] For critical discussions of the primacy of autonomy in bioethics in the context of genomics, see, *inter alia*, Bartha M. Knoppers and Ruth Chadwick, 'Human genetic research: Emerging trends in ethics' (2005) 6 *Nature Reviews Genetics* 75–9; Michael J. Sandel, *The Case Against Perfection: Ethics in the Age of Engineering* (Cambridge, MA: Harvard University Press, 2007); Heather Widdows, *The Connected Self. The Ethics and Governance of the Genetic Individual* (Cambridge: Cambridge University Press, 2013).

[30] Mary A. Glendon, *Rights Talk: The Impoverishment of Political Discourse* (New York, NY: Free Press, 1991); Costas Douzinas, 'The paradoxes of human rights' (2013) 20(1) *Constellations* 51–67.

[31] Margaret J. Radin, *Contested Commodities: The Trouble with Trade in Sex, Children, Body Parts, and Other Things* (Cambridge, MA: Harvard University Press, 1996); Donna Dickenson, *Body Shopping: The Economy Fuelled by Flesh and Blood* (Oxford: Oneworld Publications, 2008).

[32] Michele Goodwin (ed.), *Baby Markets: Money and the New Politics of Creating Families* (New York, NY: Cambridge University Press, 2010); Britta van Beers, 'Is Europe "giving in to baby markets?" Reproductive tourism in Europe and the gradual erosion of existing legal limits to reproductive markets' (2014) 23(1) *Medical Law Review* 103–34.

the datafication of healthcare.[33] One of the aspirations of this book is also to contribute to academic reflection on these important themes.

Moreover, although it is true that the chapters in this book generally focus on Me Medicine's more problematic aspects, it would be too easy to conclude that the book's central message is that personalised medicine is bad news and that efforts in this field should therefore be abandoned. Instead, it is our hope that, by exploring the frictions between Me Medicine and We Medicine, between *individual choice* and the *common good*, this book can fuel and stimulate the debate about personalised medicine and enable its participants to come to a more balanced understanding of the interests and values at stake.

---

[33] Jonathan H. Chen and Steven M. Asch, 'Machine learning and prediction in medicine – Beyond the peak of inflated expectations' (2017) 376 (26) *New England Journal of Medicine* 2507-9; K. A. Oye, G. Jain, M. Amador et al., 'The next Frontier: Fostering innovation by improving health data access and utilization' (2015) 98 (5) *Clinical Pharmacology & Therapeutics* 514-21.

Personalised Medicine and the Politics of Human Nuclear Genome Transfer

FRANÇOISE BAYLIS AND ALANA CATTAPAN

2.1 Introduction

In the autumn of 2016, media outlets around the world reported the first live birth of a healthy child following the experimental use of human nuclear genome transfer (so-called *mitochondrial replacement*).[1] This novel technology involves the transfer of the nucleus from the egg of one woman into the enucleated egg of another woman. It is often referred to as 'three-person IVF' or 'three-parent IVF' because the technology requires use of in vitro fertilisation (IVF) and results in the creation of a human with DNA from three individuals.

In this first case, the aim was to avoid the birth of a child with Leigh syndrome – a rare, fatal neurological disorder caused by dysfunctional

---

[1] Gina Kolata, 'Birth of baby with three parents' DNA marks success for banned technique' (27 September 2016) *The New York Times*, sec. Health, www.nytimes.com/2016/09/28/health/birth-of-3-parent-baby-a-success-for-controversial-procedure.html;
Jessica Hamzelou, 'World's first baby born with new "3 parent" technique' (2017) *New Scientist*, www.newscientist.com/article/2107219-exclusive-worlds-first-baby-born-with-new-3-parent-technique. Much has been written criticising the description of human nuclear genome transfer as 'mitochondrial replacement therapy', 'mitochondrial manipulation' or 'mitochondrial donation'. These terms variously suggest that the technology involves the replacement of mitochondria, when the technology actually involves the transfer of the nucleus from the egg of one woman into the enucleated egg of another woman. As Nisker explains, 'mitochondrial replacement' is a camouflage term that works to buttress support for the technology, framing it entirely as therapy for mitochondrial disease, rather than presenting it, more controversially as a germline modification. See Jeff Nisker, 'The latest thorn by any other name: Germ-line nuclear transfer in the name of "mitochondrial replacement"' (2015) 37(9) *Journal of Obstetrics and Gynaecology Canada* 829–31; Françoise Baylis, 'Human nuclear genome transfer (so-called mitochondrial replacement): Clearing the underbrush' (2017) 31(1) *Bioethics* 7–19; Erica Haimes and Ken Taylor, 'Sharpening the cutting edge: Additional considerations for the UK debates on embryonic interventions for mitochondrial diseases' (2017) 13(1) *Life Sciences, Society and Policy*.

mitochondrial DNA. Using a technique known as maternal spindle transfer, the nucleus was removed from the unfertilised egg of the woman carrier of Leigh syndrome and transferred to the enucleated unfertilised egg of a woman with healthy mitochondrial DNA. The reconstructed egg was then fertilised and transferred to the uterus of the woman who provided the nucleus. The embryo was created by a team of researchers in the United States led by Dr John Zhang, and a child was born in Mexico in April 2016 to a Jordanian couple.[2] The birthplace was chosen because of the absence of legislation governing the use of this technology.[3]

Soon after, the procedure started to be profiled as a specialised reproductive technology, not only for women at risk of having children with a mitochondrial disease, but also for women experiencing infertility. In January 2017, a child created using pronuclear transfer (another nuclear genome transfer technique) was born in Ukraine as part of fertility treatment.[4] In February 2017, the United States National Academies of Science, Engineering and Medicine issued a report that endorsed the use of human nuclear genome transfer under specified conditions and made mention of its potential future use for age-related fertility treatment.[5] Later, in June 2017, Zhang announced that his new start-up company Darwin Life would provide human nuclear genome transfer to older infertile women (between the ages of 42–47) as a way of prolonging natural fertility at a cost of between US$80,000 and 120,000.[6] According to Zhang, 'Everything we do is a step toward

---

[2] John Zhang et al., 'Live birth derived from oocyte spindle transfer to prevent mitochondrial disease' (2017) 34(4) *Reproductive Biomedicine Online* 361–8. www.rbmojournal .com/article/S1472-6483(17)30041-X/pdf.

[3] Hamzelou (see footnote 1). At the time, the only country with clear legislation permitting human nuclear genome transfer (referred to as mitochondrial donation) was the United Kingdom. This technology was legalised in 2015 for the sole purpose of preventing 'the transmission of serious mitochondrial disease from a mother to her child'.

[4] Henry Bodkin, 'Three-parent baby born to infertile couple in world first', *The Telegraph*, 18 January 2017, www.telegraph.co.uk/science/2017/01/18/three-parent-baby-born-infertile-couple-world-first; Michelle Roberts, 'IVF: First three-parent baby born to infertile couple', *BBC News*, 18 January 2017, sec. Health, www.bbc.com/news/health-38648981.

[5] Anne Claiborne, Rebecca English and Jeffrey Kahn, *Mitochondrial Replacement Techniques: Ethical, Social, and Policy Considerations*, ed. National Academies of Sciences, Engineering, and Medicine et al. (Washington, DC: National Academies Press, 2016).

[6] Emily Mullin, 'The fertility doctor trying to commercialize three-parent babies' (13 June 2017) *MIT Technology Review*, www.technologyreview.com/s/608033/the-fertility-doctor-trying-to-commercialize-three-parent-babies.

designer babies'.[7] And with this statement, Zhang crystallised the status of human nuclear genome transfer as personalised medicine – a technology that can readily be customised to meet individual desires.

In this chapter, we reflect on the emergence of human nuclear genome transfer as a form of personalised medicine akin to private umbilical cord blood banking and direct-to-consumer genetic testing. We do so using the framework developed by Donna Dickenson in *Me Medicine vs We Medicine: Reclaiming Biotechnology for the Common Good*.[8] Herein, Dickenson identifies four possible reasons (hypotheses) for the rise in personalised medicine: (1) threat and contamination, (2) narcissism and 'bowling alone', (3) corporate interests and political neoliberalism and, finally, (4) the sacredness of personal choice.

As applied to human nuclear genome transfer, the framework translates as follows: (1) For women at risk of having children with mitochondrial disease, there is the threat of serious (sometimes fatal) illness to potential offspring. As well, there is the risk of familial genetic contamination with the use of third-party eggs, which is one of the proposed alternative 'treatments'. This risk applies not only to women at risk of having children with a mitochondrial disease, but also to women with age-related infertility. (2) For both groups of women there is the widely touted 'need' for genetically related children vested in a selective understanding of the importance of nuclear DNA. (3) There is disproportionate (nearly exclusive) attention to the personal interests of families and children yet to be born with nary a word about the corporate interests being served. And (4) reproductive choice is championed as a fundamental right that undergirds women's right to avail themselves of nuclear genome transfer. In closing, we briefly comment on the implications of human nuclear genome transfer as a form of personalised medicine, drawing attention to the consequences for our genetic and reproductive futures.

2.2   Me Medicine, We Medicine and the Governance of Biotechnologies

In *Me Medicine vs We Medicine*, Dickenson critically examines the move to personalised medicine. This is a relatively new approach to healthcare centred on the customisation of treatment based on a patient's predicted response to particular interventions. The tailoring of treatment occurs

[7] Ibid.   [8] Dickenson, *Me Medicine vs We Medicine*.

through a combination of available medical and genetic information, including population-based studies of genomics, that can determine the likelihood that people of certain ages, genders and ethno-cultural backgrounds, who have engaged in certain behaviours, will get certain diseases, and may react in discrete ways to relevant interventions.

In her critique, Dickenson challenges the underlying assumption that for too long medicine has relied on a 'one size fits all approach' to healthcare that fails to account for the particular patient.[9] In so doing, she focuses on biotechnologies that have been lauded as revolutionary personalised medical interventions as evidence of a move away *from* medicine as a collective endeavour with an eye to the public good *to* medicine as a private, personalised encounter that is primarily (if not exclusively) responsive to individual needs and desires. Dickenson's aim is to expose the changing sociocultural priorities that have enabled the emergence of personalised medicine. These priorities include increased concern about threat and contamination, increasing narcissism and a move away from communal identity, the ascendency of a neoliberal politics and a commitment to personal choice above all other logics of decision-making.

First, regarding threat and contamination, Dickenson addresses a range of ways in which individuals come to perceive themselves as vulnerable and begin to look inward for medical solutions. There is, for example, the perception that communal medical resources like the blood supply may be limited and less safe than individual resources and repositories. This perception has given rise to the practice of storing one's own blood in private blood banks, not only to ensure ready access but also to avoid the risk of contamination. As well, and most relevant in the context of 'treatment' for mitochondrial disorders, there is the perception that potential genetic anomalies might be addressed most effectively by genetic screening and expensive, targeted genetic and genomic technologies. As to the latter, threat takes on yet another meaning, insofar as the rising costs of healthcare mean that many focused genetic and genomic technologies very likely will only be available privately and thus will be inaccessible to those without significant economic resources. Targeted technologies, developed with public funding in the name of benefiting the many, thus become an exclusive benefit for the wealthy.

Second, on narcissism, Dickenson highlights the possibility that the emergence of personalised medicine is closely linked to an indulgent,

---

[9] Ibid., 10.

self-involved view of the world, a 'narcissistic culture' in which individuals worry about their health and well-being, and seek to maximise personal interests over shared interests (i.e. the interests of the collective). Dickenson does not explicitly link this narcissism to the ascendency of neoliberalism, but she does identify the increased focus on the individual and on personal responsibility for health as contributing factors in the rise of personalised medicine.

Third, on neoliberal politics and corporate interests, Dickenson points to the ever-growing, entanglements of biomedical science and corporate interests as a site of concern, especially as public resources are increasingly repurposed for private profit. She argues that the use of publicly funded scientific research to advance corporate interests results in the privileging of technologies and pharmaceuticals that generate the highest market value over those that might result in greater health benefits for a broader public.

Fourth and finally, in ways closely intertwined with the other three priorities, Dickenson identifies the primacy of autonomy – the 'sacredness of personal choice'[10] – as contributing to the emergence and acceptance of personalised medicine. According to Dickenson, in recent years there has been an overemphasis on autonomy in medicine and this has undermined the possibility of addressing other equally important ethical principles such as the principle of social justice.

Taken together, Dickenson's critiques of personalised medicine highlight a broader concern about the shrinking state and the increasing understanding of individuals as the primary site of political intervention. On this view, the public sector looks to corporations to establish the agenda for biomedical and biotechnological advancements, leaving the state and its citizens to 'shoulder the risks for the private sector'.[11] The move toward personalised medicine may be beneficial in many ways, but as Dickenson identifies, it is informed by politics that shift our attention and our efforts away from thinking about medicine as a public good.

2.3 Mitochondrial Diseases and the Emergence of Human Nuclear Genome Transfer

Genes are subunits of DNA and there are two kinds of DNA. There is *nuclear DNA* (nDNA), located in the nucleus of the cell, and there is

---

[10] Ibid., 10.   [11] Ibid., 180.

DNA in mitochondria (*mitochondrial DNA* or mtDNA), found in the material that surrounds the cell's nucleus. MtDNA is largely responsible for cellular function. Whereas nDNA is inherited from both parents, mtDNA is only passed down from mothers to their children (both sons and daughters).

Mitochondrial diseases (sometimes referred to collectively as *mitochondrial disease*) are a group of heterogeneous disorders caused by mutations in mtDNA.[12] Because mtDNA mutations are many and varied, mitochondrial diseases are notoriously difficult to diagnose. The onset of medical problems may occur early in life or in adulthood, and symptoms may range from mild to very severe. Functions of the body that might be affected also vary widely, including the brain, nerves and muscles, heart, liver, ears, eyes, kidneys and pancreas, with several organs or systems typically affected.[13]

The contemporary history of disease caused by dysfunctional mtDNA begins with the discovery of Luft disease. In a groundbreaking 1962 paper, a Swedish team of researchers led by Rolf Luft described an unusual case in which a patient, a woman in her thirties, had an unexplained, extraordinarily high metabolic rate. From the age of seven, she had been sweating profusely, was thirsty and hungry all the time, and was exceptionally tired. Building on their research on mitochondrial function,[14] Luft and his team established that dysfunctional mtDNA could be the cause of disease. Since then, there have been several important advances in knowledge about mitochondrial disease. And in 1988, two critical papers confirmed that mutations in mtDNA could cause cellular dysfunction, and subsequently disease.[15] By 2010, more than 250 different types of mtDNA mutations had been

---

[12] Maurizio Moggio et al., 'Mitochondrial disease heterogeneity: A prognostic challenge' (2014) 33(2) *Acta Myologica* 86–93; Patrick F. Chinnery, 'Mitochondrial disorders overview' in Roberta A. Pagon et al. (eds.), *GeneReviews* (Seattle, WA: University of Washington, Seattle, 1993), www.ncbi.nlm.nih.gov/books/NBK1224.

[13] Ainsley J. Newson, Stephen Wilkinson and Anthony Wrigley, 'Ethical and legal issues in mitochondrial transfer' (2016) 8(6) *EMBO Molecular Medicine* 589–91.

[14] Lars Ernster, Denis Ikkos and Rolf Luft, 'Enzymatic activities of human skeletal muscle mitochondria: A tool in clinical metabolic research' (1959) 184 *Nature* 1851–54; Rolf Luft et al., 'A case of severe hypermetabolism of nonthyroid origin with a defect in the maintenance of mitochondrial respiratory control: A correlated clinical, biochemical, and morphological study' (1962) 41(9) *Journal of Clinical Investigation* 1776–1804.

[15] I. J. Holt, A. E. Harding and J. A. Morgan-Hughes, 'Deletions of muscle mitochondrial DNA in patients with mitochondrial myopathies' (1988) 331 *Nature* 717–19; Douglas C. Wallace et al., 'Mitochondrial DNA mutation sssociated with Leber's hereditary optic neuropathy' (1988) 242(4884) *Science* 1427; see also Dorothy R. Haskett,

identified.[16] At the present time, there is no treatment for mitochondrial disease other than the management of symptoms.[17]

In the 1990s, researchers in the United States led by Jacques Cohen developed a fertility treatment they called *cytoplasmic transfer*. This technology involved injecting the non-nuclear contents of a cell (i.e. the cytoplasm) from one woman's egg into the egg of an infertile woman undergoing IVF. The first successful birth following human cytoplasmic transfer was reported in 1997.[18] By 2001, Cohen's research team had fifteen live births – about half of the estimated number of such babies born worldwide.[19] Available preliminary data suggested that the transfer of mitochondria might work to prevent offspring from getting some forms of heritable mitochondrial disorders. At this time, the United States Food and Drug Administration (FDA) informed Cohen and his team that they needed an investigational new drug exemption to continue their research. Then, in 2002, the FDA determined that additional preclinical data was needed before further clinical trials could proceed. These decisions by the FDA effectively stopped the practice of cytoplasmic transfer.

Since then, three different techniques for conducting human nuclear genome transfer have been developed. Maternal spindle transfer and pronuclear transfer are two of these techniques, both of which involve the transfer of the nucleus from one woman's egg into the enucleated egg of another woman. A third option is polar body transfer, involving either the transfer of the first polar body into an enucleated unfertilised egg or the transfer of the second polar body into an enucleated fertilised egg. The primary benefit of these transfers is that woman with dysfunctional mtDNA might be able to have genetically related children who may not suffer from mitochondrial disease.

In the case of maternal spindle transfer (which involves the transfer of a nucleus from the egg of one female into the enucleated unfertilised egg

---

'Mitochondrial diseases in humans' (2014) *The Embryo Project Encyclopedia*, http://embryo.asu.edu/pages/mitochondrial-diseases-humans.

[16] Helen A. L. Tuppen et al., 'Mitochondrial DNA mutations and human disease' (2010) 1797(2) *Biochimica et Biophysica Acta – Bioenergetics* 113–28; Shoukhrat Mitalipov and Don P. Wolf, 'Clinical and ethical implications of mitochondrial gene transfer' (2014) 25(1) *Trends in Endocrinology and Metabolism* 5–7.

[17] Lyndsey Craven et al., 'Mitochondrial DNA disease: New options for prevention' (2011) 20(R2) *Human Molecular Genetics* R168–174.

[18] Jacques Cohen et al., 'Birth of infant after transfer of anucleate donor oocyte cytoplasm into recipient eggs' (1997) 350(9072) *Lancet* 186–7.

[19] Jason A. Barritt et al., 'Mitochondria in human offspring derived from ooplasmic transplantation' (2001) 16(3) *Human Reproduction* 513–16.

of another), early attempts occurred around 2000, when scientists in China reported that they were able to transfer nuclei between the egg cells of mice, resulting in viable offspring.[20] Then, in 2012, a team in Oregon led by Shoukhrat Mitalipov reported that the same was possible in rhesus macaques.[21]

In the interim, work continued with human embryos. In 2003, a team of researchers from China led by John Zhang reported that five human embryos had been transferred to the uterus of a woman being treated for infertility following pronuclear transfer. Although three embryos were successfully implanted, there were no live births.[22] In 2005, a team from Newcastle University in the United Kingdom obtained a license to conduct research on nuclear genome transfer using human embryos.[23] In 2010, they reported that the technique was possible in human embryos, and again successfully applied for a research license, observing embryo growth for six to eight days.[24] Finally, in March 2017, the Newcastle team received a license to carry out human nuclear genome transfer (referred to as *mitochondrial donation*) on a case-by-case basis.[25] In conjunction with this license, the Newcastle team (along with the Newcastle-upon-Tyne Hospitals NHS Foundation Trust) also received funding for a five-year clinical trial to track the health outcomes of children conceived following nuclear genome transfer.[26] As yet, no live

---

[20] Min-Kang Wang et al., 'In vitro fertilisation of mouse oocytes reconstructed by transfer of metaphase II chromosomes results in live births' (2001) 9(1) *Zygote* 9–14.

[21] Masahito Tachibana et al., 'Mitochondrial gene replacement in primate offspring and embryonic stem cells' (2009) 461(7262) *Nature* 367–72; Masahito Tachibana et al., 'Towards germline gene therapy of inherited mitochondrial diseases' (2013) 493(7434) *Nature* 627–31; Hyo-Sang Lee et al., 'Rapid mitochondrial DNA segregation in primate preimplantation embryos precedes somatic and germline bottleneck' (2012) 1(5) *Cell Reports* 506–15.

[22] John Zhang et al., 'Pregnancy derived from human nuclear transfer' (2003) 80 *Fertility and Sterility* 56; John Zhang et al., 'Pregnancy derived from human zygote pronuclear transfer in a patient who had arrested embryos after IVF' (2016) 33(4) *Reproductive Biomedicine Online* 529–33.

[23] Lyndsey Craven et al., 'Research into policy: A brief history of mitochondrial donation' (2016) 34(2) *Stem Cells* 265–7.

[24] Lyndsey Craven et al., 'Pronuclear transfer in human embryos to prevent transmission of mitochondrial DNA disease' (2010) 465(7294) *Nature* 82–5.

[25] HFEA Statement on Mitochondrial Donation, 15 March 2017, www.hfea.gov.uk/about-us/news-and-press-releases/2017-news-and-press-releases/hfea-statement-on-mitochondrial-donation.

[26] Katie Forster, 'First "three-parent babies" to be born this year as licence approved for new fertility technique' (16 March 2017) *The Independent*, www.independent.co.uk/life-style/health-and-families/health-news/three-3-parent-babies-latest-licence-approved-ivf-fertility-technique-hfea-dna-mitochondrial-a7632916.html; Clive Cookson, 'UK researchers secure

birth has been announced by the Newcastle team. Meanwhile, as discussed above, in September 2016, John Zhang announced the birth of a child in Mexico via maternal spindle transfer to avoid mitochondrial disease, and in January 2017, news reports emerged that a child conceived via pronuclear transfer had been born in the Ukraine, as part of fertility treatments.[27]

Human nuclear genome transfer has been positively described as the 'poster child' for personalised medicine[28] given the relatively rare incidence of mitochondrial diseases, their heritability (and therefore their ties to genetic testing) and the need for new interventions that look beyond contemporary practices. Further, as argued in subsequent sections, when examined with reference to Dickenson's four possible hypotheses for the rise in personalised medicine – threat and contamination (Section 2.4), narcissism (Section 2.5), corporate interests and political neoliberalism (Section 2.6) and the sacredness of personal choice[29] (Section 2.7) – the relationship between human nuclear genome transfer and personalised medicine becomes clear.

2.4 On Threat and Contamination: The Potential Eradication of Mitochondrial Disorders

In *Me Medicine vs We Medicine*, Dickenson describes how understandings of threat and contamination inform the uptake of personalised medicine. In her view, the rise of personalised medicine is bound up with the desire to control one's fate – and more specifically, to take responsibility for one's health – because the threats and risks of contamination are too many and too overwhelming not to do so. By way of illustration, in her discussions of cord blood banking and retail, mail-order genetics, she identifies the ways that threat of potential disease is often reimagined as promise of a cure, or hope to avoid disease altogether.

In the case of human nuclear genome transfer, the technology represents the promise of healthy children, a future unburdened by concern

licence for "three-parent" baby procedure' (16 March 2017) *Financial Times*, www.ft.com /content/a4c7e0ba-0a41-11e7-ac5a-903b21361b43.
27 Bodkin, 'Three-parent baby born to infertile couple in world first'; Roberts, 'IVF'.
28 Marni J. Falk, Alan Decherney and Jeffrey P. Kahn, 'Mitochondrial replacement techniques – implications for the clinical community' (2016) 374(12) *The New England Journal of Medicine* 1103–6.
29 Dickenson, *Me Medicine vs We Medicine*, 10.

for the effects of mitochondrial anomalies on one's descendants, and protection from the genetic contamination of one's familial DNA (one's 'blood line') were it otherwise necessary to use third-party eggs to conceive a child. The link between these hoped-for benefits and human nuclear genome transfer is tenuous, however, for at least three reasons.

First, most mitochondrial disorders are the result of anomalies in nDNA for which human nuclear genome transfer is irrelevant. Only 15–20 per cent of mitochondrial disorders occur as a result of mutations in mtDNA.[30]

Second, few women with dysfunctional mtDNA who might benefit from the technology are likely to do so. Estimates from the research team at Newcastle suggest that if all women in the United Kingdom between the ages of 15 and 44, at risk of transmitting mitochondrial disease, were to avail themselves of nuclear genome transfer, about 150 births a year might be positively affected.[31] The fact is, however, that not all such women will choose to use this technology. For example, some at-risk women may not want children, and among those at-risk women who do want children, some may prefer less risky ways of family-making (albeit, ways that preclude genetic-relatedness). There are, for example, risks associated with the IVF that is required to achieve a pregnancy following human nuclear genome transfer. These risks are in addition to those associated with pregnancy for women with mitochondrial disease.[32] Moreover, it is important to note that some women who are at risk of transmitting mitochondrial disease will not know they are at risk (and therefore would not be thinking of nuclear genome transfer when making reproductive choices). Among such women are those who are asymptomatic carriers, who will not know that they are likely to pass on mitochondrial mutations until after they have had a child with a mitochondrial disease.[33] Further, if human nuclear genome transfer is offered as a matter of private-for-profit medicine, the number of potential beneficiaries likely will be small, as few women will be able to

---

[30] Salvatore DiMauro and Guido Davidzon, 'Mitochondrial DNA and disease' (2005) 37(3) *Annals of Medicine* 222–32.

[31] Gráinne S. Gorman et al., 'Mitochondrial donation – How many women could benefit?' (2015) 372(9) *New England Journal of Medicine* 885–7; Cathy Herbrand, 'Mitochondrial replacement techniques: Who are the potential users and will they benefit?' (2017) 31(1) *Bioethics* 46–54.

[32] Rebecca E. Say et al. 'Mitochondrial diseases in pregnancy: A systematic review' (2011) 4(3) *Obstetric Medicine* 90–4.

[33] Herbrand, 'Mitochondrial replacement techniques'; Baylis, 'Human nuclear genome transfer (so-called mitochondrial replacement)'.

purchase the technology.[34] It follows that potential benefits will accrue to a very small number of people, the threat of mitochondrial disease will continue, and the chance of achieving the promise of a future without mitochondrial disease will be slim. As such, the potential benefits of human nuclear genome transfer are vastly overestimated.

Third, among those women who might use the technology, there is the risk of genetic drift,[35] whereby dysfunctional mtDNA is carried over to the healthy enucleated egg. As a result, mitochondrial disease might nonetheless continue in the family. In April 2017, Zhang and his team published the details of the first birth following maternal spindle transfer to avoid the transmission of Leigh syndrome. In this case, some dysfunctional mtDNA was transmitted to the child. The hope (expectation) is that, given the relatively small number of mtDNA mutations, the child may not display any symptoms of mitochondrial disease, but this is unknown.[36]

Finally, there is one other way in which the language of threat in debates about human nuclear genome transfer mirrors debates in personalised medicine. In her discussion of cancer, for example, Dickenson examines the complex two-faced nature of threat, whereby would-be patients must weigh the threat of disease against the threat of treatment.[37] In the case of nuclear genome transfer, the threat of mitochondrial disease must be weighed against the unknown threat of using this novel technology. Debates about its use in both the United Kingdom and the United States have circled around the risks of intervening, and the risks of not doing so. Ultimately the decision to proceed with human nuclear genome transfer in both of these countries – albeit tentatively – suggests that the risks of experiencing mitochondrial disease are, from the perspective of clinician-scientists and some prospective end-users,

[34] Considering these factors, the potential 150 births per year in the United Kingdom that might be positively affected by the use of human nuclear genome transfer is a very high estimate. Françoise Baylis has suggested that the maximum benefit would be fewer than 22 births per year. See Baylis, 'Human nuclear genome transfer (so-called mitochondrial replacement)'.

[35] Mitsutoshi Yamada et al., 'Genetic drift can compromise mitochondrial replacement by nuclear transfer in human oocytes' (2016) 18(6) Cell Stem Cell 749–54.

[36] Sara Reardon, 'Genetic details of controversial "three-parent baby" revealed' (6 April 2017) 544(7648) Nature News 17. See also Louise A. Hyslop et al., 'Towards clinical application of pronuclear transfer to prevent mitochondrial DNA disease' (2016) 534 (7607), Nature 383–6.

[37] Erica Haimes and Ken Taylor, 'Rendered invisible? The absent presence of egg providers in UK debates on the acceptability of research and therapy for mitochondrial disease' (2015) 33(4) Monash Bioethics Review 360–78.

greater than the risks of the technology. This is problematic, however, given that there are other ways in which to avoid mitochondrial disease, and given that nuclear genome transfer is neither treatment nor cure.[38]

On contamination, the purported benefit of human nuclear genome transfer is that familial nDNA is uncontaminated by third-party nDNA as this technology only requires the use third-party mtDNA. This perceived benefit rests on the belief that, while mtDNA is important, the traits that 'constitute the core of genetic relatedness in terms of physical and behavioural characteristics' are in the nDNA and it is this DNA that ought not to be contaminated by third-party genetic material. On this view, donor mtDNA is not a contaminant, it is a genetic 'treatment' for a disorder that does not yet exist, in a person not yet conceived.

2.5   On Narcissism: Human Nuclear Genome Transfer as a Much-Needed Technology

Dickenson's second hypothesis, on narcissism, is directly relevant to the emergence of human nuclear genome transfer as personalised medicine. Here, Dickenson explores the rise of a 'narcissistic culture' that privileges the realisation of individual desires and its implications for biotechnologies. Medical interventions are justified because they may help patients achieve the life that they want.

Nuclear genome transfer is not a lifesaving technology insofar as there are no living persons to be 'saved' by this technology. The potential benefit of this technology is the benefit of a new life free of mitochondrial disease – a benefit to people yet to be conceived, and their families. This benefit could more easily and assuredly be achieved by other means, however, including adoption, co-parenting, use of eggs provided by a third party, or conceiving naturally and using prenatal genetic testing and abortion. The usual objection to these reproductive strategies, however, is that all but the last strategy do not ensure the birth of genetically-related children. This objection makes explicit the prioritisation of genetic relatedness (through nDNA) above other important factors. The desire to engage in biological, genetic reproduction can readily be understood as a form of narcissism: a desire to see oneself in the world, quite literally as a love of one's own reflection.

[38] Nuclear genome transfer is neither treatment nor cure as it does not treat a person with dysfunctional mtDNA, but rather aims to ensure the birth of a different person, hopefully one that who will not have dysfunctional mtDNA. See Tina Rulli, 'What is the value of three-parent IVF?' (2016) 46(4) *Hastings Center Report* 38–47.

The perceived 'unique and special' value of one's own nDNA fuels the rhetoric around a perceived 'need' rather than a 'want' or desire for human nuclear genome transfer.[39] Proponents of this technology do not merely perceive its use as desirable, but rather as imperative because having genetically related children is positioned as superior to having non-genetically related children. This perception is well entrenched in popular culture and has been leveraged effectively by those who insist that human nuclear genome transfer responds to an important need, not merely a desire.

The view that human nuclear genome transfer is imperative to both ensure genetic relatedness and to ensure that children with certain genetic anomalies are not born raises important concerns about the rights of people with disabilities. While mitochondrial anomalies some-times result in fatal diseases, some people with dysfunctional mtDNA live very fulfilling lives, albeit with some measure of disability. The idea that people can and should use human nuclear genome transfer to avoid genetically transmitted disorders is likely to have been influenced by the life-shortening, very challenging nature of many of the relevant disorders. However, the suggestion that mitochondrial anomalies *need* to be eradicated is informed by assumptions about what kinds of lives are worth living (see 'The Best Me I Can Possibly Be', Van Beers' chapter in this volume). If nuclear genome transfer becomes widely available, there may be increased pressure on women to use the technology to ensure that their children do not experience mitochondrial disorders. Women who cannot afford nuclear genome transfer or its alternatives (i.e. adoption; assisted reproduction using third-party eggs), but wish to bear children, may one day be chastised as irresponsible for not having prevented the birth of children with mitochondrial disease. As Dorothy Roberts points out, poor women and women of colour will be increasingly compelled to use certain reproductive and genetic technologies to conceive 'the children that the state believes would be less of a burden on it'.[40]

Further, the desire to use nuclear genome transfer to select out certain genes in order to produce genetically related children hinges on a paradoxical view of genetic relatedness. On this view, some genes (i.e. those located in the nucleus of the cell – nDNA) are relevant to genetic relatedness, while other genes (i.e. those located in the mitochondria –

---

[39] Baylis, 'Human nuclear genome transfer (so-called mitochondrial replacement)'.
[40] Dorothy Roberts. Webinar on Gene Editing and the Future of Reproductive Justice, 13 June 2017. See www.geneticsandsociety.org/multi-media/gene-editing-and-future-reproductive-justice.

mtDNA) are not. It is not obvious, however, why genetic relatedness associated with nDNA should be thought of as more important than genetic relatedness associated with mtDNA. The selective nature of the desire for a certain kind of genetic relatedness is based on a complex conflation of genetics, kinship, eugenics and disability.

2.6   On Political Neoliberalism: Balancing Public Costs with Potential Benefits

Dickenson's third, and most convincing, hypothesis explaining the rise of personalised medicine is the ascendency of neoliberalism as a sociopolitical ethos. Here, she suggests that, although proponents of personalised medicine emphasise the potential health benefits to a small number of patients, the truly significant benefits, namely profits, accrue to pharmaceutical and biotechnology firms. This marks a transfer of public resources to private corporations, as the knowledge developed in publicly funded university systems comes to be commercialised and resold to the public for a profit. This is evident in the case of most pharmaceutical research, and particularly in the field of pharmacogenetics, which aims to develop targeted pharmaceutical interventions for disorders based on research derived from publicly funded genetic databases. The disproportionate emphasis on potential health benefits to patients also works to obscure the significant and often disproportionate risks downloaded to other parties, including already marginalised groups such as women, racialised people and people experiencing socioeconomic disadvantage.

In the case of human nuclear genome transfer, a great deal of public resources (derived from university budgets, charitable trusts and public research councils) have contributed to its development.[41] It is nonetheless the private-for-profit fertility industry that will capitalise on these investments. This marks a transferring of 'public wealth' to private corporations, through the development of biotechnologies in universities that are eventually owned by private individuals and corporations, and paid for a second time by the public, either when they access care through the public healthcare system or through individually purchased private healthcare services.

The stated goals of relevant researchers – to avoid mitochondrial disease and to ensure the safe use of human nuclear genome transfer

---

[41] Ewen Callaway, 'UK sets sights on gene therapy in eggs' (26 January 2012) 48(7382) *Nature News* 419.

when and where it is used – are important. At the same time, the public costs of developing technological interventions for this relatively rare group of disorders have been high, particularly given that claims about how human nuclear genome transfer will save money overall by reducing the incidence of catastrophic, expensive-to-treat mitochondrial disorders are overstated. As noted above, a very small number of people are likely to use human nuclear genome transfer to avoid mitochondrial disease, and the technology addresses disorders in people not-yet-conceived that can otherwise be avoided.

Here, it is perhaps worth noting that human nuclear genome transfer is poised to become widely available as a highly profitable technique for age-related infertility. This use of nuclear genome transfer is currently banned in many countries, including the United Kingdom, where the technology is only allowed under license for the prevention of mitochondrial disease. Yet, as noted above, in June 2017, Zhang began marketing human nuclear genome transfer explicitly for age-related infertility,[42] for which he has since been reprimanded by the FDA.[43] Nonetheless, heritable genetic modification is touted by many as the new horizon of (highly profitable) commercial infertility treatments, and the legal and regulatory frameworks being developed for the use of human nuclear genome transfer for mitochondrial disease are paving the way.

In addition to the transfer of public funds to the private sector, a core feature of neoliberalism is the redistribution of risk and vulnerability. The children conceived following nuclear genome transfer and their families are one key group, but important risks are also borne by the women who provide the third-party eggs used in nuclear genome transfer – the so-called 'mitochondrial donors'.[44] The process of providing

---

[42] Mullin, 'The fertility doctor trying to commercialize three-parent babies'.

[43] The reprimand, issued as a letter to Zhang's company, Darwin Life, was based on Zhang's creation of a 'genetically modified embryo' within the United States (followed by its exportation to Mexico). Both the marketing and export of the technology contravened elements of the FDA's regulations. The FDA also made clear that it would not be engaging in the pre-investigational new drug (IND) meetings necessary to approve a new drug, device or technology as it will not do so for interventions 'that involve "a human embryo . . . intentionally created or modified to include a heritable genetic modification"'. Letter to Dr John Zhang from Mary A. Malarkey, Director of the Office of Compliance and Biologics Quality, Center for Biologics Evaluation and Research of the United States Food and Drug Administration (FDA), 4 August 2017. www.fda.gov/downloads/BiologicsBloodVaccines/ GuidanceComplianceRegulatoryInformation/ComplianceActivities/Enforcement/ UntitledLetters/UCM570225.pdf.

[44] Françoise Baylis, 'The ethics of creating children with three genetic parents' (2013) 26 Reproductive Biomedicine Online 531–34.

eggs for human nuclear genome transfer (and the research that has informed its development) is time-consuming and invasive, including medical screening, daily hormonal injections for approximately four weeks, monitoring and transvaginal surgical extraction. Like egg provision for IVF, egg provision for human nuclear genome transfer also involves considerable risks, the most significant of which is hyperstimulation of the ovaries. Severe ovarian hyperstimulation syndrome can result in respiratory distress, blood clots, stroke, kidney failure and ovarian rupture resulting in haemorrhage. If untreated, it can be life-threatening or fatal.[45]

By and large, the contributions of the women who provide the egg cells (from which the nucleus is removed in order to receive the nDNA of another woman who hopes to conceive a child without a mitochondrial disorder) are 'rendered invisible'.[46] This was certainly the case, for example, in the United Kingdom in the media and policy debates that preceded the legalisation of human nuclear genome transfer (referred to as *mitochondrial donation*).[47] Egg providers were generally viewed as minimal contributors to the process, and peripheral to the conception of the offspring. Future risks were typically understood in terms of potential harms to the children yet to be conceived of the technology, and the unknown risks of altering the human genome. And although the language of the 'three-parent baby' and 'three-person IVF' was (and continues to be) widely used, when egg providers were explicitly mentioned in the parliamentary debates as part of a genetic triad, it was largely to dismiss their contributions by referring to how few genes were involved

---

[45] Selma Mourad, Julie Brown and Cindy Farquhar, 'Interventions for the prevention of OHSS in ART cycles: An Overview of Cochrane Reviews' in *Cochrane Database of Systematic Reviews* (John Wiley & Sons Ltd, 2017); Joint Society of Obstetricians and Gynaecologists of Canada-Canadian Fertility Andrology Society Clinical Practice Guidelines Committee et al., 'The diagnosis and management of ovarian hyperstimulation syndrome' (2011) 33(11) *Journal of Obstetrics and Gynaecology Canada* 1156–62; The Practice Committee of the American Society for Reproductive Medicine, 'Ovarian Hyperstimulation Syndrome' (2008) 90(S1) *Fertility and Sterility*. See also Vanessa Gruben, 'Women as patients, not spare parts: Examining the relationship between the physician and women egg providers' (2013) 25(2) *Canadian Journal of Women and the Law* 249–83; Alison Motluk, 'Is egg donation dangerous?' (2012) 46 *Maisonneuve* 26–33; Kanna Jayaprakasan et al., 'Estimating the risks of ovarian hyperstimulation syndrome (OHSS): Implications for egg donation for research' (2007) 10(3) *Human Fertility* 183–7.

[46] Haimes and Taylor, 'Rendered invisible?'

[47] See also Donna L. Dickenson, 'The commercialization of human eggs in mitochondrial replacement research' (2013) 19(1) *The New Bioethics: A Multidisciplinary Journal of Biotechnology and the Body* 18–29.

(mtDNA contains 37 genes), and how few of a child's personal characteristics, including personality, intelligence and appearance, might be affected by these genes.[48]

The risks and rewards of using human nuclear genome transfer were, and continue to be, understood in terms of moving science forward to address mitochondrial disease. The rhetorical construction of nuclear genome transfer has focused almost exclusively on future risks – to would-be offspring and to the human genome – positioning moving forward with nuclear genome transfer (as well as other new genetic technologies) as a step that biomedical science can and should take, albeit with caution. The real risks to women providing eggs are 'vanished',[49] presenting human nuclear genome transfer as relatively benign.

2.7   The Right to Choose Human Nuclear Genome Transfer

Dickenson's fourth and final hypothesis explaining the rise of personalised medicine is the primacy of autonomy. In recent years, in the context of Western medicine, the principle of autonomy has come to be narrowly understood in terms of informed choice. In time, in both subtle and not so subtle ways, this principled commitment has morphed into what Dickenson refers to as the 'sacredness of personal choice'.[50] Here, choice and entitlement become one: patients should be able to get what they want. On this view, once there are reasonable assurances (preferably through clinical trials) that a novel technology is safe (and hopefully effective) the only remaining issue regarding the ethical use of the technology is freedom of choice.

The privileging of personal choice above all is particularly apparent in the case of human nuclear genome transfer. It is widely argued that if women at risk of transmitting mitochondrial disease to their offspring want to use nuclear genome transfer in the hope of having genetically related children free of mitochondrial disease, they should be able to choose to do so (even when safer and more effective alternatives are available). In response to media queries about the first birth via maternal spindle transfer in Mexico, the clinic responded that 'patients come

---

[48] Haimes and Taylor, 'Rendered invisible?' 371.

[49] Dickenson, 'The commercialization of human eggs in mitochondrial replacement research'; Donna L. Dickenson, 'The lady vanishes: What's missing from the stem cell debate' (2006) 3(1–2) *Journal of Bioethical Inquiry* 43–54.

[50] Dickenson, *Me Medicine vs We Medicine*, 10.

first'.[51] In the context of limited research about the short- and long-term effects of human nuclear genome transfer, the absence of any kind of regulatory oversight and a move across international borders to avoid professional, regulatory or legal ramifications, this statement provides clear evidence of the 'sacredness of personal choice'.

This narrow focus on personal choice is worrisome insofar as the prioritisation of patient desires may culminate in the acceptance and widespread use of technologies with complex, intractable, intergenerational effects. The alteration of the genome for the eradication of mitochondrial disease may quickly give way to its use for other reasons. If, in time, Zhang's plans to use maternal spindle transfer for age-related infertility are widely implemented, it is possible that nuclear transfer from one woman to another will become mundane, and women will take for granted that they will be able to conceive easily at an older age, using the eggs of another woman. Technologies that enable conception at an older age are already occurring through the use of donor eggs and the proliferation of egg freezing technologies, but the possibility of using human nuclear genome transfer in order to have a genetically related child (with the mtDNA of another woman) may enable women to make reproductive decisions even later than egg freezing currently makes possible.

Even more worrisome, however, is Zhang's statement that his work is 'a step toward designer babies'.[52] The potential that human nuclear genome transfer (in conjunction with other technologies like CRISPR-Cas9) may be used to engage in the selection of particular genetic traits and unfettered alteration of the genome is of particular concern. Consider, for example, the potential for class-based genetic stratification that may subsequently emerge. This could have critical implications for social justice in future generations. Of particular interest, though, are the ways in which contested practices are normalised, as occurred, for example, in the case of prenatal genetic testing for genetic anomalies. Initially, these tests were simply made available to women for the detection of 'serious genetic disorders', but increasingly women are expected to use these tests to avoid not only 'serious genetic disorders' but also a range of anomalies, some of which are not seriously harmful. And while the emergence of human nuclear genome transfer for the creation of

---

[51] Jennifer Couzin-Frankel, 'Unanswered questions surround baby born to three parents' (27 September 2016) Science|AAAS, www.sciencemag.org/news/2016/09/unanswered-questions-surround-baby-born-three-parents.

[52] Mullin, 'The fertility doctor trying to commercialize three-parent babies'.

'designer babies' may still be distant, the 'sacredness of personal choice' may mean that, once it is available, people will be able – and compelled – to use it, no matter the societal outcomes.

2.8   Conclusion

Human nuclear genome transfer is profiled by its proponents as a reproductive technology aimed at helping specific women with dysfunctional mtDNA to have genetically related children free of mitochondrial disease. From this view, which effectively positions the technology in the realm of personalised medicine, human nuclear genome transfer is similar to other reproductive technologies insofar as it is up to eligible women (alone or with their partners) to decide if they want to partake. To this end, human nuclear genome transfer is distanced from any assessment of whether it serves (or could serve) the common good.

As Dickenson's framework on the emergence of personalised medicine elucidates, the successful positioning of human nuclear genome transfer as a form of personalised medicine is possible because of a number of cultural and societal features. First, there are the ways in which fear of mitochondrial disease as a threat to children not yet conceived has been used to allay fears about potential threats to the human genome (even though very few people at risk of having children with mitochondrial disease will benefit from human nuclear genome transfer). Second, there is the oft-repeated claim that, as compared with available alternatives for childbearing and childrearing, human nuclear genome transfer better responds to a (potentially narcissistic) desire to perpetuate certain genes and to ensure a genetic relationship with one's child. Third, human nuclear genome transfer involves a great deal of potential profit for corporate interests while downloading the financial costs of development to the public, and the risks of engagement to egg providers, the women seeking to use the technology and children yet to be conceived. Finally, like other forms of personalised medicine, the emphasis is on the choices of individual patients – in this case, personal reproductive choices – to the exclusion of broader considerations of social justice.

In closing, the emergence of human nuclear genome transfer as a form of personalised medicine is consistent with other efforts to undermine the idea of the human genome as something 'we all hold in common'.[53] This involves a shift from thinking about the human genome as a site of

[53] Dickenson, *Me Medicine vs We Medicine*, 193.

shared interest – a genetic commons – to one of personal property focused on one's descendants, and a desire to produce genetically-related offspring. And so it is that contemporary debates about the use of human nuclear genome transfer have pitted collective interests in preserving the integrity of the genome against its overt manipulation, in the name of helping individuals realise personal reproductive desires including the potential mitigation of serious mitochondrial disease. As the use of human nuclear genome transfer inches towards broader genomic alterations and 'designer babies', the framing of this technology as a matter of individual choice, and of personalised medicine that is part of the new bioeconomy, must be weighed substantively against the costs for our genetic and reproductive futures.

3

Stem Cell-Derived Gametes and Uterus Transplants

Hurray for the End of Third-Party Reproduction! Or Not?

HEIDI MERTES

3.1 Introduction

Although third party reproduction has become increasingly accepted, it remains a last resort and a suboptimal option for most people, which is often only taken into consideration when reproduction with one's own gametes or own womb has proven to be impossible.[1] The paradigmatic cases for people who cannot become genetic or gestational parents/ mothers are people who lack (functional) gametes and women who lack a uterus, either from birth or due to disease. In an effort to make genetic and gestational parenthood possible for these two groups, research is being conducted aimed at deriving gametes from stem cells matched to the patient and clinical trials are ongoing for uterus transplantation. Both are examples of what Donna Dickenson has called 'Me Medicine': medical interventions focusing on individual interests rather than on the common good.[2] However, are these also worrisome examples of Me Medicine? And is an alternative, We Medicine, approach possible?

3.2 The Science

3.2.1 Stem Cell-Derived Gametes

In order to produce gametes in vitro containing the genetic material of the patient, several steps are needed, which are all technically difficult and

---

[1] Elia Wyverkens, Veerle Provoost, An Ravelingien et al., 'The meaning of the sperm donor for heterosexual couples: confirming the position of the father' (2015) 56 *Family Process* 203–16.

[2] Donna Dickenson, *Me Medicine vs We Medicine: Reclaiming Biotechnology for the Common Good* (New York, NY: Columbia University Press, 2013).

at present experimental. First, a stem cell line needs to be created matching the patient's genome. This can currently be done in two ways. The first technique – called *somatic cell nuclear transfer* (SCNT) or 'therapeutic cloning' – involves the transfer of the cell nucleus of a somatic cell of the patient (e.g. a skin cell) into an enucleated egg cell. The egg cell will then erase the epigenetic marks on the nuclear DNA, and on activation an embryo can be grown which is genetically identical to the patient (not taking the mitochondrial DNA into consideration). When this embryo reaches the blastocyst stage (after five days), the inner cell mass can be extracted and cultured, resulting in an embryonic stem cell line. The second technique is direct reprogramming, resulting in induced pluripotent stem cells (iPS cells). In this scenario, somatic cells are reverted to their embryonic state by adding a small number of specific factors, a technique for which the Nobel prize in physiology/medicine was awarded to Sir John Gurdon and Shinya Yamanaka in 2012. Once a stem cell line has been established containing the DNA of the patient, gametes (ideally sperm or egg cells, or precursors of those cells) need to be derived from those stem cells. In the mouse model, significant progress has been made in the last decade, resulting in the creation of functional sperm cells in vitro, which produced live offspring in 2016.[3] Before transferring this science to clinical trials in humans, much research remains to be done regarding the safety of the procedure. Given the profound manipulations, the residual risks for the children who are conceived with these stem cell-derived gametes due to genetic, epigenetic, transcriptomic and imprinting problems are likely to remain higher than for the established option of donor conception, even after preclinical animal and embryo research. Moreover, follow-up over several generations will be necessary in order to confirm that the technology is really safe.

---

[3] Karin Hübner, Guy Fuhrmann, Lane K. Christenson et al., 'Derivation of oocytes from mouse embryonic stem cells' (2003) 300 *Science* 1251–6; Yayoi Toyooka, Naoki Tsunekawa, Ryuko Akasu et al., 'Embryonic stem cells can form germ cells in vitro' (2003) 100 *Proceedings of the National Academies of Sciences of the United States of America* 11457–62; Niels Geijsen, Melissa Horoschak, Kitai Kim et al., 'Derivation of embryonic germ cells and male gametes from embryonic stem cells' (2004) 427 *Nature* 148–54; Karim Nayernia, Jessica Nolte, Hans W. Michelmann et al., 'In vitro-differentiated embryonic stem cells give rise to male gametes that can generate offspring mice' (2006) 11 *Developmental Cell* 125–32; Katsuhiko Hayashi, Sugako Ogushi, Kazuki Kurimoto et al., 'Offspring from oocytes derived from in vitro primordial germ cell-like cells in mice' (2012) 338 Science 971–5; Quan Zhou, Mei Wang, Yan Yuan et al., 'Complete meiosis from embryonic stem cell-derived germ cells in vitro' (2016) 18 *Cell Stem Cell* 330–40.

3.2.2   Uterus Transplantation

Unlike stem cell-derived gametes, uterus transplantation is already in the phase of clinical trials. After unsuccessful clinical trials in Saudi Arabia and Turkey, several children have been born thanks to uterus transplantation in a Swedish clinical trial involving nine patients, and recently the first birth in the US was reported in the media.[4] A uterus transplantation involves an extensive surgical procedure for both the donor and the recipient. Donor surgery typically lasts between 10 and 13 hours and recipient surgery between four and six hours (there does not seem to be a learning curve yet).[5] One reported donor complication is ureterovaginal fistula (one case). Postoperative recipient complications include thrombosis or infections, which led to the removal of the transplanted uterus in two cases, pleural fluid (which was spontaneously resorbed) and a haematoma (requiring blood transfusion).

After the transplantation, the recipient needs to take immunosuppressive drugs in order to avoid rejection. Johansson et al. report rejection episodes in five of seven recipients (some had multiple rejection episodes).[6] All but one were classified as mild and all rejection episodes were without clinical symptoms. Immunosuppression implies that patients are more susceptible to, for example, viral infections and certain cancers. For the foetus, several immunosuppressive regimens are considered to be safe,[7] although caution and follow-up are warranted as there is still a great deal of conflicting evidence.[8]

All officially reported deliveries were preterm Caesarean sections. In the first case reported, the mother developed pre-eclampsia in the

[4] Mats Brännström, Liza Johannesson, Hans Bokström et al., 'Livebirth after uterus transplantation' (2015) 385 *The Lancet* 607–16; Mats Brännström, Hans Bokström, Pernilla Dahm-Kähler et al., 'One uterus bridging three generations: First live birth after mother-to-daughter uterus transplantation' (2016) 106 *Fertility and Sterility* 261–6; Alexandra Sifferlin, 'Exclusive: First US Baby Born After a Uterus Transplant' (2017) *Time*, Published 1 December 2017. Available at: http://time.com/5044565/exclusive-first-u-s-baby-born-after-a-uterus-transplant/
[5] Mats Brännström, Liza Johannesson, Pernilla Dahm-Kähler et al., 'First clinical uterus transplantation trial: A six-month report' (2014) 101 *Fertility and Sterility* 1228–36.
[6] Liza Johannesson, Niclas Kvarnström, Johan Mölne et al., 'Uterus transplantation trial: 1-year outcome' (2015) 103 *Fertility and Sterility* 199–204.
[7] Lisa A. Coscia, Serban Constantinescu, John M. Davison et al., 'Immunosuppressive drugs and fetal outcome' (2014) 28 *Best Practice & Research Clinical Obstetrics & Gynaecology* 1174–87.
[8] Giuseppe Benagiano, Laurens Landeweerd and Ivo Brosens, 'Medical and ethical considerations in uterus transplantation' (2013) 123 *International Journal of Gynecology & Obstetrics* 173–7.

32nd week of pregnancy; in the second case, the delivery was preterm due to cholestasis.[9] The weight of the children was low due to the preterm birth, but – fortunately – well within the average weight range for their gestational age.

A category of patients with absolute uterine factor infertility who might benefit from uterus transplantation are patients with Mayer–Rokitansky–Küster–Hauer (MRKH) syndrome, with congenital absence of uterus and vagina. This syndrome is also oftentimes accompanied by renal problems such as kidney malformation, single kidneys or pelvic kidneys, which can cause additional risks during pregnancy and delivery: for example, pre-eclampsia. Eight out of the nine patients in the Swedish clinical trial are MRKH patients.[10]

In short, we can say that although there is proof of principle that it is possible to deliver a healthy baby after a uterus transplantation, these are high-risk pregnancies which require invasive surgical procedures for the patient and the healthy research participant (the uterus donor). In other words, it is *not* a proof of principle that uterus transplantation is safe. Attempts have been made to use a uterus from a deceased donor (in order to avoid harming at least one of the participants in these experiments), which has both advantages and disadvantages from a technical perspective. At the time of writing, there have been several successful transplants from deceased donors, but no live births have been reported.[11]

3.3   Why Do We Transplant Uteri? Why Do We Attempt to Make Eggs and Sperm in Vitro?

Uterus transplantation and in vitro gametogenesis are not among the usual examples of personalised or 'Me' medicine, which is often identified with genomic medicine (see the introduction to this volume). Yet they certainly fit within the broader paradigm: they are very individualistic solutions for very personal desires. Also, as will be argued below, although research in these areas may further the interests of individual

---

[9] Brännström, Johannesson, Bokström et al., 'Livebirth after uterus transplantation'; Brännström, Bokström, Dahm-Kähler et al., 'One uterus bridging three generations'.

[10] Brännström, Johannesson, Dahm-Kähler et al., 'First clinical uterus transplantation trial: A six-month report'.

[11] Omer Ozkan, Munire Erman Akar, Ozlenen Ozkan et al., 'Preliminary results of the first human uterus transplantation from a multiorgan donor' (2013) 99 *Fertility and Sterility* 470–6; Giuliano Testa, Tiffany Anthony, Gregory J. McKenna et al., 'Deceased donor uterus retrieval: A novel technique and workflow' (2017) *American Journal of Transplantation*. doi: 10.1111/ajt.14476.

patients, the balance in terms of overall healthcare benefit may turn out to be negative rather than positive. It is therefore unsurprising that the four possible drivers of personalised medicine (at the expense of We Medicine), as discerned by Donna Dickenson, can also be applied to the contexts of gamete derivation and uterus transplantation: (1) threat and contamination, (2) narcissism and 'bowling alone', (3) corporate interests and political neoliberalism, and (4) the sacredness of personal choice.

First, threat and the fear of contamination can be linked to fear of third party involvement in the formation of a family. In the case of adoption, parents may wonder if the child has been psychologically damaged by being abandoned by its parents. In the case of surrogacy, parents may he worried about the impact of the behaviour of the women carrying their child (Does she drink alcohol? Does she eat healthily? Does she take folic acid?) and about the possibility that there may be an emotional bond between her and their child. In the case of donor conception, parents may worry about the donor being perceived as the 'real parent' or about 'flaws' in their children due to the donor's contribution.

Second, narcissism and bowling alone are reflected in the importance that is attached to genetic parenthood. This is not only important in the context of stem cell-derived gametes, but also plays a role in the enthusiasm surrounding uterus transplantation, as surrogacy (which is the only alternative option if a genetic link is to be established) is not an available alternative in many countries. As mentioned, in Sweden, where the successful clinical trial for uterus transplantation is taking place, surrogacy is prohibited. In *Me Medicine vs We Medicine: Reclaiming Biotechnology for the Common Good*, Dickenson links narcissism with the 'genetic mystique' (giving DNA a soul-like status) and genetic determinism (believing that we are determined by our genes).[12] These phenomena may indeed do much of the explanatory work of why people think it is so important to pass on their genes to their children and why they want to avoid genes from strangers entering 'their' gene pool.

Third, corporate interests might reinforce the technological imperative of moving these new technologies to the clinic as fast as possible. Offering the newest technology to patients can be perceived by the latter as a sign of excellence, of being a state-of-the-art clinic. We will, however, not discuss this element any further.

---

[12] Dickenson, *Me Medicine vs We Medicine*, p. 15.

Finally, the sacredness of personal choice is very prominent in this debate. Under the flag of reproductive liberty or reproductive autonomy, it is insinuated that everyone has the right to have genetically related children and that every woman has the right to gestate her own children (if at all possible). If one accepts this premise (which sounds deceptively self-evident to many) and if one takes as a given that, for some people, the only option of granting this right is by uterus transplantation or gamete derivation, then it logically follows that people have the right to have access to uterus transplantation and stem cell-derived gametes.

These three reasons why uterus transplantation and SCD gametes are so welcome – the avoidance of third party involvement, the importance of genetic and gestational parenthood and the emphasis on reproductive rights – will be further elaborated on in the following sections.

3.4   Threat and Contamination: 'Third Party Reproduction is Problematic'

There are different ways of making this argument, some more convincing than others.

First, some people question the morality of any kind of third party reproduction in favour of the traditional family unit (one father and one mother). This can be based on a number of grounds, both religious and secular. Some religions equate sperm donation with adultery or claim that third party involvement in reproduction violates the holy union between husband and wife and the sacred act of conception. The Catholic Church and Sunni Muslims, for example, do not approve of donor conception.[13] On the secular side, objections that donor conception is unnatural and concerns for the welfare of the future child are voiced, as third party reproduction would, for example, impact on their identity formation.[14]

Second, for the parents, the involvement of an outsider in the creation of their family can be emotionally troubling. The romantic image of creating a new individual by joining characteristics of two partners into

---

[13] Marcia C. Inhorn, 'Making Muslim babies: IVF and gamete donation in Sunni versus Shi'a Islam' (2006) 30 Culture, Medicine and Psychiatry 427–50; Julie H. Rubio, 'Family ties: A Catholic response to donor-conceived families' (2015) 21 Christian Bioethics 181–98.

[14] Amanda J. Turner and Adrian Coyle, 'What does it mean to be a donor offspring? The identity experiences of adults conceived by donor insemination and the implications for counselling and therapy' (2000) 15 Human Reproduction 2041–51.

one and/or of carrying a partner's child to term is shattered, which may result in a sense of failure. Moreover, the donor presents a threat to the family unit and more specifically to the legitimacy of the parental role of the 'social parent', or is at least perceived as such.[15] This fear is possibly even greater in jurisdictions where donor anonymity has been lifted. Surrogacy may involve the fear that the surrogate will become emotionally attached to the child and claim a parental role. Also, it is difficult for a couple to start bonding with their child before birth and the intended parents may disagree with the surrogate about permissible lifestyle habits or more profound decisions regarding the pregnancy (such as a reduction of a multiple pregnancy, for example).

Third, the practical implications of third party reproduction have proven to be an ethical minefield. Concerns for exploitation and commodification are linked to oocyte donation and surrogacy, there is fierce ongoing debate worldwide about the acceptability of donor anonymity, there have been sporadic reports of custodial battles, abandoned and stateless children and of embryo trading, there are concerns about sperm donors transmitting genetic diseases, etc.[16]

Against this backdrop, it is unsurprising that many research efforts are aimed at methods to avoid third party involvement in reproduction. However, while uterus transplantation and in vitro gametogenesis avoid some of the objections to surrogacy and donor conception mentioned above, it does not logically follow that they are more acceptable and less problematic, as they present their own ethical concerns, primarily in terms of safety, as mentioned above. Also, even if – under certain

---

[15] Wyverkens, Provoost, Ravelingien et al., 'The meaning of the sperm donor for heterosexual couples'.

[16] Nicole Bromfield and Karen Smith Robati, 'Global surrogacy, exploitation, human rights and international private law: A pragmatic stance and policy recommendations' (2014) 1 *Global Social Welfare* 123–35; I. Glenn Cohen, 'Sperm and Egg Donor Anonymity' in Leslie Francis (ed.), *The Oxford Handbook of Reproductive Ethics* (Oxford: Oxford University Press, 2016); Donna Dickenson, *Property in the Body: Feminist Perspectives* (Cambridge: Cambridge University Press, 2017, 2nd ed.), pp. 65–87; Anders Hansen, 'Danish sperm donor passed neurofibromatosis on to five children' (2012) 345 *British Medical Journal (Online)* e6570; Mark Henaghan, 'International surrogacy trends: How family law is coping' (2013) 7(3) *Australian Journal of Adoption*. Available at: www.nla .gov.au/openpublish/index.php/aja/article/view/3188; Barry J. Maron, John R. Lesser, Nelson B. Schiller et al., 'Implications of hypertrophic cardiomyopathy transmitted by sperm donation' (2009) 302 *Journal of the American Medical Association* 1681–4; Usha R. Smerdon, 'Crossing bodies, crossing borders: International surrogacy between the United States and India' (2008) 39 *Cumberland Law Review* 15–85; Stephen Wilkinson, 'The exploitation argument against commercial surrogacy' (2003) 17 *Bioethics* 169–87.

circumstances – they would be the better option to achieve the goal of parenthood as compared to third party reproduction (or in some jurisdictions the only legal option), that does not automatically legitimise them, as will be discussed below.

3.5   Narcissism and 'Bowling Alone': 'Genetics/Gestation is Very Important'

Both genetics and gestation tend to be portrayed in terms of basic human needs, rather than in terms of personal desires. This portrayal makes it easier to argue for investments in reproductive medicine in general and paves the way for greater acceptance of costly high-tech innovations in this domain, as has been remarked by Françoise Baylis and Alana Cattapan in the context of human nuclear genome transfer.[17]

A first way of addressing the claim that genetics and gestation are very important in family relationships is to refer to family functioning. However, family functioning in families created through third party reproduction has been reported to be well within the normal range.[18] Moreover, even in those cases where family functioning *is* affected, or where higher levels of stress and anxiety are reported, one can wonder whether this is due to the absence of the genetic/gestational link in itself or due to the narratives that accompany alternative ways of family creation. For example, it is very unlikely that the absence of a genetic link would have any effect on family functioning as long as the parents were unaware of the fact that they are not the genetic parents of the child (e.g. after an IVF mix-up). As previously argued, *genetic* parenthood is not the objective, biological concept that it once was or that we take it to be, as illustrated by debates over who the genetic parents of clones would be and whether mitochondrial transfer really generates 'three-parent babies'. Also, although it is unsurprising from an evolutionary perspective that we have a preference for raising genetically related children, this does not

---

[17] Françoise Baylis, 'Human nuclear genome transfer (so-called mitochondrial replacement): Clearing the underbrush' (2017) 31 *Bioethics* 7–19. Also see the chapter in this volume by Françoise Baylis and Alana Cattapan, 'Personalised Medicine and the Politics of Human Nuclear Genome Transfer'.

[18] Susan Golombok, Jennifer Readings, Lucy Blake et al., 'Families created through surrogacy: Mother–child relationships and children's psychological adjustment at age 7' (2011) 47 *Developmental Psychology* 1579–88; Lucy Blake, Vasanti Jadva and Susan Golombok, 'Parent psychological adjustment, donor conception and disclosure: A follow-up over 10 years' (2014) 29 *Human Reproduction* 2487–96.

explain why we legitimise this evolutionary urge: why a genetic link to our children *should* matter.[19]

Note that the latter question only becomes relevant when other issues are in the balance, for instance, safety for the resulting children. If I have an irrational, evolutionary urge to have genetically related children and I harm no-one in the process of pursuing that urge, there is not a problem. This changes when I request a medical treatment that puts other individuals in harm's way (e.g. a uterus donor) or that has a higher chance of resulting in the birth of a child with a disability than available alternatives (e.g. conception with SCD-gametes as opposed to donor gametes). In these cases I will need to back up my desire with good reasons, justifying why the (moral) benefits of gratifying my desire for a genetic child outweigh the (moral) disadvantages. While acknowledging that the absence of genetic parenthood – when desired – *can* lead to a decrease in subjective well-being and to a sense of loss of purpose in life, and that this suffering can justify public funding of medical interventions such as IVF, it does not necessarily justify the risks involved in reproduction with SCD-gametes or in uterus transplantation.

Concerning the importance of *gestational* parenthood, a first observation is that essentialist discourse about what it means to be a mother tends to incorporate pregnancy. However, this is but one possible discourse, which is challenged by adoption and 'queer motherhood'.[20] Moreover, a simple but strong counterargument against the belief that pregnancy is of such great importance that it would justify the introduction of uterus transplantation into the clinic is that the male half of the world's population is not capable of bearing children and yet, this is not problematised at all. We do not regard the father as being less of a parent because he does not gestate children, so consistency demands that a mother who does not gestate her children is not regarded as less of a parent either. One might reply that gestation is not a crucial facet of *parent*hood, but that it is a crucial facet of *mother*hood. Indeed, it is right that not gestating deprives a woman of a facet that is typical of motherhood. However, does this deprivation carry much moral weight? And if so, why? A woman who delivers her child through a Caesarean section instead of a natural birth is also deprived of a typical feature of

[19] Heidi Mertes, 'Gamete derivation from stem cells: Revisiting the concept of genetic parenthood' (2014) 40 *Journal of Medical Ethics* 744–7.
[20] Elisabeth A. Suter, Leah M. Seurer, Stephanie Webb et al., 'Motherhood as contested ideological terrain: Essentialist and queer discourses of motherhood at play in female–female co-mothers' talk' (2015) 82 *Communication Monographs* 458–83.

motherhood, but one would think that the other aspects of parenthood and motherhood easily trump this missing feature. The same can be said about gestation: is the experience of pregnancy really worth risking prematurity, pre-eclampsia or thrombosis? Moreover, on a more practical note, the experience of a pregnancy with a transplanted womb as compared to one's own womb differs significantly as the nerves are not connected and therefore the pregnant woman will not feel much of the foetal movements or contractions.

In short, it is far from obvious that the desire for genetic or gestational parenthood can trump considerations for the welfare of the future child, for the safety of the other parties involved (in the case of uterus transplantation) or that it can justify resource allocation to these new reproductive technologies.

3.6   Sacredness of Personal Choice: 'Everyone Has the Right to Reproduce'

The most straightforward answer to this claim is that the right to reproduce is a liberty right instead of a claim right, which therefore does not amount to a duty on society to accommodate that right. This counterargument is well rehearsed in the legal and ethics literature on reproductive medicine.[21] Moreover, rights are always to be balanced against other people's rights, for example, the right not to be harmed. Both in the case of uterus transplantation and of gamete generation, there is a trade-off between the prospective parents' desire for (genetic/gestational) parenthood on the one hand and the welfare of the donor, recipient and resulting children. In transplantation medicine, living organ donation always involves invasive surgical procedures on healthy people without a direct benefit to the donor. This appears to violate the physician's oath to 'do no harm', but in many jurisdictions, this infraction is accepted in cases where the donor provides her informed consent and when the intervention can save the life of the recipient. However, in uterus transplantation, the bar is set lower: the transplant is not aimed at the survival of the recipient or a profound increase in her quality of life.

---

[21] Carter J. Dillard, 'Rethinking the procreative right' (2007) 10 *Yale Human Rights and Development* 1; John A. Robertson, 'Embryos, families, and procreative liberty: The legal structure of the new reproduction' (1985) 59 *Southern California Law Review* 939–1041; Laura Shanner, 'The right to procreate: When rights claims have gone wrong' (1995) 40 *McGill Law Journal* 823–74.

Besides concerns for the donor's welfare, respecting reproductive autonomy does not mean that doctors should always cater to patient demand, especially in domains as emotionally charged as reproduction. Infertile women have previously been reported to be particularly vulnerable to the appeal of the technological imperative.[22] For many women, it is important for their peace of mind that they 'did everything they could', regardless of the clinical, financial and emotional repercussions, almost as if they do not want to abandon a child that is waiting somewhere to be brought into existence. It is therefore all too easy for physicians to say that the procedure is legitimised by the patient's informed consent, as the validity of that informed consent can be seriously contested and as the establishment of high risk pregnancies, even with a woman's consent, can hardly be considered as good clinical practice. Several authors have referred to the danger of the therapeutic misconception, both in the minds of doctors/researchers and patients/participants, in the context of uterus transplantation clinical trials.[23] Ideally, the prime motivation of participants in clinical trials should be to advance knowledge about the safety and feasibility of new medical procedures. However, in the context of uterus transplantations, this requirement is completely unrealistic. The primary motivation for women to participate in these clinical trials is their desire to gestate a baby and become a parent. There are no clinical trials set up recruiting women without a desire for motherhood, merely studying survival of the graft, and it would be very unlikely that such trials would be approved by ethics committees. The therapeutic misconception is therefore not a misconception in the sense that the aim – even in the clinical trials – is primarily therapeutic. Yet it remains important that participants are warned that while a therapeutic benefit is possible and aimed at, it is not likely and that they may end up worse off after completion of the trial than they were before.

One can also legitimately wonder whether the welfare of the future child has received adequate consideration in the ongoing clinical trials of uterus transplantation. Despite the births of several healthy children, it

---

[22] Judith C. Daniluk, "'If we had it to do over again...'": Couples' reflections on their experiences of infertility treatments' (2001) 9 *The Family Journal* 122–33; Tjeerd Tymstra, "'At least we tried everything": About binary thinking, anticipated decision regret, and the imperative character of medical technology' (2007) 28 *Journal of Psychosomatic Obstetrics & Gynecology* 131.

[23] Kavita Shah Arora and Valarie Blake, 'Uterus transplantation: The ethics of moving the womb' (2015) 125 *Obstetrics & Gynecology* 971–974; Arthur L. Caplan, Constance M. Perry, Lauren A. Plante et al., 'Moving the womb' (2007) 37 *Hastings Center Report* 18–20.

might be only a matter of time before a baby gestated in a transplanted uterus suffers lifelong consequences of prematurity or other pregnancy complications linked to the transplant. Some might invoke the non-identity problem[24] to argue for a very low threshold of well-being in the case of stem cell-derived gametes: the resulting children are not harmed as they would not have existed without this technology, unless if their lives are not worth living (the wrongful life standard). Technically speaking, this argument does not apply in the context of uterus transplantation. The future children growing from the transferred IVF-embryos have better prospects if they are carried to term by a healthy gestational carrier, than if they are carried to term in a transplanted uterus (although this interpretation was challenged by John Robertson[25]). They can therefore be said to be harmed – or at least put into harm's way – by being the subject of an experimental procedure.

Despite the non-identity problem (in the case of SCD gametes), other ethical principles give reason for a cautious approach when risks for the future children are present. First, when aspiring parents need to choose between two modes of conception, all other things being equal, it is better to choose the one that is most likely to result in healthy children (i.e. they should choose those children who are most likely to suffer the least), although it is not necessarily immoral to take limited risks in regard to the future child's well-being.[26] Second, it has been argued that the most appropriate welfare standard for future children is the 'reasonable welfare standard', meaning that '[t]he provision of medical assistance in procreation is acceptable when the child born as a result of the treatment will have a reasonably happy life'.[27] Third, physicians and parents have a shared responsibility regarding the welfare of the children who are created by means of assisted reproduction. The physician therefore needs to make his or her own assessment of the harms and benefits involved for all parties. After decades of successful efforts to make pregnancy and childbirth safer for both mother and child, uterus transplantation and reproduction by stem cell-derived gametes seem to be a step back, rather than a step forward.

---

[24] Derek Parfit, *Reasons and Persons* (Oxford: Oxford University Press, 1984).

[25] John A. Robertson, 'Impact of uterus transplant on fetuses and resulting children: A response to Daar and Klipstein' (2016) 3 *Journal of Law and the Biosciences* 710.

[26] Julian Savulescu and Guy Kahane, 'The moral obligation to create children with the best chance of the best life' (2009) 23 *Bioethics* 274–90.

[27] Guido Pennings, 'Measuring the welfare of the child: In search of the appropriate evaluation principle' (1999) 14 *Human Reproduction* 1146–50.

Importantly, it is dishonest to weigh the efforts and risks for mother, child and donor against the birth of a healthy baby. The healthy live births that are reported are not the only attempts made to establish pregnancies through uterus transplantation. The hardship endured by all the couples in the clinical trial whose desire for a child was not met should therefore also be taken into account. This new innovation may provide hope to many involuntarily childless women with uterine factor infertility, but for most of them – and even many of the ones who have access to the technology – this hope will turn out to be false hope, and for some of them, their adventure may end in tragedy in case of serious morbidity. This is a factor that should also be incorporated into the equation and that is easily forgotten in the excitement of a success story.

Also, on a more speculative note, the fact that there is a proof of principle that women without a uterus are able to gestate their child, but that this treatment option is out of reach for the great majority of women, may hinder the coping process of that majority and lead to additional frustration. Therefore, if the group of patients as a whole is considered, the cost–benefit analysis may turn out to be very grim. The same reasoning would apply for patients 'needing', but not having access to, SCD-gametes. In the latter context, it has been noted that by developing the technology of in vitro gametogenesis, needs are being created for categories of people that currently are not labelled as infertile (such as same-sex couples or postmenopausal women), but at the same time these needs are not met.[28] Paradoxically, a focus on reproductive liberty may therefore lead to a frustration of that same liberty.

3.7 The Common Good and We Medicine

Moreover, as repeatedly pointed out by Dickenson,[29] an increased focus on individual rights in biotechnology and bioethics has diverted attention away from the common good. While this is not – and should not be – an either–or story, it is interesting to consider how we might approach the given problem (grief caused by the inability to achieve genetic/gestational parenthood) from a common good perspective. In any case, taking a broader perspective does not mean that the personal suffering caused by

---

[28] Anna Smajdor and Daniela Cutas, 'Will artificial gametes end infertility?' (2015) 23 *Health Care Analysis* 134–47.

[29] Dickenson, *Me Medicine vs We Medicine*; Donna Dickenson, 'The common good' in Roger Brownsword, E. Scotford and K. Yeung (eds.), *The Oxford Handbook of Law, Regulation and Technology* (Oxford: Oxford University Press, 2017), p. 135.

infertility should be minimised. It has been well established that people
who are faced with a diagnosis of infertility suffer tremendously. As an
indication: the same degree of depression is reported in infertility
patients as in cancer patients.[30] The no-treatment option is not an option.
People who suffer from infertility should receive appropriate care.

However, this does not equate to giving them what they want (a baby),
regardless of the risks, efforts and of whether society can afford it. If we
take a step back and look at infertile people as a group, they may be very
ill served by constantly confirming and thereby reinforcing the idea that
one is only 'truly' a mother if one has gestated her own child and that one
is only 'truly' a parent if one is a genetic parent. Many people are excellent
parents to children whom they did not gestate and who did not spring
from their genes. I am not only referring to third party conception here,
but also to adoption, foster care, stepparents and even involved aunts and
uncles. Moreover, many people lead a perfectly happy and satisfying
child-free life. In terms of well-being, there have been numerous studies
showing that there is no positive correlation between having children and
happiness or life satisfaction.[31] The message that genetics and gestation
are *not* necessary components of parenthood and that parenthood is *not*
a necessary requirement for a meaningful life should receive adequate
attention, despite the fact that patients are unreceptive to this message.
Let us not forget that, at present, a large percentage of women who get on
the ART-rollercoaster end up childless (e.g. for US patients receiving IVF
with their own gametes in 2014: 30 per cent of patients below 35,
42 per cent of patients between 35 and 37, 59 per cent of patients between
38 and 40, 78 per cent of patients between 41 and 42 and 93 per cent of
patients above 42 years are unsuccessful[32]). All these women and their
partners balance several years between hope and despair and are left
empty-handed. It is often only at this point of their journey – if at all –
that they will get the message that life is possible without (genetically
related / personally gestated) children, after years of receiving the opposite message.

---

[30] Alice D. Domar, Patricia C. Zuttermeister and Richard Friedman, 'The psychological
impact of infertility: A comparison with patients with other medical conditions' (1993) 14
Journal of Psychosomatic Obstetrics and Gynaecology 45.

[31] Thomas Hansen, 'Parenthood and happiness: A review of folk theories versus empirical
evidence' (2012) 108 *Social Indicators Research* 29–64.

[32] Society for Assisted Reproductive Technology, 'National Summary Report'. Available at:
www.sartcorsonline.com/rptCSR_PublicMultYear.aspx?reportingYear=2014

Thus, if we look at the group of infertile people, are they really helped by ever new options that provide hope for all, but only a child for the happy few? Perhaps we need a new approach, whereby we content ourselves with the idea that we attempt to satisfy the desire for parenthood within certain safety limits and within certain financial constraints and that those who fall outside these limits are helped in a different way. Specifically, this would mean helping them find out what it is they are looking for in genetic parenthood or gestational parenthood and try to accommodate these desires in a different, safer, manner and/or by helping them cope with infertility.

3.8 Conclusion

Faced with the hope and hype surrounding stem cell-derived gametes and uterus transplantation, we need to stop and wonder whether the goal of assisting people in their reproductive endeavours is blinding us to the 'collateral damage' that it is causing. If fertility clinics are really interested in helping *all* infertile people, the right approach is not to invest in high-tech solutions that are likely to remain elite-medicine for many years and help only a limited number of people. Rather, efforts are needed to replace Me Medicine by We Medicine when possible. One way of doing this is by critically questioning the beliefs on which the patient request is based, rather than accommodating and thereby confirming and reinforcing them. It should be brought to patients' attention that genetics and gestation are not essential elements of parenthood; that third party reproduction is not necessarily problematic or inferior; that the desire for genetic and gestational parenthood or an appeal to reproductive autonomy does not automatically justify the risks of uterus transplantation and reproduction through SCD gametes; and that parenthood is not a necessary requirement for a happy, meaningful or satisfying life. Although changing people's beliefs takes time, tackling these myths will in the long run have a bigger chance of reducing the suffering of people faced with infertility than reinforcing them.

4

Personalising Future Health Risk through 'Biological Insurance'

Proliferation of Private Umbilical Cord Blood Banking in India

JYOTSNA AGNIHOTRI GUPTA

4.1 Introduction

In her book *Me Medicine vs We Medicine*, [1] Donna Dickenson expresses her concern that Me Medicine is eclipsing We Medicine, 'so that we're losing sight of the notion that biotechnology can and should serve the common good'. In her view 'it would be wrong to prioritize personalized health technologies at the expense of public health measures, which have brought us comparative freedom from the ill health that plagued our ancestors. I see a pattern here – not only a similarity among all the apparently disparate forms of personalized medicine but also a familiar political formula: "private good, public bad"'.[2] There are two unchallenged assumptions, she writes, 'that "individual" is better than "social" and that we are on the cusp of a "true revolution in medicine" to make it more individualized'. She is sceptical whether these are justified.[3] Dickenson voices the need for 'a disinterested and balanced critique of personalised medicine's origins, the commercial interests that lie behind it, and the dynamics of its marketing', as what she terms *'retail therapy*, that is medical treatment ... conceived as consumer goods'.[4] This is imperative as '... what may look like innocent individual consumer choices will shape how we as a society assure our health and that of future generations'.[5]

One of the examples Dickenson uses to illustrate this concept of 'Me Medicine vs We Medicine' is that of the increasing proliferation of

[1] Donna Dickenson, *Me Medicine vs We Medicine: Reclaiming Biotechnology for the Common Good* (New York, NY: Columbia University Press, 2013).
[2] Ibid., pp. 2–3.   [3] Ibid., p. 4.   [4] Ibid., p. 4.   [5] Ibid., p. 3.

private umbilical cord blood (UCB) banks. Inspired by Dickenson's work, I discuss the proliferation of private UCB banks in India. I identify the strategies used by private UCB banks to recruit pregnant women and explore what this means for pregnant women's decision-making, as UCB banks lay the onus for the future health and treatment of their child on them, and the factors and actors and values used to influence their decision whether to bank or not. I establish that private UCB banks in India are driven by corporate interest and political neo-liberalism (two of the four phenomena mentioned by Dickenson as possible explanations for the rise of 'Me Medicine') while offering 'choice' to pregnant women.

4.2   Umbilical Cord Blood Banking

In the late 1980s and early 1990s scientists began to realise the importance of blood from the human umbilical cord and placenta as a rich source of haematopoietic stem cells which can be harvested and cryo-preserved for transplantation to treat certain blood cancers and immune system disorders.[6] The first public and private UCB banks were established in the USA in 1993.[7] During the 1990s, most developed nations organised public systems for the collection of cord blood, which were built over previous bone marrow registries or blood collection services. The public systems are based on donation of cord blood for research and therapy on an 'allogeneic' (self-to-other) rationale, i.e. on the transplantation of cord blood from a related or unrelated tissue-matched donor to an immunologically compatible host. The first transplant from an unrelated donor was carried out in 1993.[8] In this system supposedly altruism and the solidarity principle prevail.

Since 2000, with the emergence of regenerative medicine as a new field of hope, the 'promissory' value of UCB has gained importance and spurred the rapid development of the private commercial sector.[9] These services offer collection, processing and private storage of UCB

[6] Pablo Rubinstein, 'Why cord blood?' (2006) 67 *Human Immunology* 398–404.

[7] Catherine Waldby, 'Umbilical cord blood: From social gift to venture capital' (2006) 1(1) *Biosocieties* 55–70.

[8] Paul Martin, Nik Brown and Andrew Turner, 'Capitalizing hope: The commercial development of umbilical cord blood stem cell banking' (2008) 27 (2) *New Genetics and Society* 127–43.

[9] Nik Brown, Alison Kraft and Paul Martin, 'The promissory pasts of blood cells' (2006) 1(3) *Biosocieties* 329–48; Nik Brown and Alison Kraft, 'Blood ties – Banking the stem cell promise' (2006) 3/4 *Technology Analysis and Strategic Management* 313–27.

just for the child's own future use or its family members': in other words, autologous donation. Sometimes, cord blood is banked with a clear intention of using it for a family member already suffering from a disease that may need bone marrow or transplant.

To date, there have been few documented cases of autologous use of cord blood, and even in these few cases, the utility of the autograft is still dubious,[10] while over 25,000 patients have been cured with allogeneic transplants.[11] But private banks, which define themselves as 'family banks', advertise their services through their websites on the Internet and base their discourse on the autologous possibility, defining the stored sample as 'a "self-repair kit" for your child' (www.stemcytefamily.com/cord_blood), and qualifying the private preservation of cord blood as a form of 'biological insurance for your child', and as a 'once in a lifetime opportunity to preserve a biomedical resource that could be a lifesaver for your child and other family members'. But importantly, more than offering an actual, therapeutic service, the commercial sector has grown through the selling, overall, of something immaterial: expectations of the future development of autologous transplantation.

4.3 State of the Art: Public and Private Initiatives in Umbilical Cord Blood Stem Cell Banking in India

India is an emerging economy, where both public and private initiatives in stem cell research exist and are proliferating, riding on the second wave of globalisation in the biomedical and IT industry. In the public sector their primary purpose is the creation of an inventory of UCB units for allogeneic use. The first private UCB bank in India was opened in Chennai, in South India, by LifeCell in 2004. The last decade has seen the establishment of several private UCB banks. The leading private players in cord blood banking in India include LifeCell International, Reliance Life Sciences, Cryobanks International India (now known under the name Cryoviva India), Cryo Stemcell Karnataka, Cordlife Sciences, Stem One, International Stemcell Services and CryoSave India. CryoSave, established in 2000, headquartered in Switzerland, claims to have banked samples from over 70 countries on six continents. It launched its operation in India in December 2008 and set up stem

---

[10] Karen Ballen, 'Challenges in umbilical cord blood stem cell banking for stem cell reviews and reports' (2010) 6(8) *Stem Cell Review and Reports* 8–14, p. 8.

[11] Karen Ballen, 'Update on Umbilical Cord Blood Transplantation' (2017) 6 *F1000Research* 1556. doi:10.12688/f1000research.11952.1.

cell storage banks in the country. In October 2017 Cryo-Save India signed a formal agreement with LifeCell International for formal transfer of all of its 18,000 cryopreserved umbilical cord units and corresponding customer agreements to LifeCell. LifeCell's storage facilities in Chennai (South India) and Gurgaon (North India) currently house more than 270,000 samples of preserved UCB and tissue stem cell units.[12] A new entrant in the UCB banking market is the Singapore-based firm Cordlife Group Limited, which has a pan-India presence. Relicord (Reliance Life Sciences Stem Cell Banking services) has established what they claim is south Asia's first, most advanced and completely automated stem cell enriched umbilical cord blood repository. This is the first cord blood repository in the world to be accorded a license by an official regulatory authority, the Food and Drug Administration of the Government of India, and is accredited by the American Association of Blood Banks. According to the Association of Stem Cell Banks of India, over 1.6 million units of cord blood are stored in 15 private banks.[13]

Many UCB banks also have a hybrid model, operating both a private and a public bank, such as Relicord (Reliance Life Sciences), Jeevan Stem Cell Bank (until 2012), South Korean Histostem Co. Ltd and StemCyte India Therapeutics Pvt Ltd, which is a joint venture between StemCyte Inc. USA, Apollo Hospitals Enterprises Ltd and Cadila Pharmaceuticals Ltd. Histostem Co. Ltd is a South Korean, US-based Biotechnology firm. Its main divisions are cell therapy research, a public cord blood bank for transplantation, and family cord blood banking providing stem cells for transplant surgeons globally. The distinction between public and private banks is not quite clear as public banks fund themselves by selling cord blood units to other banks on a global scale.[14] Most cord blood banking companies and research centres have formal tie-ups with prestigious hospitals in big cities in India. In India UCB transplantation is in its infancy. There are very few reports of applications in case of acquired and constitutional haematological disorders and none for metabolic

---

[12] Times News Network, 11 October 2017.
[13] www.womensweb.in/articles/cord-blood-banking-in-india. Accessed 5 January 2018.
[14] Nik Brown, Laura Machin and Danae McLeod, 'The immunitary bioeconomy: The economisation of life in the international cord blood market' (2011) 30 *Social Science and Medicine* 1–8; Christine Hauskeller and Lorenzo Beltrame, 'Hybrid practices in cord blood banking. Rethinking the commodification of human tissues in the bioeconomy' (2016) 35(3) *New Genetics and Society* 228–45; Dickenson, *Property in the Body*.

disorders. By 2011, around 13 cases of thalassaemia had been treated using UCB transplantation.[15]

Of India's population of nearly 1.3 billion, nearly 70 per cent live in rural areas where basic healthcare services are unavailable, inadequate or inequitably distributed, with class and literacy/education being important factors determining access to medical settings. Only 60 per cent of rural women and 86 per cent of urban women receive antenatal check-ups.[16] Of the approximately 26 million births a year 60 per cent of deliveries still take place at home under the supervision of trained and untrained birth attendants (50:50 ratio) (www.unicef.org/infobycountry/india). India is in a transitional phase from home-based deliveries to institutional deliveries. Most of the UCB banks are located in urban metropolises. According to Asim Ghazi, Director of Marketing at Cryobanks International, 'Counsellors sit in birth centres, any place where births take place. UCB collection centres have been set up also in small towns'.[17]

Umbilical cord blood has become a commodity in the international 'bioeconomy' which is flourishing by commodifying body parts, tissues and fluids.[18] With the increase in medical tourism to India, the country could be the largest potential supplier of UCB in the world; 600,000 are potential customers.[19] The UCB banking market is worth US$750 million per year. India has a major share of the projected market.[20] However, the global 'immunitary bioeconomy' rewards rareness of the blood type rather than size of the supply.[21] India has ethnic diversity in terms of Aryan, Dravidian and Mongoloid populations.

Cord blood is collected after the umbilical cord has been clamped before being cut during the process of giving birth. This can be done either while

---

[15] David McKenna and Jayesh Sheth, 'Umbilical cord blood: Current status & promise for the future' (2011) 134 (3), *Indian Journal of Medical Research* 261–69.

[16] M. B. Agarwal, 'Umbilical cord blood transplantation: Newer trends' (2006) 54 *Journal of the Association of Physicians of India* 143–47, p. 144.

[17] Nancy Singh, *C(h)ords of Life* (2010), www.chillibreeze.com/articles_various/Umbilical-cord-banking-in-India-310.asp. Accessed 20 December 2012.

[18] Dickenson, *Me Medicine vs We Medicine*; Dickenson, *Property in the Body*.

[19] Singh, *C(h)ords of Life.*

[20] Shashank S. Tiwari, *The Ethics and Governance of Stem Cell Clinical Research* (2013) PhD Thesis, University of Nottingham, Institute for Science and Society, www.eprints.nottingham.ac.uk/14585/1/602957. Accessed 20 September 2016.

[21] Brown et al., The immunitary bioeconomy.

the placenta remains attached to the uterine wall (*in utero*), or after delivery of the placenta (*ex utero*). UCB stem cells can be banked in a private, public or hybrid bank. According to Dr P. Srinivasan, Chairman of the Jeevan Stem Cell Bank in Chennai, 'Availability or the willingness of people to donate for public storage is not a problem, but it is the funds required for collecting, testing and storing the units that will be the limiting factor'.[22] On average it costs between 75,000–90,000 Indian rupees (approximately US$1,200–1,500)[23] to collect and process cord blood; these costs are covered by the public cord blood bank. Public banks charge approximately 170,000 rupees for each sample released for transplant. A limited number of hospitals offer public donation. Many clients and even clinicians are not aware of the existence of public UCB banks, as they do not advertise aggressively.

For the most part, donating UCB to a public bank does not cost the family anything. The obstetrician/gynaecologist doing the collection may charge a small fee, which in some cases may be covered by medical insurance. Private UCB banks, however, charge a fee for collection, processing and storage of UCB. The cost of banking per umbilical cord at a private bank is approximately 75,000 Indian rupees all-in, or a one-time payment of 27,000 rupees for enrolment and processing fees plus 3,000 rupees per year for 21 years. Various options are available, such as only cord blood stem cells preservation, cord blood stem cells and cord tissue, cord blood stem cells and 1 million cord tissue stem cells harvested and preserved, and cord blood stem cells and 50 million cord tissue stem cells harvested and preserved, with the price going up to 119,900 rupees (promotional flyer LifeCell). Another fee is often charged when a sample is removed for testing or treatment. Stem cells derived from the UCB are initially to be stored for 21 years, after which the individual would get to decide about further storage of her/his cells. Some UCB banks offer 'pocket-friendly payment options' (payment in instalments).[24]

Undoubtedly, this is a huge sum of money for the vast majority of Indians who live on less than US$2 per day. However, there is a sharp growth in the numbers of the Indian middle class, which has reaped the benefits of globalisation and the neo-liberal market economy in India.

[22] R. Prasad, 'Public cord-blood banking becomes a reality in Chennai,' *The Hindu*, 1 January 2009.
[23] Exchange rate of approximately US$ 1 = 64 INR.   [24] Cryobanks information leaflet.

This category looks to the West for inspiration in lifestyle; these are the main targets of the UCB banks. Celebrities such as Bollywood film stars and cricketers (who often serve as role models and 'brand ambassadors') were some of the first parents who banked the cord blood of their newborns and have since been followed by many other well-to-do parents who see it as rational and responsible behaviour and an investment in the future health of their progeny and perhaps of the whole family.

UCB banking is advertised as a kind of personal biological life insurance for your child (as one bank puts it) based on the expectations of a future development of 'autologous', or self-to-self, transplantation. Viewing the promise of cord blood stem cells as a form of biological health insurance, about 5 per cent of parents now bank their newborn's cord blood, with about 80 per cent of that going to private banks for the child's/family's own possible use and about 20 per cent going to public banks.

UCB banking is poised to grow in the years to come for three reasons: a) more and more cord banking companies are operating actively; b) more Indians are increasingly aware of this facility and are keen on ensuring their child's lifelong health (although, relatively speaking, it is a miniscule proportion of the large Indian population); and c) the process of UCB banking has been granted regulatory approval. A high growth rate is expected, but it is subject to various factors such as successful stem cell research, government policy, etc. The Indian Council of Medical Research (ICMR) and the Department of Biotechnology (DBT) established Guidelines for Stem Cell Research and Therapy in 2007. 'These cord blood banking guidelines, which became effective in 2012, are applicable to cord blood units intended for autologous and allogeneic use and are designed to provide a framework for facilities to obtain a license to manufacture and distribute cord blood in India. The guidelines outline the collection, processing, testing, storage, banking, and release requirements for umbilical cord blood'.[25] These guidelines were revised in October 2017.[26]

---

[25] www.aabb.org/advocacy/regulatorygovernment/ct/international/Pages/india.aspx. Accessed 15 September 2016.
[26] ICMR and DBT, *National Guidelines for Stem Cell Research* (New Delhi: Indian Council for Medical Research and Department of Biotechnology, October 2017).

4.4   Approach

4.4.1   Theoretical and Conceptual Framework

In addition to Dickenson's concept of 'Me Medicine vs We Medicine', I will discuss the marketing of UCB within the framework of 'risk' theory, and concepts such as 'manufactured risk' and 'risk society'.[27] There is a construction of a new kind of patient, the 'at-risk individual' who needs 'personalised medicine'.

4.4.2   Research Methodology and Methods

This chapter is based on pilot research and reflects work in progress. It is part of a study on the proliferation of private UCB banking in India. Qualitative research methods, such as literature research for theoretical understanding of the issue and analysis, and fieldwork were adopted. Initially, an analysis of media coverage on UCB banking was done to map the field. Also, promotional material of UCB banks (including information on websites), was collected and scrutinised.

Empirical research using qualitative research methods, including semi-structured interviews, was conducted in phases in Delhi and its suburban towns (Noida and Gurgaon), in February 2010, February 2011, October 2012, February 2013 and November 2013, with various stakeholders such as: (a) directors and managers of private UCB banks, (b) gynaecologists and (c) pregnant women. Interviews with women were conducted to assess their knowledge, attitude and willingness to bank. Twenty-five interviews were conducted in the gynaecology department of Sir Ganga Ram Hospital, a private charitable hospital in Delhi. Also, eight interviews with women who had delivered recently were conducted by telephone. This had to do with the fact that these women were too busy at work and/or with the care of the newborn, and apparently could not spare time for the researcher's visit, but they were prepared to answer a few questions on the telephone while the baby slept. These respondents were identified using a snowball approach. Besides this, two participant

---

[27] Ulrich Beck, *Risk Society: Towards a New Modernity* (New Delhi: Sage, 1992); Ulrich Beck, *World Risk Society* (Cambridge: Polity Press, 1999); Anthony Giddens, *The Consequences of Modernity* (Cambridge: Polity Press 1991); Anthony Giddens, 'Risk and Responsibility' (1999) 62(1) *Modern Law Review* 1–10; Deborah Lupton, *Risk* (London: Routledge, 1999); Nikolas Rose, 'The politics of life itself' (2001) 18(6) *Theory, Culture and Society* 1–30; John Tullock and Deborah Lupton, *Risk and Everyday Life* (London: Sage, 2003).

observation sessions at antenatal clinics attended by 10 and 18 pregnant women, respectively, in Delhi and Noida were held.

4.5   Laypersons' Knowledge Regarding UCB Banking

From time to time the print media covers developments in science and technology, including stem cell technology in the science section of newspapers or in the economics section mentioning growth figures of corporations. There are only a few studies[28] on the social and ethical aspects of developments and applications of stem cell research in general, or on UCB banking in particular in India[29] from the viewpoint of (prospective) clients/donors. Information on advances in medicine and therapies is available through the media to people with higher education levels and access to the Internet, or through gynaecologists and maternity departments of some hospitals.

Health risk perception is dependent on knowledge and access to information, which often correlates with (higher) economic status in the Indian context. Genetic literacy is not only a complex issue for the (semi-)literate, but even for the educated. Due to a lack of public information and discussion on UCB banking one does not know what the knowledge base regarding UCB banking is among laypersons. The perceived use of UCB as a source of stem cells may affect parents' willingness to bank.

4.6   Strategies of Private UCB Banks to Recruit Potential Clients

Various strategies are used by private UCB banks to enrol clients. Direct-to-consumer advertising via the Internet is one of the primary sources of information on UCB banking and recruitment. Another important source comprises flyers, leaflets and posters which are distributed in gynaecology/maternity wards of hospitals to recruit 'mothers-to-be' as prospective clients. Private UCB banks offer free antenatal classes at

---

[28] Aditya Bharadwaj, *Local Cells, Global Science: The Proliferation of Stem Cell Technologies in India* (London: Routledge, 2009); Tiwari, 'The ethics and governance of stem cell clinical research'.

[29] Diksha Pandey, Simar Kaur and Asha Kamath, 'Banking Umbilical Cord Blood (UCB) Stem Cells: Awareness, Attitude and Expectations of Potential Donors from One of the Largest Potential Repository (India)' (2016) 11(5) *PLoS One* e0155782. doi:10.1371/jour nal.pone.0155782; Prasanna Patra and Margaret Sleeboom-Faulkner, 'Following the banking cycle of UCB in India: The disparity between pre-banking persuasion and post-banking utilization' (2016) 35(3) *New Genetics and Society* 267–88.

private hospitals/gynaecology clinics comprising pre- and post-natal care advice, viz. exercises during pregnancy to ease labour during childbirth, nutrition and dietary advice, and answering frequently asked questions about pregnancy during interactive sessions attended by pregnant women and their husbands or other family members. At the end of the session refreshments are served and information kits (containing brochures, DVDs and CDs) are distributed (source: participant observation by researcher).

Some companies also distribute exciting gifts and freebies to all expectant parents attending the antenatal classes.[30] Appointments are made for home visits to make presentations and hand over information and cord blood collection kits. In the opinion of one of my interviewees, 'Private UCB banks chase prospective clients rather aggressively to make an appointment for a home visit' (A.C. interview 2011). The companies offer attractive deals. If a pregnant woman brings along or introduces two friends, she gets a discount on banking charges for her own UCB.

Marketing representatives of private cord blood banks admit that they are getting good support from doctors, whereas some of my requests to interview their patients were turned down. Gynaecologists are allowing them to approach prospective parents directly. Marketing representatives try to convince them through presentations and counselling as well as common sessions for pregnant women and their spouses. The companies are also organising continuous medical education programmes.[31]

All pregnant women visiting her clinic are informed about cord blood banking, says Dr Nandita Palshetkar, consultant gynaecologist at Lilavati Hospital, Mumbai. 'And 70 per cent of my patients go for it.' She says, 'There is definitely an increase in the trend. Currently, the prohibitive factor is the cost, but once it goes down the demand will rise'.[32]

4.6.1   UCB Advertising (websites and information packs/leaflets)

In the following sections I use excerpts from some of the freely distributed publicity material which I examined in order to understand what kind of information is being provided in the promotional literature.

---

[30] www.cordlifeindia.com/News_Events/Antenatal_Classes.php. Accessed 13 December 2012.
[31] Snehlata Shrivastav, 'Cord blood banking takes off in Nagpur', Times News Network, 16 May 2012.
[32] Deepa Suryanarayan, 'Young Mumbai women go for cord blood banking', Mumbai Agency: Daily News and Analysis (DNA), 9 May 2010.

In general the information consists of: What are cord blood cells, and their therapeutic uses? UCB is (incorrectly) classified as biomedical waste that would otherwise be discarded. This is erroneous,[33] just like the claim that UCB cells can provide a cure for about 75 life-threatening diseases, although scientific progress may increase the range of diseases and conditions which can be treated by using stem cells in the future. Some private UCB banks mention briefly that UCB can be banked either in public or private banks, elaborate on the advantages of banking in private banks and then go into the details of why theirs is the best choice. Each UCB bank claims to offer world-class state-of-the-art (cost, safety and quality norms) facilities. The information is addressed to potential mothers/parents, calling upon the parental responsibility for the future health of the child and its family members with the stipulation that it is a once-in-a-lifetime chance not to be missed. Often testimonials by public figures and celebrities such as actors, sports personalities and high-placed officials are used on websites and in information material to recruit clients. Also used are testimonials by medical experts and former clients:

Medical experts' (paediatricians' and gynaecologists') testimonials proclaim.

> Preserving stem cells is the wisest decision that parents can take during the birth of their baby. Parents who have stored their baby's cells can be part of a medical revolution and will have more medical options available to them...
>
> (Cordlife)

4.6.2   Using Patient/Client Testimonials

> 'Mothers Speak' testimonials are used to convince, reassuring parents for lifelong [sic].
>
> (Cryobanks)

These are some examples from the promotional material of LifeCell:

---

[33] Nicholas M. Fisk and Ifat Atun, 'Public–private partnership in cord blood banking' (2008) 336 *British Medical Journal* 642–44.

'Storing umbilical cord blood is similar to taking out life insurance. It's the greatest gift you could give.'

(Priya Dutt, Member of Parliament)

'My kids are my precious little gifts from God and I want the best for them. I've gifted Rashaa something extremely precious – a life filled with health and happiness, by storing her stem cells with LifeCell.'

(Raveena Tandon, Actor)

'From our first contact to the sample collection, the team was efficient, prompt and professional. Post collection, the follow-ups were regular. We are therefore pleased we selected LifeCell.'

(Ajith Agarkar, Cricketer)

'LifeCell is a life saver.'

(R. Madhavan, Actor)[34]

'Stem Cell banking is an essential modality of healthcare for newborns. With many recent advances in the field of stem cell therapies, I believe it has enormous advantages in the future, especially for diseases which cannot be treated in the present day. Cordlife was the most reliable and obvious choice to store my baby's cord blood.'

(Hesiba Jacob, Hyderabad)[35]

'In India, when a child is born, the parents open a savings bank account to ensure the financial and educational future of the newborn. In my opinion, banking the stem cells of the newborn is equally important as it helps in insuring the medical future of the child. It is a boon and the best gift we can give our children – the miracle of good health.'[36]
Also, success stories of patients *cured* by stem cell therapy are included.

'Umbilical cord stem cell banking is an essential aspect for every child since every parent holds the responsibility of securing their child's health for the future. I have benefitted by getting myself completely cured by this revolutionary concept of umbilical cord blood stem cell banking and I insist that every parent should consider in the future interest of their child.'

(Mr Vigneshwaran, Cord blood stem cell transplant beneficiary)[37]

[34] www.Lifecellinternational.com. Accessed 12 December 2010.
[35] www.cordlifeindia.com/testimonial. Accessed 12 September 2016.
[36] www.CryoSave.com. Accessed 11 October 2017.
[37] www.cordlifeindia.com/testimonial. Accessed 12 September 2016.

4.6.3   Promotion and Offers

NOW YOU RECEIVE GIFTS FOR JUST MEETING US

> Sometimes good things in life are just a click away. Celebrations have no avenues as CordLife brings to you more than one reason to stay stylish, beautiful and always charming. All you got to do is just meet us to learn more about protecting your family with your baby's stem cells and get the following gift vouchers absolutely FREE![38]

Since June 2016 LifeCell has been offering a BabyMoon vacation package worth 20,000 rupees to customers enrolling to bank with it. With over 25 exotic destinations in India to choose from, LifeCell offers 'a vacation to enjoy the joyous moments of pregnancy with your spouse before you welcome your baby home'. It is meant to be an ideal vacation to relish in nature's serene beauty and enjoy blissful moments of togetherness, time to relax, rejuvenate and connect with each other.[39]

4.6.4   Banking Your Hopes and Parental and Familial Responsibility

The message that is transmitted through the information packs is on the benefits of UCB banking couched in the language of parental and familial responsibility.

> 'Decision to save your Baby's cord blood cells is very crucial step in ensuring your entire family's health. Cord Blood banking has become more important protection to your family compared with other ways like home or auto insurance.'
> 'Stem cells . . . offer a lifeline to your child should he or she be afflicted by disorders later. Bank your child's placenta; save your child.'
> 'Now your family's future lies in your hands.'
> 'You have only one chance, at birth, to collect the cord blood cells. Missing this would mean losing out on a precious potentially life-saving opportunity, FOREVER.'
> 'Bank your hopes with cord of life. . .'
> 'As a proud parent-to-be, you are obviously planning ahead for your little one's future. While money, name and fame can be earned by your child, there are some things that only you can give – like the security of parental love and the legacy of cord blood: a potential lifeline for your child's future.' (Relicord, promotional brochure)

[38] www.cordlifeindia.com. Accessed 12 September 2016.
[39] www.lifecell.in/services/babycord/greetings/offers/baby-moon/baby-moon.php. Accessed 12 September 2016.

4.7 Preliminary Findings

4.7.1 Playing on Emotions and Hope

Websites and flyers, posters and information kits (including CDs and DVDs) provide interesting material regarding recruitment practices and strategies used by UCB banks to enrol customers. 'The private banks encourage parents to bank cord blood through a series of promissory, practical and moral arguments.'[40] A comparison is made with depositing money in the bank as an investment plan on the birth of a child. In a Zee TV news item a medical specialist said it would not be a misnomer to call cord blood *'Sanjivani'*. This was a reference to *'Sanjivani Booti'* – the almost magical medicinal herb which saved the life of the severely wounded Lakshman, younger brother of Lord Rama in the epic *Ramayana*, a popular story known to almost every Indian. The flyer of LifeCell has as its opening sentence the commonly given blessing to a child, *'Ayushman Bhav'* (May you live long!), adding that this 'is no longer a prayer for your newborn. LifeCell can help make it come true'.

Most UCB banks call upon the parental responsibility for the future health of the child and its family members as well to take timely action by not missing the once-in-a-lifetime chance to bank the cord blood on delivery of the child. Often the language of the 'gift' is also used.

'Your baby got a gift from heaven ... Preserve it!! – Preserve Umbilical Cord Blood Stem Cells & save your loved ones from life threatening diseases.'

'Storing your own baby's cord blood is a first gift from your side to your baby. No doubt is left regarding the importance and medical value of Cord blood banking. More than 20 companies now offer this service either for donation or private storage. It is a hard to believe fact that in spite of global acceptance of Cord blood importance, very few expectant parents in India know about this 'God gift' and this is thrown into dustbins. Is not it an injustice to innocent newly born baby?'

(Cryobanks India promotional flyer)

In general, a lot of misinformation was present among pregnant women and family members regarding the benefits of UCB banking. There was much hype and speculation regarding possible future therapies. Preliminary research shows that there is much in the promotional literature which is misleading, selling hope concerning therapies derived

---

[40] Martin et al., Capitalizing hope, p. 139.

from cord blood stem cells in case they are needed by the child or its family in the distant future, although these promises are built on as yet unproven clinical efficacy: UCB banking for autologous use is associated with even greater uncertainty than for allogeneic use.

Most pregnant women I interviewed at SRGH Hospital were unaware of the concept of UCB banking; they would often ask me for information about it and expressed the opinion that their gynaecologists should provide them more information ('hold classes') on this subject. Some had heard that, like blood, UCB can be banked for later use. Some professional women had heard of it through newspaper articles, the Internet or from a friend/colleague who had banked, yet they had only a vague idea of what it really entailed. In such cases, they contacted a UCB bank themselves. Many of my respondents (expectant mothers) were undecided whether they would bank. Some indicated a positive response/willingness to bank. It was seen as a good/wise investment by expectant women/ couples, mostly from higher income groups due to the cost factor.

Some women even expressed anticipated regret:

> 'Having missed the chance, do I need to regret it? I think I was careless. I will certainly bank if pregnant again.'
>
> (AJ, MBA, telephone interview, 22 February 2011)

Others were happy to have taken the decision to bank in spite of the cost:

> 'We're quite contented with the decision to bank. We'll see 10 less movies, but bank.'
>
> (pregnant woman, engineer, telephone interview, 29 February 2012)

> 'It's more like a precaution than a cure. Our baby will have an option, also in case of a second child, the sample will be useful for both.'
>
> (GT, pregnant woman, 11 November 2013)

> 'It's not a proven technology. Moreover, it is not that ubiquitous. There has to be a balance between how much safety you want and the money you spend.'
>
> (JB, pregnant woman, post-graduate, 25 November 2013)

> 'Everyone should do it for the future of the baby, if finances allow it.'
>
> (pregnant woman, ophthalmologist, 26 November 2013)

None were aware of any risks to mother or child associated with UCB collection, particularly with early clamping of the umbilical cord, as noted by some researchers.[41]

4.7.2   Opinions of Medical Professionals

Among the gynaecologists and obstetricians interviewed I encountered varying opinions on UCB banking; some placed their hope in stem cell technology, while others were critical even of members of their own profession who support UCB banking as well as of their patients/clients. Dr V. K. Khanna, Head Thalassaemia Unit of the SGRH Hospital is in favour of UCB banking:

> 'I tell all my thalassaemia patients to go for it. The problem is when you store, the yield is less. The quantity is less than in bone marrow transplant. If after five years they can find the cells can be multiplied in vivo, we may have a cure. Many people have done it, and left it because of less [sic] success rates. In the conventional bone marrow transplant dose the number of cells is more. At this time it is private banking. The government should take the initiative. So many deliveries are taking place in government hospitals. You will get better match.' (interview, 27 November 2013).

> 'We can help other family members. Family relations can be stronger. But, not every family thinks like this. If we counsel, as a gynaecologist I think, we can help promote this. I would like to tell my patients about it. For any procedure we discuss benefits and risks. We should also think about affordability, keep in mind that if you don't bank, you're not losing on something.'

> (pregnant woman, herself a gynaecologist, interview 7 November 2013)

> 'There are only two public banks – Stemocyte and Reliance. Public banking is more recent. I do recommend in cases of blood disorders. It's a good thing if family can afford it … It's a cord and placenta which will otherwise be thrown away. At the moment they can preserve for only twenty-one years. After twenty years the contract is transferred to the child. When the contract expires, will he be able to get it, that question they can't answer.'

> (Dr V., gynaecologist, interview 16 February 2011)

---

[41] David Hutchon, 'Commercial cord blood banking – immediate clamping is not safe' (2006) 333 *British Medical Journal* 919.

My preliminary findings are largely corroborated by Pandey et al.,[42] who conducted a pioneering study to assess current awareness and attitudes, in a sample population of potential donors from one of the largest potential UCB repositories in India. They write:

> We established only 26.5% of pregnant women in our study population knew what exactly is meant by UCB. A large proportion (55.1%) was undecided on whether they want to bank UCB or not. Women were more aware of the more advertised private cord blood banking compared to public banking. More than half of the pregnant women expected their obstetrician to inform them regarding UCB. One-third of the women in our population had undue expectations from banking of the UCB.

4.8   Discussion

4.8.1   Truth versus Hope

Public and private cord blood banks draw on different 'biosocialities',[43] with very few points in common: what Santoro[44] refers to as clearly two opposite models, not only at the point of arrival – that is, where the UCB is finally preserved – but in the whole process of collection and preservation. It is important to remember that UCB banking is based mainly on the future development of stem cell-based therapies. 'The banking of UCB rests on current applications of stem cell-based therapies and the future potential of regenerative medicine and marks the capitalization of human tissues within a future-oriented regime of hope'.[45] Prainsack[46] discusses 'the process of biomedicalization, in which market rationalities have led to new narratives of hope and promise, both in terms of increased health and increased profits'.

UCB banking for autologous use is associated with even greater uncertainty than for allogeneic use. The type of disorder and the need for autologous cells versus allogeneic cells determines the actual potential use of these cells. The likelihood of a child requiring a transplant with its

[42] Pandey et al., *Banking Umbilical Cord Blood (UCB) Stem Cells.*
[43] Paul Rabinow, 'Artificiality and Enlightenment: From Sociobiology to Biosociality.' in *Essays on the Anthropology of Reason* (Princeton, NJ: Princeton University Press, 1996).
[44] Pablo Santoro, 'From (public?) waste to (private?) value. The regulation of private cord blood banking in Spain' (2009) 22(1) *Science Studies* www.sciencetechnologystudies.org/system/files/Santoro.pdf. Accessed 10 December 2012.
[45] Martin et al., Capitalizing hope, p. 127.
[46] B. Prainsack, "Negotiating Life": The regulation of human cloning and embryonic stem cell research in Israel' (2006) 36(2) *Social Studies of Science* 173–205, p. 176.

own cord blood is small: from a 1:400 to 1:200,000 chance over the child's lifetime,[47] and thus private UCB banking is currently not even cost effective.[48] In fact, there are certain instances in which the use of one's own umbilical cord blood is contraindicated, as in cases when the defect is of a genetic origin. For example, autologous cord blood stem cells cannot be used to treat malignant cancers such as leukaemia because the genetic mutations for the cancer already exist in the DNA of the cord blood. Using one's own stem cells would be, in effect, contaminating oneself with the same disease process.[49] None of this information is to be found in the promotional flyers and information packs.

The American Academy of Pediatrics[50] states that the use of banked umbilical cord blood as 'biological insurance' is unwarranted, noting that many of the claims of private cord blood banks are unfounded. Unlike the American College of Obstetricians and Gynecologists,[51] the AAP recommends cord blood collection and banking for all families, but stipulates that all cord blood should be banked in public banks for use by the general population. It recommends private cord blood banking *only* if a full sibling has a medical diagnosis for which stem cells are currently being used for treatment.

The unproven clinical efficacy of UCB banking signifies, as several authors have noted, the increasing dependence of emerging bioeconomies on a promissory future economic value and potential rather than present use. This has come to signify shifts from 'regimes of truth' (linked to established practice and proven evidence), to 'regimes of hope'.[52] Martin et al. write about how publics are mobilised as active consumers within neo-liberalised bioeconomies. There is a 'construction of expectations', expectations which have links with markets and 'promissory capital'. These bioeconomies depend upon the participation of multiple constituencies collaborating in the establishment of 'communities of promise'.[53] They are founded on the 'political economy of hope',

[47] M. J. Sullivan, 'Banking on cord blood stem cells' (2008) 8 *Nature Reviews Cancer* 554–63.
[48] A. J. Kaimal, C. C Smith, R. K. Laros Jr et al., 'Cost-effectiveness of private umbilical cord blood banking' (2010) 11(5) *Obstetrics and Gynecology* 1090.
[49] B. Percer, 'Umbilical cord blood banking: Helping parents make informed choices' (2009) 13(3) *Nursing for Women's Health* 216–23.
[50] American Academy of Pediatrics (AAP), 'Policy statement: Cord blood banking for potential future transplantation' (2007) 119(1) *Pediatrics* 165–70.
[51] American College of Obstetricians and Gynecologists (ACOG), *Committee Opinion 648*, December 2015.
[52] Martin et al., 'Capitalizing hope,' p. 128.   [53] Ibid., p. 129.

on 'capitalizing hope': narratives promising hope in terms of improved health and increased lifespan.[54] Brown and Kraft[55] write about active consumers and responsible parents who are mobilised through commercial UCB banks. The Internet plays a crucial role in this.

As Pablo Santoro[56] observes:

> The language of insurance and precautionary investment permeates the marketing of commercial services. Even if the potential applications of autologous transplantation remain mainly unproven, preserving UCB is offered as the gate to a potential, though unequal, double future: that of the child or a family member developing a disease and that of the biomedical evolution, in which a whole new generation of stem cell therapies will be developed.

4.8.2   Risk and Uncertainty

It is useful to discuss the marketing of UCB within the framework of 'risk' theory, which includes concepts such as 'manufactured risk' and 'risk society',[57] and 'manufactured uncertainty'/'fabricated uncertainty'.[58] In his various writings Ulrich Beck analyses how science and technology, mediated through market relations and various social institutions under industrial modernity, are shaping the future – one dominated by the matrix of risk and the requirements of risk management, creating a 'world risk society'. According to Rose,[59] 'Risk here denotes a family of ways of thinking and acting, involving calculations about probable futures in the present followed by interventions into the present in order to control that potential future.' Beck writes about self-generated manufactured uncertainties in modern societies and distinguishes between 'decision-dependent *risks* that can in principle be brought under control, and *dangers* that have escaped or neutralized the control requirements of industrial society'.[60] Various authors have attempted to make a distinction between 'risk' and 'uncertainty' in that the former concerns

---

[54] Nikolas Rose and C. Novas, 'Biological citizenship' in A. Ong and S.J. Collier (eds.) *Global Assemblages: Technology, Politics, and Ethics as Anthropological Problems* (Malden: Blackwell, 2005), 439–64.

[55] N. Brown and A. Kraft, *Blood Ties*.

[56] Santoro, 'From (public?) waste to (private?) value'. p. 9.

[57] Beck, *Risk Society*; Beck, *World Risk Society*; Giddens, *The Consequences of Modernity*; Giddens, 'Risk and responsibility'; Lupton, *Risk*; Tullock and Lupton, *Risk and Everyday Life*; Rose, 'The politics of life itself'.

[58] Beck, *World Risk Society*; Giddens, *The Consequences of Modernity*.

[59] Rose, 'The politics of life itself', p. 7.   [60] Beck, *World Risk Society*, p. 31.

future probabilities that can be calculated, whereas the latter represents ones that cannot be. 'Manufactured uncertainty' means a *mélange* of risk, more knowledge, more unawareness and reflexivity, and *therefore* a new type of risk'.[61] 'The sociology of risk is a science of potentialities and judgments about probabilities.'[62] There is a significant level of human agency operating in the production and mitigation of 'manufactured risks'.

In modern industrialised societies, new types of uncertainties arise which Giddens[63] and Beck[64] call 'manufactured uncertainties'. Scientific experts participate in the role of producers, analysts and profiteers from risk definitions by bringing risk into being and 'selling risk'.[65] The shift from countable risk to uncountable uncertainty is a shift that implies a parallel change from 'rational' prevention to uncertain precaution.[66] It also marks a transition from the exercise of a 'pastoral power' by the state to the precautionary action of the 'somatic individual'.[67]

4.8.3 Governmentality and Individual Responsibility

Exponents of the 'risk society' thesis argue that in late modernity there is a trend towards individualisation, in that individuals are positioned as choosing agents who can exercise a great deal of control over the course of their own lives. 'Risk is primarily understood as a human responsibility, both in its production and management, rather than the outcome of fate or destiny, as was the case in pre-modern times'.[68]

Using the 'governmentality'[69] approach, several authors have drawn attention to the importance placed upon the self-management of risk and the increasing 'privatisation' of risk, according to Lupton.[70] Prainsack[71] argues: 'The regulation of population takes place by devolving a significant amount of agency to individuals.' Recent trends within healthcare to strengthen the autonomy of patients encourage a shift

---

[61] Ibid., p. 112.   [62] Ibid., p. 136.   [63] Giddens, 'Risk and responsibility'.
[64] Beck, *World Risk Society*, p. 140.   [65] Lupton, *Risk*.
[66] H. Gottweis, 'Governing genomics in the 21st century: Between risk and uncertainty' (2005) 24(2) *New Genetics and Society* 175–94.
[67] Rose, 'The politics of life itself'.   [68] Lupton, *Risk*, p. 4.
[69] Michel Foucault, 'Governmentality' in Graham Burchell, Colin Gordon and Peter Miller (eds.), *The Foucault Effect: Studies in Governmentality* (London: Harvester Wheatsheaf, 1991), 87–104.
[70] Lupton, *Risk*.
[71] Barbara Prainsack, '"Negotiating life": The regulation of human cloning and embryonic stem cell research in Israel' (2006) 36 (2) *Social Studies of Science* 173–205, p. 195.

from being a passive patient to being a responsible consumer and active in assuming responsibility for health (also see the chapters by Huijer and Detweiler, Zwart and van Beers in this volume).

Lupton[72] points out that 'the theorization of risk has tended to neglect the insights offered by contemporary feminist theory and the sociology of the body in understanding the links between gender, embodiment, subjectivity and risk'. According to the 'governmentality' perspective, the pregnant body is 'an intensely governed body, both on the part of medicine and on the part of the woman herself as an autonomous, self-regulating citizen seeking her own best interests (and, even more importantly these days, those of the foetus)'.[73] Parallels can be drawn here with women's use of prenatal diagnosis technologies to ensure the health of the foetus, the future child. 'Public awareness regarding the role of genes in the incidence of disease and the possibility of making use of PNT is increasing; it is associated with modernity and good parenthood.'[74] With the principle of informed choice and the ethical imagining of the pregnant woman as an autonomous individual, the woman is perceived as responsible for this choice and thereby also for the possible future of the child and the family unit, the prevailing theme in the advertising of commercial services. Once again, as with other reproductive technologies (such as contraceptives or prenatal testing technologies), the onus is laid on women. There is an imperative to choose in favour of technology when women find themselves in the risk trap, and anticipated regret if they do not bank. For this reason, some women whom I interviewed expressed feelings of guilt and a sense of regret if UCB had not been banked in an earlier pregnancy. This is also reported by Fernandez et al.[75] based on their study among Canadian pregnant women. As Helén[76] warns in the context of prenatal genetic testing, it is a case of 'risk individualized' and 'responsibilization', leaving the ethical responsibility with 'the mother' and, in doing so, imposing an existential condition.

The AAP made a strong case for public cord blood banking in 2007. In Europe and the USA, professional bodies actively discourage private

---

[72] Lupton, *Risk*, pp. 7–8. [73] Lupton, *Risk*, p. 8.
[74] Jyotsna A. Gupta 'Exploring Indian women's reproductive decision-making regarding prenatal testing' (2010) 12(2) *Culture, Health and Sexuality* 191–204, p. 192.
[75] C. V. Fernandez, K. Gordon, M. Van den Hof, S. Taweel and F. Baylis, 'Knowledge and attitudes of pregnant women with regard to collection, testing and banking of cord blood stem cells' (2003) 168(6) *Canadian Medical Association Journal* 695–98.
[76] I. Helén, 'Risk management and ethics in high-tech antenatal care', in R. Bunton and A. Petersen (eds.), *Genetic Governance: Health, Risk and Ethics in the Biotech Era* (London: Routledge, 2005), 47–63, pp. 55–6.

UCB banking for self-use or for use by a family member at a later date, and instead recommend publicly funded banks that collect voluntary donations.[77] When the number of units stored in public banks increases, the chances of finding a matching unit also increase. If most parents bank their babies' UCB privately there will not be enough supply for public banks for the general public to draw from. Although therapeutic claims relating to UCB stem cells are still doubtful, questions of access to banking facility through public banks for the less well-off need to be considered as private UCB banks are proliferating. Private UCB banks threaten the solidarity principle as equity and access to future therapies may be limited to the few who can afford private UCB banking. Private and public banking reflect the wider gap between private and public healthcare in India.

There is much controversy surrounding the efficacy of stem cell-based treatments. There is a lack of knowledge and a lot of misinformation present among pregnant women and family members in India regarding the benefits of UCB banking. Most of the respondents thought that the therapies were already available or would be shortly available for over 45 diseases and medical conditions, and since one or more family members suffered from various diseases they would be able to benefit. Some of the statements made by private cord blood banks are outright misleading.[78] This has to do with misleading advertising which builds on the promissory value of stem cells derived from UCB rather than proven therapies. 'Lothian and DeVries[79] reinforce the AAP's position that expectant families are vulnerable to the marketing strategies of private cord blood banks. The authors go on to say that expectant parents should know that banking UCB does not guarantee a cure. Likewise, there is no guarantee that a private UCB bank will be able to adequately preserve the cord blood until a time when it is needed. One potential reason for being unable to preserve the cord blood is that the private UCB bank could go out of business. The shelf-life of UCB is uncertain; currently it is

---

[77] American Academy of Pediatrics (AAP), 'Policy statement: Cord blood banking for potential future transplantation' (2007) 119(1) *Pediatrics* 165–70; D. McKenna and J. Sheth, 'Umbilical cord blood: Current status and promise for the future' (2011) 134(3) *Indian Journal of Medical Research* 261–69; American College of Obstetricians and Gynecologists (ACOG). *Committee Opinion 648*, December 2015.

[78] N. S. Fox, C. Stevens, R. Cuibotariu, P. Rubinstein, L. B. McCullough and F. A. Chervenak, 'Umbilical cord blood collection: Do patients really understand?' (2007) 35 *Journal of Perinatal Medicine* 314–21.

[79] J. Lothian and C. De Vries, *The Official Lamaze Guide: Giving Birth with Confidence* (New York, NY: Meadowbrook Press, 2010, 2nd ed.).

estimated that its efficacy ranges from 15 to 18 years, but it is unknown if the cells would be preserved over the entire lifetime of a person. Also, this may vary from unit to unit, or from one bank to another.

One may also ask how informed is informed consent in the case of women who do decide to bank. As research in other settings has revealed,[80] my respondents also appeared to be underinformed about UCB banking. They do not seem to be aware that the success rates described for UCB relate to haematological disorders within the family (usually sibling donations), whereas the usefulness of autologous UCB in other disorders is still under trial.

4.9   Public Banking Favoured

There are now two international registries: NETCORD, which lists cord blood units only, and Bone Marrow Donors Worldwide, which lists both bone marrow and cord blood donors.[81] Private (commercial) UCB banks threaten the solidarity principle, equity and access to future therapies. When well-intentioned parents bank cord blood privately, it removes another unit from the public supply – potentially harming everyone in the end, including their own baby. In the extreme case, if the private bank goes out of business, the cord blood is lost to the parents too. 'Me Medicine, in this guise, isn't even good for the individual, let alone the collective', says Dickenson.[82] Weighing the pros and cons of private and public UCB banking she makes a strong case for public banking. She quotes from an editorial in the American College of Obstetricians and Gynaecologists journal which states, 'We argue for public umbilical cord blood banking as a matter of good public health and economic sense.'[83]

Donation to a public bank is widely regarded as an altruistic act of civic responsibility that qualifies one as a 'good citizen',[84] whereas paying to store UCB may be regarded as a 'unique opportunity' to provide 'insurance' for the child's future.[85] Based on their findings from a survey of

---

[80] Fox et al., 'Umbilical cord blood collection'.
[81] M. G. Butler and J. E. Menitove, 'Umbilical cord blood banking: An update' (2011) 28 Journal of Assisted Reproduction and Genetics 669–676. doi:10.1007/s10815-011-9577-x.
[82] Dickenson, *Me Medicine vs We Medicine*, p. 92.   [83] Ibid., p. 96.
[84] Waldby, 'Umbilical cord blood: From social gift to venture capital'.
[85] M. Porter, I. H. Kerridge and C. F. C. Jordens, '"Good Mothering" or "Good Citizenship"? Conflicting values in choosing whether to donate or store umbilical cord blood' (2012) 9 *Bioethical Inquiry* 41–7, p. 41.

Australian women, Porter et al. conclude that mothers are faced with competing discourses that force them to choose between being a 'good mother' and fulfilling their role as a 'good citizen'. In India this dichotomy is not experienced by pregnant women as the clientele of public and private banks is based on whether women give birth in a public or private hospital, which in turn is based on financial affordability. The main motivation for those who can afford to bank at a private UCB bank is to serve the future medical needs of their child or a family member if needed. Public donation of stem cells increases our national supply of cord blood samples to help save people needing a suitable stem cell match. Considering the huge ethnic diversity in the country many more units would be required to give patients a reasonable chance of finding a match. 'The major problem faced in India is collection of UCB due to high cost and comparatively less functional public banks. In addition, considering a large population with deliveries in public hospital due to low cost, UCB storage in India needs increased public-private partnership model where UCB can be stored by affordable and non-affordable people as well.'[86]

The shift from 'We Medicine' to 'Me Medicine', characterising the trend in late modernity towards individualisation, also marks a transition from the exercise of a 'pastoral power' by the state to the precautionary action of the 'somatic individual'.[87] Private storage of cord blood is thus marketed, in accordance with neo-liberal principles, as a form of speculative 'biological insurance': the cord blood 'account' offers the client personal bio-security and personal risk management.[88] 'Unlike financial types of insurance, biological insurance of the type promoted by private banks does not protect people by sharing individual risk across a population. Instead of pooling risk, this type of biological insurance operates by placing greater responsibility on individuals to manage future harm'.[89] Further, it exonerates the state from investing in preventive public health measures and public health services for the benefit of all its citizens, while shifting the responsibility to private individuals for circumventing health risk and investing in the future health of their progeny.

[86] McKenna and Sheth, 'Umbilical cord blood: Current status and promise for the future', p. 264.
[87] Rose, 'The politics of life itself'.
[88] Waldby, 'Umbilical cord blood: From social gift to venture capital', p. 64.
[89] J. Haw, 'The trouble with biological insurance,' Impact Ethics, 4 November 2013.

As private UCB banking is proliferating fast in India, an important issue to consider is how to ensure that the information is balanced (educating) and not biased (persuading) in favour of aggressive marketing and profit motivations of private enterprise or the ambitions of researchers so that pregnant women can make well-informed decisions whether to bank or not, and also to choose between public and private UCB banks.

Acknowledgements

This work was supported by the National Research Foundation of Korea Grant (NRF-2013S1A3A2054579) funded by the Korean Government.

My sincere thanks to Dr Indrani Ganguli, Head of Gynaecology and Obstetrics at Sir Ganga Ram Hospital in Delhi, for allowing me access to her patients, and the (pregnant) women and other respondents who consented to speak to me.

Combating the Trade in Organs

Why We Should Preserve the Communal Nature of Organ Transplantation

KRISTOF VAN ASSCHE

5.1 Introduction

Organ transplantation is often considered as one of the miracles of modern medicine. Patients suffering from end-stage organ failure used to face a certain, untimely and agonising death before medical break-throughs made it possible to replace a damaged organ with an organ from another person.[1] Since the first successful kidney transplant in 1954, solid organ transplantation has become a global success. In 2016, 98,531 solid organ transplants were performed worldwide, including 62,333 kidney and 21,802 liver transplant procedures.[2] From its outset the transplant system has been governed by the key principles of voluntariness and altruism. These principles are deemed crucial to safeguard the integrity of the transplant system, since continued public support for organ trans-plantation depends on confidence that organs will be ethically obtained and equitably distributed.

At a more fundamental level, the principle of altruism is essential because organs are too integral to personhood to allow their commodi-fication. Treating organs as articles of commerce would undermine the value of the persons who sell them and, in a broader perspective, would debase humanity in general. Relatedly, altruism in organ donation is important because it allows persons to express and foster communal virtues. Therefore, allowing market norms to invade the interpersonal context of organ donation would irreversibly damage the quality of

---

[1] Peter J. Morris, 'Transplantation – A medical miracle of the 20th century' (2004) 351 *New England Journal of Medicine* 2678–80.
[2] Data from Global Observatory on Donation and Transplantation (GODT).

relationships, community identification and notions of shared obligations essential to a flourishing society.[3]

Since altruism and solidarity remain the guiding principles, Donna
Dickenson rightly emphasises that the transplant system has come to
'symbolize We Medicine at its noblest'.[4] However, she warns that,
with the advent of 'market triumphalism' and the concomitant
exaltation of personal choice, we are currently witnessing an (allegedly) unstoppable movement towards claiming property rights in
human body parts. The examples given by Dickenson, such as
DNA samples, oocytes and umbilical cord blood, and her discussion
about collecting, storing, using and patenting human tissues in the
context of biobanks expose what she calls a new 'enclosure movement' that is targeting human body material.[5]

The aim of this chapter is threefold. First, I will show that, just like
the other human biotechnologies considered by Dickenson, organ
transplantation has come under intense pressure from free-market
economics. The focus here will be both on the existing black market
in organs and on proposals to establish a regulated organ market in
developed countries. Second, I will examine and reject both the claims
made by proponents of a regulated organ market and the validity of the
utilitarian theory of property, which is – albeit generally uncon-
sciously – invoked by these advocates to substantiate their claims.
Third, building in part on the ethical considerations put forward by
Dickenson, I will examine the value of the personhood theory of
property and demonstrate that it is *essential* to preserve the altruistic
nature of organ transplantation so as to prevent dehumanisation and
the further erosion of our social fabric.

5.2   The Spectre of the Black Market

Contrary to general belief, attempts to trade in organs are not new.
In fact, the buying and selling of organs emerged as a fairly widespread

---

[3] The arguments and the literature to substantiate these claims will be provided further on in
this chapter.

[4] Donna Dickenson, *Me Medicine vs We Medicine: Reclaiming Biotechnology for the
Common Good* (New York, NY: Columbia University Press, 2013), p. 72.

[5] See also Donna Dickenson, 'Commodification of human tissue: Implications for feminist
and development ethics' (2002) 2(1) *Developing World Bioethics* 55–63; Donna Dickenson,
Property in the Body: Feminist Perspectives (Cambridge: Cambridge University Press,
2007); Donna Dickenson, *Body Shopping: The Economy Fuelled by Flesh and Blood*
(Oxford: Oneworld Publications, 2008).

phenomenon immediately after it became technically possible to receive an organ from an unrelated donor. Back in 1985, two years after cyclosporine was released for general use in the prevention and treatment of organ rejection, the first cases were reported of kidney patients from wealthy countries travelling to developing countries to purchase a kidney from destitute persons. Patients in need of an organ soon learned that they could circumvent the prohibition of commercialisation in their countries of origin and, if they could afford it and had no ethical objections, could buy an organ in countries where this prohibition was poorly enforced or where transplant legislation was marred by loopholes. This phenomenon of 'transplant tourism' was quickly and universally condemned by international organisations.[6] Despite significant successes in curbing transplant tourism – a practice which in 2000 was subsumed under the general heading of 'human trafficking (for organ removal)' – the international black market involving the payment and outright exploitation of organ donors has proven very difficult to eradicate.[7]

Due to its illegal and dynamic nature, the exact extent of the international black market in organs is unknown. According to broad estimates by the World Health Organization (WHO), transplantation of organs purchased from destitute populations in the developing world accounts for up to 10 per cent of all transplant activities performed worldwide. Australia, Canada, Japan, South Korea, the USA and countries in Western Europe and the Middle East have been identified as the main countries of origin of transplant tourists.[8] By contrast, the countries of destination are to be found in the developing world and include Bolivia, Brazil, China, Colombia, Costa Rica, Egypt, India, Iraq, Moldova, Nepal, Pakistan, Peru, the Philippines, Sri Lanka and Turkey.

Building on pioneering reports from anthropologists Nancy Scheper-Hughes and Debra Budiani-Saberi, a clear picture of the international

---

[6] World Medical Association Statement on Live Organ Trade, Brussels, October 1985; World Medical Association Declaration on Human Organ Transplantation, Madrid, October 1987; 3rd Conference of European Health Ministers, Organ Transplantation, Paris, 16–17 November 1987, Appendix II, Para. 16; Resolution WHA42.5 on Preventing the Purchase and Sale of Human Organs, Geneva, 15 May 1989.

[7] United Nations, Protocol to Prevent, Suppress and Punish Trafficking in Persons, Especially Women and Children, Palermo, 15 November 2000.

[8] Yosuke Shimazono, 'The State of the international organ trade: A provisional picture based on integration of available information' (2007) 85(12) *Bulletin of the World Health Organization* 955–62.

black market in organs has only recently emerged.[9] Research reveals an enormous discrepancy between what the recipient has to pay (between $100,000 and $200,000) and what the organ vendor eventually receives (between $500 and $10,000).[10] Therefore, it comes as no surprise that this trade in organs is considered as one of the most lucrative of black markets, with strong incentives on the part of brokers and collaborating healthcare professionals to continue their illegal activities.[11]

One of the most disturbing findings of these reports is that, invariably, organ vendors come from the poorest strata of society and only cooperate because of their desperate financial situation and because they are misled about the nature of the surgical procedure and the consequences of giving up a kidney. Trafficking networks ruthlessly exploit the position of extreme vulnerability, lack of alternatives and lack of education of their victims to maximise their own profits. Due to their precarious situation, victims generally have no real and acceptable choice but to submit to this very serious violation of their physical integrity.[12] Several studies highlight that a huge majority of organ vendors later express serious regrets, stating that they would certainly not have agreed to the transaction if

---

[9] See Debra A. Budiani-Saberi and Francis L. Delmonico, 'Organ trafficking and transplant tourism: A commentary on the global realities' (2008) 8(5) *American Journal of Transplantation* 925–9; Debra A. Budiani-Saberi, 'Organ trafficking and transplant tourism' in Vardit Ravitsky, Autumn Fiester and Arthur L. Caplan (eds.), *The Penn Center Guide to Bioethics* (New York, NY: Springer, 2009), pp. 699–708; Debra A. Budiani-Saberi and Kabir Karim, 'The social determinants of organ trafficking: A reflection of social inequity' (2009) 4(1) *Social Medicine* 48–51; Debra A. Budiani-Saberi and Amr Mostafa, 'Care for commercial living donors: The experience of an NGO's outreach in egypt' (2011) 24(4) *Transplant International* 317–23; Nancy Scheper-Hughes, 'The global traffic in human organs' (2000) 41(2) *Current Anthropology* 191–224; Nancy Scheper-Hughes, 'Keeping an eye on the global traffic in human organs' (2003) 361(9369) *The Lancet* 1645–8; Nancy Scheper-Hughes, 'Black market organs: Inside the trans-atlantic transplant tourism trade' *LIP Magazine* 3 June 2005.

[10] Marta López-Fraga, Kristof Van Assche, Beatriz Domínguez-Gil et al., 'Human trafficking for the purpose of organ removal' in Ryszard Piotrowicz, Conny Rijken and Baerbel H. Uhl (eds.), *Routledge Handbook of Human Trafficking* (London: Routledge, 2017), pp. 120–134; Assya Pascalev, Jessica de Jong, Frederike Ambagtsheer et al., 'Trafficking in human beings for the purpose of organ removal: A comprehensive literature review' in Frederike Ambagtsheer and Willem Weimar (eds.), *Trafficking in Human Beings for the Purpose of Organ Removal: Results and Recommendations* (Lengerich: Pabst, 2016), pp. 15–68; Scheper-Hughes, 'The Global Traffic'.

[11] Jeremy Haken, *Transnational Crime in the Developing World* (Washington, DC: Center for International Policy, 2011).

[12] United Nations Office on Drugs and Crime, *Issue Paper: Abuse of a Position of Vulnerability and other 'Means' within the Definition of Trafficking in Persons* (New York, NY: United Nations, 2013).

their situation had not been so hopeless and if they had been properly informed about the consequences.[13]

To make matters even worse, intimidation and coercion are frequently used to force reluctant or unwilling victims to cooperate and to dissuade them from later alerting law enforcement officials. Moreover, organ vendors are further exploited in that the sum they eventually receive generally is much less than what had been promised.[14] Shockingly, some cases have even been reported of blatant organ theft from persons undergoing unrelated surgery or from patients in psychiatric institutions. There is even some anecdotal evidence of persons, including children, having been abducted, sold and killed for their organs.[15]

Even apart from their exploitation at the moment of recruitment and organ removal, victims of the black market in organs suffer from very negative post-operative consequences. Their hope of paying off crippling debts and securing a minimum level of subsistence through selling an organ quickly proves illusory. Few, if any, vendors manage to improve their financial situation in the medium term. On the contrary, they are back in significant debt within a couple of years and experience a significant decline in household income, attributed to a deterioration in their physical status, which prevents them from sustaining the demands of hard physical labour. A large majority of vendors even report that their health worsened significantly, due to mediocre initial health, lack of post-operative care and a continuing unhealthy lifestyle or environment. Because of the unavailability of medical assistance, or the inability to pay for it, many of these vendors in time suffer organ failure,

---

[13] Debra A. Budiani-Saberi and Seán Columb, 'A human rights approach to human trafficking for organ removal' (2013) 16(4) *Medicine, Health Care, and Philosophy* 897–914; Budiani-Saberi and Delmonico, 'Organ trafficking and transplant tourism'.

[14] See Organization for Security and Co-operation in Europe, *Trafficking in Human Beings for the Purpose of Organ Removal in the OSCE Region: Analysis and Findings*, Occasional Paper Series 6 (Vienna: Office of the Special Representative and Co-ordinator for Combating Trafficking in Human Beings, 2013); United Nations Office on Drugs and Crime, *Assessment Toolkit: Trafficking in Persons for the Purpose of Organ Removal* (New York, NY: United Nations, 2015). See also Alexis A. Aronowitz, *Human Trafficking, Human Misery: The Global Trade in Human Beings* (Greenwood Publishing Group, 2009); Elaine Pearson, *Coercion in the Kidney Trade? A Background Study on Trafficking in Human Organs Worldwide* (Deutsche Gesellschaft für Technische Zusammenarbeit, 2004).

[15] Vivek Chaudhary, 'Argentina uncovers patients killed for organs' (1992) 304(5834) *British Medical Journal* 1073–4; Nancy Scheper-Hughes, 'Commodity fetishism in organs trafficking' in Nancy Scheper-Hughes and Loïc Wacquant (eds.), *Commodifying Bodies* (London: Sage, 2002), pp. 31–62.

which most likely results in early death. Furthermore, vendors suffer from stigmatisation and social isolation and many of them mention suffering severe depression and anxiety.[16]

In the context of the international black market in organs, the introduction of rampant market forces has resulted in a complete and intentional disregard for even the most basic interests of organ vendors. Their desperation is unscrupulously exploited to make huge profits and they are left even worse off. Moreover, the interests of the recipients, whose own desperation fuels the demand that drives the black market, are frequently also negatively affected. Compared to transplantation within the regulated domestic system, transplant tourists run significantly higher mortality and morbidity risks. More specifically, data reveal a heightened frequency of complications, due to a higher incidence of unconventional, often life-threatening infections, resulting in a significantly lower patient and graft survival rate. The reasons for this poor outcome are multifactorial: worse initial health of recipients, who are generally older or occasionally even excluded from their domestic waiting list for medical reasons; the inadequacy of pre-transplantation health screening of donors; substandard medical facilities; abbreviated and deficient medical aftercare; and compromised follow-up at home, due to scarce and often unintelligible medical documentation.[17]

[16] See Nasrollah Ghahramani, S. Adibul Hasan Rizvi and Benita Padilla, 'Paid donation: A global view: Outcomes of paid donation in Iran, Pakistan and Philippines' (2012) 19(4) Advances in Chronic Kidney Disease 262-8; Madhav Goyal, Ravindra L. Mehta, Lawrence Schneiderman and Ashwini R. Sehgal, 'Economic and health consequences of selling a kidney in India' (2002) 288(13) Journal of the American Medical Association 1589-93; S. Naqvi, S. Rizvi, M. Zafar et al., 'Health status and renal function evaluation of kidney vendors: A report from Pakistan' (2008) 8 American Journal of Transplantation 1444-1450; Imran Sajjad, Lyndsay S. Baines, Prem Patel et al., 'Commercialization of kidney transplants: A systematic review of outcomes in recipients and donors' (2008) 28 (5) American Journal of Nephrology 744-54; Allison Tong, Jeremy R. Chapman, Germaine Wong et al., 'The experiences of commercial kidney donors: Thematic synthesis of qualitative research' (2012) 25 (11) Transplant International 1138-49.
[17] See Ashley E. Anker and Thomas H. Feeley, 'Estimating the risks of acquiring a kidney abroad: A meta-analysis of complications following participation in transplant tourism' (2012) 26(3) Clinical Transplantation E232-41; N. Inston, D. Gill, A. Al-Hakim et al., 'Living paid organ transplantation results in unacceptably high recipient morbidity and mortality' (2005) 37(2) Transplant Proceedings 560-2; Meng-Kun Tsai, Ching-Yao Yang, Chich-Yuan Lee et al., 'De novo malignancy is associated with renal transplant tourism' (2011) 79(8) Kidney International 908-14; Yarkin K. Yakupoglu, Ender Ozden, Melda Dilek et al., 'Transplantation tourism: High risk for the recipients' (2010) 24(6) Clinical Transplantation 835-8.

Combined with the enormous financial sacrifice required to obtain an organ, recipients may thus run a real risk of being exploited themselves.

'Transplant tourism' not only negatively affects the interests of both vendors and recipients, but it also creates significant negative externalities, in that it may result in major costs and harms that have to be borne by third parties. In this respect, it has to be noted that both the lost productivity of vendors and the possible medical costs exceeding their financial ability will have to be shouldered by local communities. In addition, the emergence of underground markets may impede the development of a regular local transplant system that would allow local residents a reasonable chance of obtaining an organ.[18] The negative externality argument equally applies to the country of origin of the transplant tourist. On their return home, the medical problems that recipients may experience as a result of the suboptimal transplant conditions associated with their illicit transplant will need to be addressed by the domestic healthcare system.[19] In addition, physicians will be forced to bear responsibility for their medical treatment.[20] Transplant tourism is also likely to have detrimental effects on the efforts to develop organ transplant programmes and attain national self-sufficiency in the country of origin, since governments may feel less responsibility if their nationals can obtain organs abroad relatively easily.[21]

5.3 The Delusion of a Regulated Organ Market

Although the principle of non-commercialisation has been upheld in clinical practice across the USA and Western Europe for a long time, as it was already specified in the first domestic transplant laws (i.e. Italy, Norway and Spain) and is enshrined in a wide range of international guidelines and legal instruments, the idea of introducing a domestic market in organs has proven difficult to resist for some.[22] Notoriously,

---

[18] Emily R. Kelly, 'International Organ Trafficking Crisis: Solutions Addressing the Heart of the Matter' (2013) 54(3) *Boston College Law Review* 1317–49.

[19] Katrina A. Bramstedt and Jun Xu, 'Checklist: Passport, Plane Ticket, Organ Transplant' (2007) 7(7) *American Journal of Transplantation* 1698–701.

[20] Budiani-Saberi and Delmonico, 'Organ Trafficking and Transplant Tourism'.

[21] George M. Abouna, 'Negative Impact of Trading in Human Organs on the Development of Transplantation in the Middle East' (1993) 25(3) *Transplant Proceedings* 2310–3; Budiani-Saberi, 'Organ Trafficking and Transplant Tourism'.

[22] International guidelines and legal instruments include Council of Europe, Convention on Human Rights and Biomedicine, Oviedo, 4 April 1997, CETS No. 164; Council of Europe, Additional Protocol concerning Transplantation of Organs and Tissues of Human

at the end of 1983, a Virginia physician established a company to broker kidney sales in the USA. Triggered by the growing demand for kidney transplants and the emergence of transplant tourism, he planned to bring in poor donors from developing countries to sell kidneys directly on American soil.[23] Fear of exploitation, inequality in allocation and erosion of the communitarian spirit of the transplant system quickly prompted the US Congress to adopt the National Organ Transplant Act, criminalising the transfer of an organ for valuable consideration.[24]

However, the general prohibition on commercialisation has not been universally well received. As a result of the increasing gap between the supply of and the demand for organs, especially in the USA, calls to relax or abandon the principle of non-commercialisation are growing louder. Proponents of an organ market point out that, as compared to the first decennia of organ transplantation, the number of patients desperately waiting for an organ is much higher and continues to grow at a much faster pace than organ donation rates and transplant activities. Recently published data on kidney transplantation indeed paint a grim picture. For instance, at the end of 2017, in the USA, 103,226 patients were waiting for a kidney, as compared to 88,867 at the end of 2012, while only 19,849 transplants were performed in 2017, up from 16,487 in 2012. In 2017, approximately 14 persons died each day while waiting for a kidney transplant. By contrast, the European Union is one of very few regions where organ shortage levels seem to have stabilised over the last few years. In 2016, in the EU 69,053 patients were on the kidney waiting

Origin, Strasbourg, 24 January 2002, CETS No. 186; Council of Europe, Convention against Trafficking in Human Organs, Santiago de Compostela, 25 March 2015, CETS No. 216; European Union, Directive 2010/53/EU on Standards of Quality and Safety of Human Organs Intended for Transplantation, Brussels, 7 July 2010; World Health Organization Guiding Principles on Human Cell, Tissue, and Organ Transplantation, Geneva, May 2010; World Medical Association Statement on Human Organ Donation and Transplantation, replaced by Statement on Organ and Tissue Donation, Bangkok, October 2012; Steering Committee of the Istanbul Summit, 'Organ Trafficking and Transplant Tourism and Commercialism: The Declaration of Istanbul' (2008) 372 (9632) *The Lancet* 5–6; The Ethics Committee of The Transplantation Society, 'The Consensus Statement of the Amsterdam Forum on the Care of the Live Kidney Donor' (2004) 78(4) *Transplantation* 491–2; The Ethics Committee of The Transplantation Society, 'The Ethics Statement of the Vancouver Forum on the Live Lung, Liver, Pancreas, and Intestine Donor' (2006) 81(10) *Transplantation* 1386–7.

[23] Margaret Engel, 'Va. Doctor Plans Company to Arrange Sale of Human Kidneys' *The Washington Post* 19 September 1983.

[24] Jed A. Gross, 'E Pluribus UNOS: The National Organ Transplant Act and Its Postoperative Complications' (2008) 8(1) *Yale Journal of Health Policy, Law, and Ethics* 145–252.

list, as compared to 69,364 in 2012. However, only 20,638 transplants were performed in 2016, up from 18,854 in 2012, and on average 5 patients died each day on the kidney waiting list.[25] On a global scale, it is estimated that the number of transplants performed represents less than 10 per cent of total transplant needs.[26]

In parallel with the worsening organ shortage in the USA, the first detailed proposals for a regulated domestic organ market were presented in the 1980s. Currently, a wide variety of proposals is circulating. Some take the form of a futures market whereby individuals would sell the right to remove and transplant their organs upon their death.[27] Others propose 'benefits' for living organ donation, such as tax credits, comprehensive life-long health coverage, disability and life insurance, tuition vouchers, a contribution to a retirement plan, or the payment of funeral and burial expenses made to families of post-mortem donors.[28] However, most proposals involve direct payment to living donors.[29] In recent years, proponents of a regulated organ market have stepped up their efforts

---

[25] Calculations on the basis of the data found in the national data reports of the US Organ Procurement and Transplantation Network and in EDQM and Council of Europe, 'International Figures on Donation and Transplantation – 2016' (2017) *Newsletter Transplant* 22.

[26] Data from Global Observatory on Donation and Transplantation (GODT).

[27] Lloyd R. Cohen, 'Increasing the Supply of Transplant Organs: The Virtues of a Futures Market' (1989) 58(1) *George Washington Law Review* 1–51; Curtis E. Harris and Stephen P. Alcorn, 'To Solve a Deadly Shortage: Economic Incentives for Human Organ Donation' (2001) 16(3) *Issues in Law & Medicine* 213–33; Andrew J. Love, 'Replacing Our Current System of Organ Procurement with a Futures Market: Will Organ Supply Be Maximized?' (1997) 37(2) *Jurimetrics* 167–86.

[28] See, for instance, Robert Arnold, Steven Bartlett, James Bernat et al., 'Financial Incentives for Cadaver Organ Donation: An Ethical Reappraisal' (2002) 73(8) *Transplantation* 1361–7; J. Randall Boyer, 'Gifts of the Heart . . . and Other Tissues: Legalizing the Sale of Human Organs and Tissues' (2012) 1 *Brigham Young University Law Review* 313–40; Joseph B. Clamon, 'Tax Policy as a Lifeline: Encouraging Blood and Organ Donation Through Tax Credits' (2008) 17(1) *Annals of Health Law* 67–99; Curtis E. Harris and Stephen P. Alcorn, 'To Solve a Deadly Shortage: Economic Incentives for Human Organ Donation' (2001) 16(3) *Issues in Law & Medicine* 213–33; Jake Linford, 'The Kidney Donor Scholarship Act: How College Scholarships Can Provide Financial Incentives for Kidney Donation While Preserving Altruistic Meaning' (2009) 2(2) *Saint Louis University Journal of Health Law & Policy* 265–326.

[29] Mark J. Cherry, *Kidney for Sale by Owner: Human Organs, Transplantation, and the Market* (Washington, DC: Georgetown University Press, 2005); Gerald Dworkin, 'Markets and Morals: The Case for Organ Sales' in Gerald Dworkin (ed.), *Morality, Harm and the Law* (Boulder, CO: Westview Press, 1994), pp. 155–61; Benjamin Hippen, 'In Defense of a Regulated Market in Kidneys from Living Vendors' (2005) 30(6) *Journal of Medicine and Philosophy* 593–626; Sally Satel (ed.), *When Altruism Isn't Enough: The Case for Compensating Kidney Donors* (Washington, DC:

considerably, imploring American political leaders to start trials to assess whether the introduction of financial incentives would increase donation rates.[30] With the election of Donald Trump as the new American president, there seems to be renewed hope among proponents that their proposals might for the first time be taken seriously at governmental level.[31]

Advocates of a regulated organ market argue that the growing organ shortage and the difficulties in curtailing transplant tourism make the introduction of financial incentives morally imperative.[32] They allege that a domestic system for 'compensated living kidney donation' can be set up with substantial safeguards that would avoid the negative effects of the black market in organs. These measures would involve safety measures for vendor protection (i.e. appropriate screening, adequate information and good post-operative follow-up), quality control of the organs and complete transparency of the market process. Crucially, the state would be the only legal buyer, would set a fixed price and would determine the conditions of sale. Moreover, strict institutional oversight

AEI Press, 2008); James S. Taylor, *Stakes and Kidneys: Why Markets in Human Body Parts Are Morally Imperative* (Burlington, VT: Ashgate, 2005).

[30] See Gary S. Becker and Julio J. Elias, 'Cash for Kidneys: The Case for a Market for Organs' *The Wall Street Journal* 18 January 2014; Nir Eyal, Julio Frenk, Michele B. Goodwin et al., 'An Open Letter to President Barack Obama, Secretary of Health and Human Services Sylvia Mathews Burwell, Attorney General Eric Holder and Leaders of Congress', 11 September 2014, available at: www.ustransplantopenletter.org/openletter.html; A. Matas, J. A. E. Ambagtsheer, R. Gaston et al., 'A Realistic Proposal – Incentives May Increase Donation – We Need Trials Now!' (2012) 12(7) *American Journal of Transplantation* 1957–8; Sally Satel and David C. Cronin II, 'Time to Test Incentives to Increase Organ Donation' (2015) 175(8) *Journal of the American Medical Association Internal Medicine* 1329–33; Working Group on Incentives for Living Donation, 'Incentives for Organ Donation: Proposed Standards for an Internationally Acceptable System' (2012) 12(2) *American Journal of Transplantation* 306–12.

[31] Sally Satel, 'You've Heard of Trump Steaks, now Trump Kidneys' *Forbes* 15 November 2016.

[32] See Frederike Ambagtsheer and Willem Weimar, 'A Criminological Perspective: Why Prohibition of Organ Trade Is Not Effective and How the Declaration of Istanbul Can Move Forward' (2012) 12(3) *American Journal of Transplantation* 571–5; Michael M. Friedlaender, 'The Right to Sell or Buy a Kidney: Are We Failing Our Patients?' (2002) 359(9310) *The Lancet* 971–3; Michael B. Gill and Robert M. Sade, 'Paying for Kidneys: The Case for Repealing Prohibition' (2002) 12(1) *Kennedy Institute of Ethics Journal* 17–46; Julia D. Mahoney, 'Should We Adopt a Market Strategy to Increase the Supply of Transplantable Organs?' in Wayne N. Shelton and John Balint (eds.), *The Ethics of Organ Transplantation* (New York, NY: Elsevier, 2001), pp. 65–88.

would be provided by a competent body and the organs would be allocated on the basis of medical need.[33]

Although these proposals might seem convincing to some, they are in fact problematic on all levels. Firstly, it should be stressed that the proposed regulated domestic organ market is bound to fail. In this respect, profound doubts have been voiced as to the feasibility of a regulated system, taking into account that it would be very difficult to prevent patients from soliciting a cheaper price and circumventing the system.[34] It is indeed highly unlikely that the envisioned oversight mechanisms would be able to regulate all market transactions effectively, because the legalisation of the market will in itself encourage desperate patients and potential vendors to negotiate a better deal. Since, as will be argued below, organ supply will eventually decrease after an initial surge, regulation will probably be gradually relaxed and ever more closely resemble an open market. This will actually invite the exploitation that the regulated market was intended to prevent in the first place.[35] At the same time, continuing shortages in organs and the possibility of obtaining cheaper organs abroad will fuel black market activities in the developing world.

Moreover, it is readily predictable that the introduction of a domestic organ market in developed countries will propel developing countries to embrace a similar model, in a vain attempt to bolster donation rates and clean up their black markets. However, in view of their regulatory difficulties in combating current abuses, it is naïve to presume that in

[33] T. Randolph Beard and Jim Leitzel, 'Designing a Compensated-Kidney Donation System' (2014) 77(3) *Law and Contemporary Problems* 253–87; Gary S. Becker and Julio J. Elias, 'Introducing Incentives in the Market for Live and Cadaveric Organ Donations' (2007) 21 (3) *Journal of Economic Perspectives* 3–24; David C. Cronin II and Julio J. Elias, 'Operational Organization of a System for Compensated Living Organ Providers' in Sally Satel (ed.), *When Altruism Isn't Enough: The Case for Compensating Kidney Donors* (Washington, DC, AEI Press, 2008), pp. 34–49; Arthur J. Matas, 'Design of a Regulated System of Compensation for Living Kidney Donors' (2008) 22(3) *Clinical Transplantation* 378–84; Arthur J. Matas, Benjamin Hippen and Sally Satel, 'In Defense of a Regulated System of Compensation for Living Donation' (2008) 13(4) *Current Opinion in Organ Transplantation* 379–85; Working Group on Incentives for Living Donation, 'Incentives for Organ Donation'.

[34] Francis L. Delmonico, Robert Arnold, Nancy Scheper-Hughes et al., 'Ethical Incentives – Not Payment – for Organ Donation' (2002) 346(25) *New England Journal of Medicine* 2002–5; Francis L. Delmonico, Gabriel M. Danovitch, Alexander M. Capron et al., '"Proposed Standards for Incentives for Organs Donation" Are Neither International Nor Acceptable' (2012) 12(7) *American Journal of Transplantation* 1954–5.

[35] Simon Rippon, 'Imposing Options on People in Poverty: The Harm of a Live Donor Organ Market' (2012) 40(3) *Journal of Medical Ethics* 145–50.

those countries a market in organs could be regulated effectively.[36] Most likely, increasing financial competition between countries will emerge, resulting in a weakly regulated, globalised organ market, with international and local bureaucracies and law enforcement having the greatest trouble preventing a race to the bottom. In the worst case scenario, the exploitative practices of current transplant tourism would become legitimate practices, legally sanctioned at a global level.[37] In short, introducing a regulated organ market might well result in the exact opposite of what it aims to achieve.

Secondly, it is similarly very doubtful that the introduction of a regulated organ market would result in a stable supply of organs that would eradicate the transplant waiting list. To substantiate their claim that it is self-evident that donation rates would increase significantly, proponents of such a market generally point to Iran, the only country in the world where an official system of compensation for living kidney donors is operational.[38] However, after an initial surge in living kidney donation rates, since 2009 numbers have declined consistently and very rapidly.[39] Although there is some discussion as to whether, as the official version goes, the waiting list for kidney transplantation had at one point indeed disappeared, there is ample evidence that currently there is a long waiting list.[40] Consequently, contrary to what proponents of a regulated organ market want to believe, data from Iran indicate that an organ market is not (necessarily) able to sustain high donation rates.

[36] Vivekanand Jha and Kirpal S. Chugh, 'The Case Against a Regulated System of Living Kidney Sales' (2006) 2(9) *Nature Clinical Practice Nephrology* 466–7; Samuel J. Kerstein, 'Autonomy, Moral Constraints, and Markets in Kidneys' (2009) 34(6) *Journal of Medicine and Philosophy* 573–85; Scheper-Hughes, 'Keeping an Eye on the Global Traffic'.

[37] Hans J. Schlitt, 'Paid Non-Related Living Organ Donation: Horn of Plenty or Pandora's Box?' (2002) 359(9310) *The Lancet* 906–7; Stephen J. Wigmore, Jen A. Lumsdaine and John L. R. Forsythe, 'Ethical Market in Organs: Defending the Indefensible' (2003) 325 (7368) *British Medical Journal* 835–6.

[38] Benjamin E. Hippen, 'Organ Sales and Moral Travails: Lessons from the Living Kidney Vendor Program in Iran' (2008) *Cato Institute Policy Analysis No. 614*; Rupert W. L. Major, 'Paying Kidney Donors: Time to Follow Iran?' (2008) 11(1) *McGill Journal of Medicine* 67–9.

[39] Data from the Global Observatory on Donation and Transplantation indicate the following numbers of living kidney donors: 2009: 1,740; 2010: 1,636; 2011: 1,502; 2012: 1,506; 2013: 1,501; 2014: 1,203; 2015: 1,098; 2016: 1,078. See www.transplant-observatory.org/summary.

[40] In 2011, 17,910 patients were waitlisted for a kidney transplant and 2,273 kidney transplants were performed. See A. H. Rouchi, F. Ghaemi and M. Aghighi, 'Outlook of Organ Transplantation in Iran' (2014) 8(3) *Iranian Journal of Kidney Diseases* 185–8. See also, Anne Griffin, 'Kidneys on Demand' (2007) 334(7592) *British Medical Journal* 502–5.

Moreover, the introduction of a regulated organ market may have severe unintended effects that could result in the collapse of altruistic organ donation. More particularly, evidence suggests that financial incentives would crowd out altruistic motivations, which currently prompt donors to make organs available. Findings from behavioural sciences show that, where intrinsic incentives to perform a certain activity are replaced by extrinsic incentives, such as financial compensation, the perception of that activity drastically changes and one's moral commitment to engage in it is weakened significantly.[41] As a result, the awareness that organs are available for sale could make potential altruistic donors reluctant to volunteer. Similarly, patients themselves could be very hesitant to expose altruistic volunteers to the risks of the intervention. Furthermore, if organ donation is no longer regarded as the ultimate act of generosity, the level of altruistic deceased donation will probably also suffer heavily, with more people opting out of donation, the next of kin less inclined to authorise organ removal and transplant coordinators finding it more difficult to request approval.[42] That these are more than theoretical considerations is confirmed by data from Israel. Before the 2008 transplant law made it much more difficult for Israelis to travel abroad to purchase an organ, transplant tourism was accompanied by a decline in living kidney donation. Predictably, since the law changed, living kidney donation rates have increased exponentially.[43]

In view of these considerations, there is a real risk that a possible increase in purchased organs will only be temporary and will be offset by a reduction in altruistically donated organs. In this context, it should be noted that a large percentage of patients on transplant waiting lists

[41] Uri Gneezy and Aldo Rustichini, 'A Fine Is a Price' (2000) 29(1) *Journal of Legal Studies* 1–17; Uri Gneezy, *The W Effect of Incentives* (University of Chicago Business School, 2003). See also Richard Titmuss, *The Gift Relationship: From Human Blood to Social Policy* (London: Allen & Unwin, 1970).

[42] James F. Childress, 'The Body as Property: Some Philosophical Reflections' (1992) 24(5) *Transplant Proceedings* 2143–8; Gabriel M. Danovitch and Alan B. Leichtman, 'Kidney Vending: The "Trojan Horse" of Organ Transplantation' (2006) 1(6) *Clinical Journal of the American Society of Nephrology* 1133–5; Sheila M. Rothman and David J. Rothman, 'The Hidden Cost of Organ Sale' (2006) 6(7) *American Journal of Transplantation* 1524–8.

[43] Data from the Global Observatory on Donation and Transplantation indicate the following numbers of living kidney donors: 2003: 71; 2004: 68; 2005: 67; 2006: 54; 2007: 57; 2008: 56; 2009: 69; 2010: 78; 2011: 111; 2012: 108; 2013: 136; 2014: 135; 2015: 174; 2016: 222. See also J. Lavee, T. Ashkenazi, A. Stoler et al., 'Preliminary Marked Increase in the National Organ Donation Rate in Israel Following Implementation of a New Organ Transplantation Law' (2013) 13(3) *American Journal of Transplantation* 780–5.

would not be helped by a system of compensated living kidney donation, because they are medically unsuitable or otherwise inactive (35 per cent), or because they are in need of extra-renal organs such as a heart, a liver or lungs (20 per cent). If, as can be expected, a system of compensated living kidney donation would indeed have a negative effect on altruistic motivations, thereby jeopardising deceased donation, patients in need of extra-renal organs would be considerably worse off than before.[44] In addition, introducing a market system may remove incentives to maximise deceased donation and to prevent organ failure. For instance, patients suffering from hypertension, obesity or diabetes may be less inclined to adapt their lifestyle so as to prevent organ failure, wrongly believing that an organ market will yield an abundance of organs.[45] Again, a regulated organ market might well result in the opposite of what it aims to achieve: a net decline in kidney donation, fewer vital organs and more patients in need of a transplant.

Thirdly, the final argument underpinning current proposals for a regulated organ market, namely that it would result in a situation that would maximally respect and benefit vendors, is also utterly unconvincing. Proponents of such a market insist that a general ban amounts to misplaced paternalism. They allege that it excludes would-be vendors from an additional source of income to maximise their welfare and is an unjustifiable interference with what they consider an individual's sovereignty over his or her body.[46] However, the idea that a regulated organ market would be more respectful of an individual's autonomy and would represent a win–win situation is misguided.

[44] Alexander M. Capron, Gabriel M. Danovitch and Francis L. Delmonico, 'Organ Markets: Problems Beyond Harm to Vendors' (2014) 14(10) *American Journal of Bioethics* 23–5; Danovitch and Leichtman, 'Kidney Vending'; John H. Evans, 'Commodifying Life? A Pilot Study of Opinions Regarding Financial Incentives for Organ Donation' (2003) 28(6) *Journal of Health Politics, Policy & Law* 1003–32.

[45] Lainie Friedman Ross, 'Saving Lives Is More Important Than Abstract Moral Concerns: Financial Incentives Should Be Used to Increase Organ Donation – Con' (2009) 88(4) *Annals of Thoracic Surgery* 1056–9.

[46] Mark J. Cherry, 'Is a Market for Human Organs Necessarily Exploitative?' (2000) 14(4) *Public Affairs Quarterly* 337–60; Charles A. Erin and John Harris, 'An Ethical Market in Human Organs' (2003) 29(3) *Journal of Medical Ethics* 137–8; Janet Radcliffe Richards, 'Nephrarious Goings On: Kidney Sales and Moral Arguments' (1996) 21(4) *Journal of Medicine and Philosophy* 375–416; Julian Savulescu, 'Is the Sale of Body Parts Wrong?' (2003) 29(3) *Journal of Medical Ethics* 138–9; Luke Semrau, 'Misplaced Paternalism and Other Mistakes in the Debate over Kidney Sales' (2017) 31(3) *Bioethics* 190–8; Taylor, *Stakes and Kidneys*; Robert M. Veatch, 'Why Liberals Should Accept Financial Incentives for Organ Procurement' (2003) 13(1) *Kennedy Institute of Ethics Journal* 19–36.

Admittedly, the possibility of selling an organ would augment the options available to individuals looking for extra income. However, a decision to sell should always be understood within a socio-economic context. As the black market in organs demonstrates, only individuals who are financially desperate are likely to consider organ sale. As a rule, they do so because they are in severe debt and have no other options to quickly raise money. They would certainly not have considered selling an organ if not pressured by poverty. Despite some of the so-called protective measures introduced in proposals for a regulated organ market, there is no reason to believe that this would be any different in a regulated market. Although vendors may know what is best for them and although their decision to sell an organ may be rational and informed, their disadvantaged position and lack of alternatives will render the prospect of financial gain irresistible, with the effect that their autonomy will be undermined. The mere fact that a seller might be marginally better off does not make the decision autonomous or the offer less exploitative. Indeed, voluntariness and autonomy fall out of the picture when an agent is only presented with objectionable alternatives and left with the choice to act upon the least noxious of them.[47] In this regard, it has been convincingly argued that a regulated organ market will turn the desperation of the poor into a medical opportunity, and may, for its proper functioning, even need to rely on this kind of exploitation.[48]

Similarly, recent disturbing findings from the black market suggest that the introduction of remuneration in fact *reduces* the autonomy of potential vendors. In some 'kidney belts' the kidney has been elevated to the status of the ultimate collateral, with which poor individuals are expected to part when economic necessity arises.[49] Even under so-called controlled circumstances, it is readily conceivable that what

---

[47] Nikola Biller-Andorno and Alexander M. Capron, '"Gratuities" for Donated Organs: Ethically Indefensible' (2011) 377(9775) *The Lancet* 1390–1; Arthur L. Caplan, 'Organ Transplantation: The Challenge of Scarcity' in Ravitsky, Fiester and Caplan, *The Penn Center Guide*, pp. 679–87; Francis L. Delmonico and Nancy Scheper-Hughes, 'Why We Should Not Pay for Human Organs' (2003) 38(3) *Zygon* 689–98; Kate Greasley, 'A Legal Market in Organs: The Problem of Exploitation' (2012) 40(1) *Journal of Medical Ethics* 51–6; Paul M. Hughes, 'Constraint, Consent, and Well-Being in Human Kidney Sales' (2009) 34(6) *Journal of Medicine and Philosophy* 606–31; Ross, 'Saving Lives'.

[48] Tarif Bakdash and Nancy Scheper-Hughes, 'Is It Ethical for Patients with Renal Disease to Purchase Kidneys from the World's Poor?' (2006) 3(10) *PloS Medicine* e349; Greasley, 'A Legal Market in Organs'.

[49] Lawrence Cohen, 'Where It Hurts: Indian Material for an Ethics of Organ Transplantation' (1999) 128(4) *Daedalus* 135–65; Javaad Zargooshi, 'Quality of Life of Iranian Kidney "Donors"' (2001) 166(5) *The Journal of Urology* 1790–9.

would initially be an *option* would transform into a *demand*. Subject to normal market dynamics, it may become a regular economic asset that can be used to pay off a loan, to finance unexpected expenses or to become eligible for social benefits. Consequently, the bargaining position of the poor will change: instead of selling an organ being a genuine choice, it will be seen as the normal expectation, leaving it up to the poor to justify why they are unwilling to sell and to bear the consequences of refusal.[50] Against this background, the notion that a regulated organ market would be more respectful of vendors' autonomy and moral agency sounds very cynical.

The assertion that a regulated organ market would amount to a win–win situation is similarly implausible. Data indicating that the risks of living kidney donation are very low only apply to donors who are generally healthy, properly screened for relevant risk factors and adequately followed up.[51] However, as black market experiences indicate, the risks significantly increase when donors are not rigorously selected, live in unsanitary conditions, maintain a poor diet and unhealthy lifestyle, and lack access to long-term healthcare. Regrettably, those are the exact circumstances that can be expected among the poor vendors in regulated organ markets. Data from Iran show a substantial deterioration of health among a majority of vendors, and there is no reason to believe that vendors in developed countries will be spared this outcome. Findings from the black market and Iran point to similar concerns with regard to the financial consequences of organ sales. Since the conditions of indebtedness that lead to organ sale do not disappear, the great majority of vendors quickly find themselves in a worse financial situation

---

[50] Richard A. Demme, 'Ethical Concerns About an Organ Market' (2010) 102(1) *Journal of the National Medical Association* 46–50; Debra Satz, 'The Moral Limits of Markets: The Case of Human Kidneys' (2008) 108(3) *Proceedings of the Aristotelian Society* 269–88; Erik Malmqvist, 'Are Bans on Kidney Sales Unjustifiably Paternalistic?' (2014) 28(3) *Bioethics* 110–8; Rippon, 'Imposing Options'; Simon Rippon, 'Organ Markets and Harms: A Reply to Dworkin, Radcliffe Richards and Walsh' (2014) 40(3) *Journal of Medical Ethics* 155–6.

[51] For instance, the perioperative mortality rate is 3.1 per 10,000 procedures. See Emanuele Cozzi, Luigi Biancone, Marta López-Fraga et al., 'Long-term Outcome of Living Kidney Donation' (2016) 100(2) *Transplantation* 270–1. The risk of developing end-stage renal disease is, although possibly slightly higher than previously thought, still extremely small. See Geir Mjøen, Stein Hallan, Anders Hartmann et al., 'Long-term Risks for Kidney Donors' (2014) 86(1) *Kidney International* 162–7; Abimereki D. Muzaale, Allan B. Massie, Mei C. Wang et al., 'Risk of End-Stage Renal Disease Following Live Kidney Donation' (2014) 311 (6) *Journal of the American Medical Association* 579–86.

than before. Absent comprehensive plans to lift vendors out of poverty and to provide long-term assistance, the same fate will await vendors in developed countries.[52]

In short, a regulated organ market would not represent a win–win situation, but rather a zero-sum game at best.[53] However, even the latter would be an unlikely scenario if we take into account that would-be vendors would be persuaded not to disclose adverse health information in order not to be rejected as candidates. This would have a detrimental effect on the quality of organs and might impose unknown risks on recipients.[54] The contention that a regulated organ market would serve the good of all becomes even more of a cruel hoax if we also factor in the other negative externalities that can be expected to arise. As indicated above, these have been well documented for the black market and are likely to also hold true for markets in developed countries. Crucially, in addition to burdening local communities and the domestic healthcare system when the situation of vendors predictably deteriorates, a regulated organ market also risks corrupting the role of doctors, potentially even causing widespread distrust and loss of prestige. The ethics of the medical profession would be severely compromised if physicians were to be forced to act as facilitators of an organ trade and to infringe upon the 'do no harm' principle at the behest of wealthy donors. Under these circumstances, it is readily conceivable that donor acceptance criteria would be relaxed unduly and that the decision to perform organ removal could go against physicians' best medical judgement.[55]

As I hope to have shown convincingly, it is to be expected that, despite the protective measures envisaged to overcome the deficiencies of the black market, a regulated organ market is unfeasible and its intended

---

[52] Capron, Danovitch and Delmonico, 'Organ Markets'; Danovitch and Leichtman, 'Kidney Vending'; Thomas George, 'The Case against Kidney Sales' (2001) XI(1) *Issues in Medical Ethics* 49–50; Julian Koplin, 'Assessing the Likely Harms to Kidney Vendors in Regulated Organ Markets' (2014) 14(10) *American Journal of Bioethics* 7–18.

[53] Rothman and Rothman, 'The Hidden Cost'.

[54] Budiani-Saberi, 'Organ Trafficking and Transplant Tourism'; Rothman and Rothman, 'The Hidden Cost'; Michael L. Volk, 'Organ Quality as a Complicating Factor in Proposed Systems of Inducements for Organ Donation' (2014) 77(3) *Law and Contemporary Problems* 337–45.

[55] Gabriel M. Danovitch, 'Who Cares? Impact of Commercialized Kidney Transplantation on the Doctor–Patient Relationship' in Willem Weimar, Michael Bos and Jan van Busschbach (eds.), *Organ Transplantation: Ethical, Legal and Psychosocial Aspects: Towards a Common European Policy* (Lengerich: Pabst, 2008), pp. 49–54; Jeffrey P. Kahn and Francis L. Delmonico, 'The Consequences of Public Policy to Buy and Sell Organs for Transplantation' (2004) 4(2) *American Journal of Transplantation* 178–80.

benefits will fail to materialise. Since there is even a real risk that such an experiment will open a Pandora's box, resulting in a collapse of current systems of donation and the generalisation of exploitative practices, such a massive gamble is ill advised. In view of grave concerns of weak agency, widespread abuse and negative externalities, the 'paternalistic' intervention to completely ban commercialisation is and remains the only solution.[56] That this conclusion is unavoidable becomes even more manifest when we will shift our focus to the enormous immaterial harms that, in the name of autonomy, would be caused to society if plans to establish a regulated organ market were carried out. First, however, we will take a look at how legal theories of property are invoked to justify enclosing organs in order to solve the organ shortage.

5.4   The Tragedy of the Commons and Utilitarian Theories of Property

Organ donation and transplantation represent a typical example of a tragedy of the commons, because all individuals meeting certain medical criteria are allowed access to an organ, but contributions to the supply are voluntary and may impose costs on the donor.[57] Since individuals will not be excluded from benefiting even when they refuse to contribute, incentives to become an organ donor are few. Foreseeably, when the demand in organs rises, the common supply risks becoming depleted. In some countries, this tragedy has been addressed by introducing presumed consent for post-mortem donation, premised upon a duty of fairness (i.e. people who benefit from cooperative social schemes have a reciprocal duty to assume some of the burdens) and a duty of easy rescue (i.e. people who can prevent serious harm to others without incurring important burdens have a moral obligation to do so).[58] In countries with explicit consent regimes, constant appeals to solidarity

---

[56] It can be argued that, even in the unlikely scenario where most would-be vendors act autonomously and do not experience any harm, concern for the welfare of the remaining vendors may be sufficient to justify a complete ban. See Malmqvist, 'Are Bans on Kidney Sales Unjustifiably Paternalistic?'; Erik Malmqvist, 'A Further Lesson from Existing Kidney Markets' (2014) 14(10) *American Journal of Bioethics* 27–9.

[57] Alexander Tabarrok, 'The Organ Shortage: A Tragedy of the Commons?' in Alexander Tabarrok (ed.), *Entrepreneurial Economics: Bright Ideas from the Dismal Science* (Oxford: Oxford University Press, 2002), pp. 107–11.

[58] Micah Hester, 'Why We Must Leave Our Organs to Others' (2006) 6(4) *American Journal of Bioethics* W23-8; Jeremy Snyder, 'Easy Rescues and Organ Transplantation' (2009) 21 (1) *HEC Forum* 27–53.

remind the public of the need to contribute and, in a few countries, priority on the waiting list has partly been made conditional upon a registered willingness to contribute.[59]

However, in some countries that are confronted with a waiting list that is getting out of control, the idea seems to be gaining ground that the sole reliance on solidarity and altruism will not solve the tragedy of the commons in organ transplantation. Instead, as indicated above, it is suggested that the tragedy can only be solved by resorting to the classical liberal solution to this type of problem: a complete 'enclosure of the commons' by converting organs into private property, which would give owners a substantial, extrinsic incentive to make their 'resource' available to others in need. Donna Dickenson's general warning against an enclosure movement targeting human body material is both apt and timely.

Importantly, compared to body material that has already come into the reach of the market, organs that are still part of the body constitute a specific category that makes them legally more resistant to commodification. This has to do with the way in which property rights can be justified theoretically. Within legal philosophy, three largely incompatible models have been developed to define private property rights: the labour theory of property, the utilitarian theory of property and the personhood theory of property. The labour theory of property, established by Locke, holds that the person who encloses a previously unclaimed resource and exerts labour upon it, becomes the exclusive owner of the resource.[60] This theory is still the fundamental basis of our property law. It can be used – and, as Dickenson emphasises, is increasingly being used – to recognise property rights in excised or extracted body material that has been manipulated by the person who claims to have legal title.[61] Similarly, in a few jurisdictions, Lockean arguments

---

[59] Jacob Lavee and Dan W. Brock, 'Prioritizing Registered Donors in Organ Allocation: An Ethical Appraisal of the Israeli Organ Transplant Law' (2012) 18(6) *Current Opinion in Critical Care* 707-11; Jacob Lavee and Avraham Stoler, 'Reciprocal Altruism: The Impact of Resurrecting an Old Moral Imperative on the National Organ Donation Rate in Israel' (2014) 17(3) *Law and Contemporary Problems* 323-36.

[60] John Locke, *Two Treatises of Government*, ed. Peter Leslett (Cambridge: Cambridge University Press, [1690] 1967).

[61] For instance, in *Moore v Regents of the University of California* 793 P 2d 479 (Cal. 1990), the Supreme Court of California recognised a rightful property claim by a physician who had developed and patented a cell line using cells from a patient (without that person's consent), because the physician had in the process mixed his labour with his patient's excised body material.

have been used to recognise substances produced by the body, such as blood, sperm and milk, as property that can be sold by the individual concerned.[62] This enclosure movement raises major concerns of its own, but it has stopped short of including the human body and those body materials, such as organs, that have not been excised or extracted and that are not products of the body.

Rather, attempts to justify private property rights in organs are usually based on utilitarian theories of property. Expanding on his idea that the greatest happiness of the greatest number should form the foundation of morality and legislation, Bentham stated that the greatest happiness in respect of resources will only occur when they are the private property of persons.[63] Along the same lines, proponents of a regulated organ market allege that aggregate welfare, in terms of utility, of all those affected would be enhanced were we to grant private property rights in organs.

Since the end of the 1960s, the utilitarian theory of property has been considerably redefined by replacing some of its moral underpinnings with purely economic ones. Under the influence of Chicago-style law and economics approaches, pioneered by Richard Posner, Gary Becker and others, the extension of property rights is presented as necessary to make better use of resources.[64] It is argued that, whenever a system of private property rights would be better at minimising costs and maximising economic efficiency, such a system is justified. Coupled with a glorification of autonomy, the emphasis on economic calculations further diminishes the importance of considerations of social justice, which still holds some relevance in classical utilitarianism. Therefore, it comes as no surprise that some of the most outspoken advocates of the idea of addressing the tragedy of the commons in transplantation through granting full property rights and establishing a regulated organ market can be found among supporters of the Chicago-style theory of property.[65]

---

[62] Kara W. Swanson, *Banking on the Body: The Market in Blood, Milk and Sperm in Modern America* (Cambridge, MA: Harvard University Press, 2014).

[63] Jeremy Bentham, *A Fragment on Government and an Introduction to the Principles of Morals and Legislation*, ed. Wilfried Harrison (Oxford: Basil Blackwell, [1789] 1967); Jeremy Bentham, *Theory of Legislation*, ed. Etienne Dumont and Richard Hildreth (Holmes Beach, FL: Gaunt, [1802] 2011).

[64] Harold Demsetz, 'Toward a Theory of Property Rights' (1967) 57(2) *The American Economic Review* 347–59; Richard Posner, *Economic Analysis of Law* (Boston, MA: Little, Brown and Company, 1972).

[65] See, for instance, Becker and Elias, 'Introducing Incentives'.

However, the utilitarian approach to the tragedy of the commons in transplantation raises a host of fundamental problems. Importantly, there is no reason to presume that pursuing the greatest happiness of the greatest number in organ transplantation necessitates a market approach.[66] On the contrary, it can be convincingly argued that benefit would be maximised and harm minimised if the main causes of the need for organs were better addressed and initiatives were taken to increase donation rates without inviting crowding-out effects. For instance, encouraging a healthy lifestyle and providing quality universal healthcare may prevent or delay the onset of organ failure. Similarly, deceased donation rates may be significantly boosted by implementing elements of the 'Spanish model' of donor identification, passing presumed consent legislation or allowing donation after circulatory determination of death.[67] The observation that in the EU organ shortages recently seem to have stabilised indicates that these shortages can be effectively reduced without having to resort to financial incentives.

In addition, as compared to ideal markets, a market in organs will be inherently marred by severe market failures. The most important one is that the supply will entirely depend on individuals in desperate financial need, characterised by compromised autonomy and, hence, weak agency. Admittedly, the market could be regulated to minimise the risk of weak agency, but proposals to do so (e.g. establishing a monopsony, setting a maximum price and rigorous selection) might in fact recreate organ shortages, because many would-be vendors would be excluded and the incentives might be insufficiently attractive. This problem could be remedied by relaxing protective measures and increasing prices, but that strategy would lead to a higher risk of exploitation and lower organ quality, which can be regarded as other undesired consequences that would negatively affect aggregate welfare.[68]

Moreover, proponents of an organ market do not sufficiently take into account that the field of organ donation has some exceptional features, which, when transformed into a market, may result in an even worse

[66] Kerstein, 'Autonomy, Moral Constraints'; Ross, 'Saving Lives'.
[67] Beatriz Domínguez-Gil, Francis L. Delmonico, Faissal A. M. Shaheen et al., 'The Critical Pathway for Deceased Donation: Reportable Uniformity in the Approach to Deceased Donation' (2011) 24(4) *Transplant International* 373–8; Rafael Matesanz, Beatriz Domínguez-Gil, Elisabeth Coll et al., 'Spanish Experience As a Leading Country: What Kind of Measures Were Taken?' (2011) 24(4) *Transplant International* 333–43.
[68] Satz, 'The Moral Limits'.

tragedy of the commons. As outlined above, disrupting a system that is so firmly built on an ethos of altruism and solidarity can be expected to crowd out the motivations that would otherwise have prompted individuals to contribute to the supply. In this way, aggregate welfare would *decrease* if full property rights in organs were awarded.

It should also be noted that utilitarian appeals stressing the benefits of an organ market neglect the importance and stringency of the background conditions that would prompt individuals to sell. As indicated above, experiences from the black market and from Iran show that, because of their situation of poverty and associated unhealthy living conditions, vendors do not benefit: frequently they are considerably worse off in the longer term, both financially and physically. Since protective measures do not target these background conditions – and doing so would pose an enormous burden that would also need to be weighed in the utilitarian calculus – the assumption that providing full property rights in organs would amount to a win–win situation proves to be false.

Futhermore, utilitarian theories are notably difficult to apply to public policy, because it is not clear how one person's gain in utility should be balanced against another person's loss in utility. More specifically, utilitarianism may endorse an organ market that imposes harm on vendors to the benefit of recipients as long as the aggregate net benefit would increase. Disconcertingly, this perspective overlooks the moral importance of whether benefits and harms accrue to different persons and whether some harms may be impermissible regardless of the net benefits of the market.[69] Although proponents of a market advocate regulation to address this concern, utilitarian reasoning could, strictly speaking, condone the outright exploitation of vendors.

5.5   Organs and Personhood

Although the aforementioned reasons overwhelmingly demonstrate that utilitarian theories of property fail to properly justify the need to assign private property rights in organs, even more is at stake than is generally acknowledged. More specifically, essential immaterial interests are fostered by keeping in place the current, altruistic system of organ donation. This is recognised in the personhood theory of property. This third

---

[69]   Rippon, 'Organ Markets and Harms'.

model of private property rights in fact denies that full property rights can be granted with regard to the human body.

The personhood theory builds on the ideas of Hegel and Kant, who claimed that, since private property involves an act of appropriation indispensable for the self-realisation of the person, it is to be considered an extension of personhood.[70] According to Kant, property rights can be extended to things but not to persons or the body. The first reason is that persons cannot dispose over themselves because they are not a thing and they are not their own property. Whereas things have a price, persons have dignity – an inner value without equivalent – as a result of their capacity for morality and rationality. Since bodies are integral to the person, they also possess dignity and they should not be treated as things. The second reason is that, for Kant, persons should never be treated (or never treat themselves) merely as a means to the goals of others. After all, respect for the dignity of persons entails a duty to treat each individual (and oneself) as having incommensurable value. An insult to human dignity arises when a non-instrumental valuation is totally absent, in that persons are denied the distinct importance of their own lives, and are instead only valued for their usefulness. According to Kant, putting a price on persons or their bodies is just such an insult, because it reduces them to something fungible, an object for use. Assimilating persons to the realm of objects is the exact opposite of what we owe to them in moral terms.[71]

Kantian notions of inherent human dignity and respect for persons also lie at the heart of general human rights, as evidenced by the pride of place given to them in international human rights instruments. As a consequence, they have become the bedrock of human rights instruments in the context of biomedicine.[72] Here, the right to respect

[70] Georg W. F. Hegel, *Elements of the Philosophy of Right*, ed. Allen W. Wood (Cambridge: Cambridge University Press, [1821] 2012); Immanuel Kant, *The Metaphysics of Morals*, ed. Mary J. Gregor (Cambridge: Cambridge University Press, [1797] 2012).

[71] Immanuel Kant, *Groundwork of the Metaphysics of Morals*, ed. Mary J. Gregor and Jens Timmerman (Cambridge: Cambridge University Press, [1785] 2012); Kant, *The Metaphysics of Morals*.

[72] Roberto Andorno, 'Human Dignity and Human Rights as a Common Ground for a Global Bioethics' (2009) 34(3) *Journal of Medicine and Philosophy* 223–40; Daniela-Ecaterina Cutas, 'Looking for the Meaning of Dignity in the Bioethics Convention and the Cloning Protocol' (2005) 13(4) *Health Care Analysis* 303–13; Susan M. Shell, 'Kant's Concept of Human Dignity as a Resource for Bioethics' in The President's Council on Bioethics (ed.), *Human Dignity and Bioethics: Essays Commissioned by the President's Council on Bioethics* (Washington, DC: 2008), pp. 333–49.

for one's dignity translates into a negative right against unwilled interventions by others and, hence, the requirement of free and informed consent. But respect for dignity is increasingly also formulated as a limiting principle invoked not to promote but to restrict the exercise of autonomy, out of concern that unlimited freedom to take advantage of newly emerging biomedical possibilities could threaten human dignity itself.[73]

Importantly, in the context of organ transplantation the commercialisation of the human body and its parts is considered a type of practice that would compromise the intrinsic worth of persons. Accordingly, the *Convention on Human Rights and Biomedicine* and its *Additional Protocol concerning Transplantation* – binding legal instruments issued at the level of the Council of Europe – contain a non-commercialisation clause stipulating that 'The human body and its parts shall not, as such, give rise to financial gain.'[74] It should be noted that the reference to 'as such' leaves open the door for the legal possibility, provided by the labour theory of property, of claiming full property rights on body material to which one has applied one's skill.[75] However, this kind of enclosure is entirely prohibited where it concerns organs, at least to the extent that they have not been excised and manipulated.

It should be noted that two valid criticisms have been levelled against Kant's idea that, since the body is integral to the person and since the person is beyond price, parts of the body cannot be sold without

[73] David Beyleveld and Roger Brownsword, *Human Dignity in Bioethics and Biolaw* (Oxford: Oxford University Press, 2001); Roger Brownsword, 'Human Dignity, Biolaw, and the Basis of Moral Community' (2010) 21(4) *Journal International de Bioéthique* 21–40. See, for a more extensive discussion, Britta van Beers, *Persoon en Lichaam in het Recht. Menselijke waardigheid en zelfbeschikking in het tijdperk van de medische biotechnologie* (Vrije Universiteit Amsterdam, PhD dissertation, 2009); Britta van Beers, Luigi Corrias and Wouter G. Werner (eds.), *Humanity across International Law and Biolaw* (Cambridge: Cambridge University Press, 2014).
[74] Council of Europe, *Convention on Human Rights and Biomedicine*, Oviedo, 4 April 1997, CETS No. 164, Article 21; Council of Europe, *Additional Protocol concerning Transplantation of Organs and Tissues of Human Origin*, Strasbourg, 24 January 2002, CETS No. 186, Article 21.
[75] Many examples of this enclosure can be found in the writings of Donna Dickenson. See also, for the patenting of human body material, Sigrid Sterckx and Julian Cockbain, *Exclusions from Patentability: How Far Has the European Patent Office Eroded Boundaries?* (Cambridge: Cambridge University Press, 2012); Sigrid Sterckx and Julian Cockbain, 'The Ethics of Patenting in Genetics – A Second Enclosure of the Commons?' in Gabriele Werner-Felmayer, Barbara Prainsack and Silke Schicktanz (eds.), *Genetics as Social Practice – Transdisciplinary Views on Science and Culture* (Farnham: Ashgate, 2014), pp. 129–44.

dehumanising the person. Firstly, Kant condemns the wilful destruction of one's own bodily integrity for unnecessary reasons, which – as evidenced by his claim that 'to give away or sell a tooth to be transplanted' is tantamount to partial suicide[76] – also means that his concept would have required the rejection of living organ donation, for the same reasons as he would have rejected the sale of an organ.[77] However, this objection can be countered by pointing out that, in line with other elements in his moral theory, for Kant living organ donation would not constitute using oneself as a mere means and would even be commendable, on the basis of the duty to treat humanity as an end in itself.[78] Secondly, there does not seem to be any obvious reason why the premise that the human body as a whole possesses dignity compels us to believe that body parts also have dignity, and that treating body parts as objects would amount to treating the person as an object.[79] This is a fair objection, but it misses the point that something more fundamental underlies Kant's position and the personhood theory of property.

For Kant, persons have a corporeal identity that is indivisible, and their attitude towards their body and parts of their body therefore reflects their notion of self. Persons who would agree that something so vital for human identity as a body part could be treated as an object would signal to others that they are open to further fragmentation of what makes them human.[80] Moreover, because persons are embedded in the moral community, each person is required to exercise his or her autonomy in a way which does not damage the context that makes the moral community

---

[76] Kant, *The Metaphysics of Morals*, p. 177.

[77] Dworkin, 'Markets and Morals'; Nicole Gerrand, 'The Misuse of Kant in the Debate About a Market in Human Body Parts' (1999) 16(1) *Journal of Applied Philosophy* 59–67; Mario Morelli, 'Commerce in Organs: A Kantian Critique' (1999) 30(2) *Journal of Social Philosophy* 315–24.

[78] Ruth F. Chadwick, 'The Market for Bodily Parts: Kant and Duties to Oneself' (1989) 6(2) *Journal of Applied Philosophy* 129–39; Cécile Fabre, *Whose Body is it Anyway? Justice and the Integrity of the Person* (Oxford: Oxford University Press, 2006); Morelli, 'Commerce in Organs'.

[79] Chadwick, 'The Market for Bodily Parts'; Fabre, *Whose Body is it Anyway?*; Stephen R. Munzer, 'Kant and Property Rights in Body Parts' (1993) 6(2) *Canadian Journal of Law and Jurisprudence* 319–41; Stephen R. Munzer, 'An Uneasy Case Against Property Rights in Body Parts' (1994) 11 *Social Philosophy and Policy* 259–86; Stephen Wilkinson, *Bodies for Sale: Ethics and Exploitation in the Human Body Trade* (New York, NY: Routledge, 2003).

[80] Immanuel Kant, *Lectures on Ethics*, ed. Peter Heath (Cambridge: Cambridge University Press, 2008).

itself possible.[81] The duty not to compromise one's own dignity is violated when persons intentionally undercut the conditions that are essential for nurturing moral aspirations. When the underpinnings of the moral community are threatened by the behaviour of one person, what seems to be that person's own interest becomes a matter in which all other persons have an investment.[82] Consequently, it is essential to prohibit the sale of a body part not only to discourage a way of thinking that (some) persons may lack value, but also to uphold the very idea and functioning of the moral community.[83]

Precisely the link between embodiment and flourishing has inspired many eminent scholars to expand upon the personhood theory of property, as applied to the human body, from the perspective of virtue ethics, feminist theories and communitarian philosophy.[84] As exemplified in the

[81] Jennifer Moore, 'Kant's Ethical Community' (1992) 26(1) The Journal of Value Inquiry 51–71; Shell, 'Kant's Concept of Human Dignity'.

[82] Roger Brownsword, 'What the World Needs Now: Techno-Regulation, Human Rights and Human Dignity' in Roger Brownsword (ed.), Human Rights (Oxford: Hart, 2004), pp. 203–34; Thomas E. Hill, Jr., Respect, Pluralism, and Justice: Kantian Perspectives (Oxford: Oxford University Press, 2000).

[83] Cynthia Cohen, 'Selling Bits and Pieces of Humans to Make Babies: "The Gift of the Magi" Revisited' (1999) 24(3) Journal of Medicine and Philosophy 288–306; Samuel J. Kerstein, 'Kantian Condemnation of Commerce in Organs' (2009) 19(2) Kennedy Institute of Ethics Journal 147–69; Stephen Wilkinson, 'Commodification Arguments for the Legal Prohibition of Organ Sale' (2000) 8(2) Health Care Analysis 189–201.

[84] See, for instance, Barbro Björkmann, 'Why We Are Not Allowed to Sell That Which We Are Encouraged to Donate' (2006) 15(1) Cambridge Quarterly of Healthcare Ethics 60–70; Michelle B. Bray, 'Personalizing Personality: Toward a Property Right in Human Bodies' (1990) 69(1) Texas Law Review 209–44; Cohen, 'Selling Bits and Pieces'; Charles Foster, Human Dignity in Bioethics and Law (Oxford: Hart, 2011); Amitai Etzioni, 'Organ Donation: A Communitarian Approach' (2003) 13(1) Kennedy Institute of Ethics Journal 1–18; Charles Foster, 'Dignity and the Use of Body Parts' (2014) 40(1) Journal of Medicine and Ethics 44–7; Kate Greasley, 'Property Rights in the Human Body: Commodification and Objectification' in Imogen Goold, Kate Greasley, Jonathan Herring and Loane Skene (eds.), Persons, Parts and Property: How Should We Regulate Human Tissue in the 21st Century? (Oxford: Hart, 2014), pp. 67–87; Suzanne Holland, 'Contested Commodities at Both Ends of Life: Buying and Selling Gametes, Embryos, and Body Tissues' (2001) 11 Kennedy Institute of Ethics Journal 263–84; Dominique Martin, Beyond the Market: A New Approach to the Ethical Procurement of Human Biological Materials (The University of Melbourne, PhD dissertation, 2011); Carolyn McLeod and Françoise Baylis, 'Feminists on the Inalienability of Human Embryos' (2006) 21(1) Hypatia 1–14; Satz, 'The Moral Limits'; Bernard Teo, 'Is the Adoption of More Efficient Strategies of Organ Procurement the Answer to Persistent Organ Shortage in Transplantation?' (1992) 6(2) Bioethics 113–39; Britta van Beers, Persoon en Lichaam; Andrew Wancata, 'No Value for a Pound of Flesh: Extending Market-Inalienability of the Human Body' (2003) 18(2) Journal of Law & Health 199–228.

work of Margaret Radin and Donna Dickenson, the personhood theory embraces an account of dignity in terms of human flourishing and a perspective on personhood that stresses physical embodiment, social interconnectedness and an ethos of care. According to Radin, private property rights should only be recognised to the extent that they promote human thriving. The body and its parts, since they are integral to the self and not detachable like objects that can be owned, should be market-inalienable (i.e. not subject to sale). If they were commodified, it would violate our sense of personhood, corrupt our attitudes towards ourselves and each other, encourage the perception that persons themselves may be regarded as objects and prevent us from engaging in gift relationships that cement communal bonds.[85]

Whereas commodification of the body is intrinsically harmful according to Kant, Radin's virtue ethics approach makes its harmfulness contingent upon its effect on flourishing. The reason why commodification of the body would be detrimental in this respect and would need to be avoided can be found in Radin's domino theory, which is largely inspired by Richard Titmuss's influential analysis of commercial blood donation.[86] The domino theory holds that, where a social interaction exists both in a market and a non-market form, market rhetoric may contaminate the non-market form, suppress its value, and ultimately make it impossible to maintain. When a non-market version is morally preferable and it is likely that the market version will change public attitudes to the point that the social interaction will eventually be perceived largely or only in market terms, the market version should be banned.[87] In the context of transplantation, altruism and solidarity are essential for fostering personhood and a flourishing society and, conversely, market rhetoric would have a degrading effect on both personhood and society; thus organ markets should be prohibited.

Along similar lines, Dickenson argues that '[t]he body both is, and is not, the person' and that, since '[o]ur consciousness, dignity, *ngeia* and human essence are all embodied', the body 'should never be only a

---

[85] Dickenson, *Property in the Body*; Margaret J. Radin, 'Market-Inalienability' (1987) 100(8) *Harvard Law Review* 1849–937; Margaret J. Radin, *Reinterpreting Property* (Chicago, IL: University of Chicago Press, 1993); Margaret J. Radin, *Contested Commodities: The Trouble with Trade in Sex, Children, Body Parts, and Other Things* (Cambridge, MA: Harvard University Press, 1996).

[86] Titmuss, *The Gift Relationship*.

[87] Radin, 'Market-Inalienability'; Radin, *Reinterpreting Property*; Radin, *Contested Commodities*.

consumer good, an obscure object of material desire, a capital investment, a transferable resource: merely a thing'.[88] Criticising the 'new enclosures' that target human tissue and genetic material used in research, procreation and medicine more generally, she acknowledges that these types of human body material contain 'elements of both person and thing, subject and object', especially 'when tissues from the body are no longer physically joined to the person'.[89] Under these circumstances, they may become the subject of full property rights under Locke's labour theory of property. Fearing that the increasing tendency to grant full property rights on human tissue and genetic material would undermine our humanity, Dickenson rightfully insists that we should reclaim the use of these materials for the common good. One fruitful avenue would be to give the persons who provide the materials limited property rights, which would give them control but not the right to sell.

As indicated earlier, Kant's personhood theory of property does not leave much room for recognising any property right in the body and its parts, leading some authors to deny that property rights can have any bearing on organs.[90] By contrast, in order to allow for altruistic donation of body parts, a quasi-property right would need to be granted that excludes commercial transactions but still allows individuals to control

[88] Dickenson, *Body Shopping*, p. 168. Note that *Ngeia* is a Tongan concept that means both 'awe-inspiring' and 'dignity'. The concept was central to the opposition of the Tongan people to attempts by Australian biotech company Autogen Ltd to collect their tissue samples and conduct genetic research on the population, after Autogen had been granted exclusive access to the Tonga gene pool in an agreement with Tonga's Ministry of Health in November 2000. See, for more information, Lopeti Senituli and Margaret Boyes, 'Whose DNA? Tonga and Iceland, Biotech, Ownership, and Consent' in James V. Lavery, Christine Grady, Elizabeth R. Wahl and Ezekiel J. Emanuel (eds.), *Ethical Issues in International Biomedical Research: A Casebook* (Oxford: Oxford University Press, 2007), pp. 53–63.

[89] Dickenson, *Property in the Body*, pp. 5–6. Some might argue that not all bodily materials are integral to the functioning of the self and that, consequently, market-inalienability should be limited even in the personhood theory of property. Although some parts of the body (e.g. hair, fingernails) are clearly not essential for personal identity, there may be discussion about the intrinsic significance of certain other parts (e.g. blood, ova, genetic material, kidneys) as compared to still others (e.g. heart, liver, brain) that clearly are central. However, even if no precise distinction could be made, it is better to be inclusive so as to avoid the slippery slope effects that may emerge when some potentially essential body parts are surrendered to the market. See also Satz, 'The Moral Limits'.

[90] Most notable, see Leon R. Kass, *Toward a More Natural Science: Biology and Human Affairs* (New York, NY: Free Press, 1985); Leon R. Kass, 'Organs for Sale? Propriety, Property, and the Price of Progress' (1992) 107 *Public Interest* 65–86; Leon R. Kass, *Life, Liberty and the Defense of Dignity: The Challenge for Bioethics* (San Francisco, CA: Encounter Books, 2004).

disposition. As a way to emphasise market-inalienability without pre-cluding transfer by gift, scholars such as Radin and Dickenson have proposed the recognition of a limited property right in relation to human body material.[91] More specifically, of all the ownership entitle-ments that constitute a full-fledged property right (including the right to income, the right to capital value and the right to transfer by sale), only those sticks in the bundle that are restricted to the notion of personal control would be retained, without establishing any right to income or sale.[92] Such a carefully limited property right was proposed to allow a measure of continuing control on the part of persons whose tissues or genetic material had been removed, stored, researched, sold and even patented, so as to address the excesses documented by Dickenson.[93] However, it is similarly useful in the context of organ donation – where, in contrast to Dickenson's main field of research, an enclosure movement on the basis of the labour theory of property is largely absent – precisely to preclude the excesses that would accompany an organ market.

[91] Dickenson, 'Commodification'; Dickenson, *Property in the Body*; Dickenson, *Body Shopping*; Radin, 'Market-Inalienability'; Radin, *Reinterpreting Property*; Radin, *Contested Commodities*. See also Bray, 'Personalizing Personality'; Jonathan Herring and Pak-Lee Chau, 'Interconnected, Inhabited and Insecure: Why Bodies Should Not Be Property' (2014) 40(3) *Journal of Medical Ethics* 39–43; Nuffield Council on Bioethics, *Human Bodies: Donation for Medicine and Research* (London: Nuffield Council on Bioethics, 2011); Wancata, 'No Value for a Pound'.

[92] Note that A.M. Honoré identifies 12 elements of full individual ownership. See A.M. Honoré, *Making Law Bind: Essays Legal and Philosophical* (Oxford: Clarendon Press, 1987). See also Dickenson, *Property in the Body*; Radin, *Contested Commodities*.

[93] In this regard, it should be noted that some have argued that a broad concept of privacy may already be sufficient and would have the added benefit of avoiding the perception of fragmentation between the body and its owner that is generated by the property para-digm. See Roger Brownsword, 'An Interest in Human Dignity as the Basis for Genomic Torts' (2003) 42(3) *Washburn Law Journal* 413–87; Graeme Laurie, *Genetic Privacy: A Challenge to Medico-Legal Norms* (Cambridge: Cambridge University Press, 2002); Graeme Laurie, Pierre Mallia, David A. Frenkel et al., 'Interests in Genetic Research? Managing Access to Biobanks: How Can We Reconcile Individual Privacy and Public Interests in Genetic Research?' (2010) 10(4) *Medical Law International* 315–37; Natalie Ram, 'Assigning Rights and Protecting Interests: Constructing Ethical and Efficient Legal Rights in Human Tissue Research' (2009) 23(1) *Harvard Journal of Law and Technology* 119–77; Rhadika Rao, 'Property, Privacy, and the Human Body' (2000) 80 (2) *Boston University Law Review* 359–460; Rhadika Rao, 'Genes and Spleens: Property, Contract, or Privacy Rights in the Human Body?' (2007) 35(3) *The Journal of Law, Medicine and Ethics* 371–82; Patricia A. Roche, 'The Property/Privacy Conundrum Over Human Tissue' (2010) 22(3) *HEC Forum* 197–209.

Interestingly, under Radin's personhood theory of property it may be allowed, and even be commendable, to establish a market in an attribute integral to the self if, by doing so, the conditions of flourishing would improve despite the degrading effects of commodification. This situation may arise due to what Radin calls the 'double bind': in the non-ideal world where the poor live under oppressive conditions that cannot quickly be ameliorated, it may be better to give them the opportunity to alleviate these conditions by selling parts of their bodies. Although the poor will be harmed by a disintegrated self-conception and by stigmatisation, allowing them to engage in degrading market transactions may increase their upward mobility in a way that would still be beneficial to their personhood. By way of example, Radin suggests that, while we consider wealth redistribution to lift them out of poverty, destitute women might be allowed to engage in prostitution so as to improve their oppressed condition.

Rather surprisingly, Radin also leaves some room to consider the establishment of a regulated organ market. Although Radin emphasises that its acceptability would depend on a number of factors, the fact that she does not immediately rule out the possibility is remarkable.[94] The suggestion that the legitimacy of organ sales can be warranted on the basis of cost-benefit calculations brings her close to the position of her utilitarian counterparts. Consequently, the similar rejoinder may be made that it is completely unrealistic to speculate that vendors would manage to improve their financial and health situation in the long term. The specific health impact and the fact that it is a one-off transaction make it even less probable that, possibly unlike prostitution, organ selling would extricate vendors from their poverty.[95] Moreover, as Radin's theory highlights, dignitary harms will inevitably accrue to both the vendors and society. The prospect of being left marginally better off by the organ sale should not obfuscate the risk that severe exploitation will take place and social inequality may worsen.[96] Finally, although under the double bind commodification would be allowed as a temporary measure, while we wait for the state to improve the undesirable circumstances that led the vendors to regard selling as a viable option, states would be disinclined to intervene after the sale of organs had been

[94] Margaret J. Radin, 'Bodies and markets: Ethical arguments and choices,' lecture at Trento, Italy, 4 June 2011.
[95] Pearson, *Coercion in the Kidney Trade?*   [96] Greasley, 'A Legal Market in Organs'.

authorised, precisely because the poor would then be perceived as having an additional source of income.

5.6 The Need to Safeguard the Communal Values in Organ Transplantation

Notwithstanding the hypothetical opening left by Radin, personhood theories of property affirm that there is much more to account for in the debate about (non-)commodification in organ transplantation than is generally acknowledged by utilitarian defenders of a regulated organ market. More specifically, severe immaterial harms would also need to be taken into the equation, making utilitarian arguments even less convincing.

If an organ market were established, organ donation would suffer from the degrading effects that typically occur when the market encroaches upon a sphere of human interaction governed by a different mode of valuation. In line with the more general concern that market expansion will increase domination (Walzer) and suffocate dimensions of value incompatible with crude self-interest (Anderson), personhood theories of property highlight that, when applied to the human body, the market would erode human flourishing (Radin) and disrupt communal purposes and interconnectedness (Dickenson).[97] On the basis of the analysis performed above, we can predict that five types of immaterial harm are likely to accrue if a market in organs were established.

First, the mere existence of a market would undermine the possibility of altruism. Attitudes to donation would no longer be the same, since every future instance of altruistic organ donation would automatically be seen in terms of its market value; the act would gradually cease to be

---

[97] See, more generally, for a defence of 'blocked exchanges' to safeguard the spheres of personal interaction: Elizabeth Anderson, 'The Ethical Limitations of the Market' (1990) 6(2) *Economics and Philosophy* 179–205; Elizabeth Anderson, *Value In Ethics And Economics* (Cambridge, MA: Harvard University Press, 1995); Allen E. Buchanan, *Ethics, Efficiency, and the Market* (Oxford: Clarendon, 1985); Neil Duxbury, 'Do Markets Degrade?' (1996) 59 *Modern Law Review* 331–48; Michael J. Sandel, *What Money Can't Buy: The Moral Limits of Markets* (London: Allen Lane, 2012); Debra Satz, *Why Some Things Should Not Be for Sale: The Limits of Markets* (Oxford: Oxford University Press, 2010); Cass R. Sunstein, 'Incommensurability and Valuation in Law' (1994) *Michigan Law Review* 779–861; Michael Walzer, *Spheres of Justice: A Defense of Pluralism and Equality* (New York, NY: Basic Books, 1983).

experienced and recognised as a generous one.[98] Some have argued that permitting the sale of organs does not prevent individuals from acting altruistically and that, on the contrary, it would give altruistic donors the opportunity to act even more generously, in that they give up not only an organ but also the payment.[99]

However, this is an impoverished understanding of what is really at stake. Knowing that the organ has become an economic asset, the purity of the motivation of altruistic donors would be tainted beyond repair. What they had planned to be an ultimate act of civic virtue, a selfless sacrifice of physical integrity for the common good, a symbol of how deeply committed they are to the well-being of others, would now inevitably appear as a market exchange, impersonal and devoid of symbolic meaning. By changing the nature of the act from intrinsically valuable to purely instrumental and only appealing to desperate individuals, a market would result in the collapse of altruistic donations. Tragically, it is to be feared that, even if the purely altruistic system were reinstated after the inevitable failure of the market experiment, it would take a very long time to revert to the old perception. Indeed, it is much more difficult to infuse a social activity with symbolic meaning, especially if that meaning had earlier been intentionally destroyed, than to drain a social activity of its symbolic meaning through market rhetoric.

Second, the importation of market values would erode the sense of community fostered by organ transplantation. As is duly recognised by Dickenson and others, organ transplantation is one of only a few remaining vital areas of social interactions that is still dominated by the ethos of the gift. It is a context in which individuals know that they mutually depend on each other's generosity and have a shared responsibility. In this way, it creates opportunities for expressing solidarity, sympathy and compassion through donation. Since the experience of altruistic behaviour itself fosters attitudes of altruism and a desire to help, a system relying on gift-giving will also sustain and even expand individuals' sense of community. Replacing it with a commercial system would

---

[98] Rothman and Rothman, 'The Hidden Cost'; Radin, *Contested Commodities*; Peter Singer, 'Altruism and Commerce: A Defense of Titmuss against Arrow' (1973) 2(3) *Philosophy and Public Affairs* 312–20.

[99] Shaun D. Pattinson, *Medical Law & Ethics* (London: Sweet & Maxwell, 2014); Marc Stauch and Kay Wheat, *Text, Cases and Materials on Medical Law and Ethics* (London: Routledge, 2015).

deprive them of these valuable interactions and undermine their vision of community.[100] Consequently, a great deal would be lost.

Third, establishing an organ market, even if it were regulated, would cause additional societal disruption because it would undoubtedly have a perverse distributive impact.[101] Poor persons would be disproportionately persuaded into selling an organ, to the extent that an increase in procurement rates, which in any case would not last long, would come at their expense. Conversely, only well-off patients would be in a position to purchase an organ. As long as aggregate welfare could be expected to increase, utilitarianism would find few problems with a market model that results in the (relatively) richer segments of society taking advantage of the poorer segments, thereby further aggravating social inequalities. However, considerations of social justice militate against initiating such an experiment.

Fourth, and relatedly, the social and personal status of individuals who would contribute to the supply side of the organ market would be degraded to an extent not witnessed since the abolition of slavery.[102] Reports from the black market and from Iran show that vendors suffer from deep shame, resentment and stigmatisation because they, and their communities, experience organ sale as a form of self-mutilation that is inherently depersonalising. Precisely because of the physical embodiment of their personality, such an irreversible surrender of their physical integrity is regarded as crossing the imaginary line of what is deserving of

---

[100] Anderson, 'The Ethical Limitations'; Lori Andrews and Dorothy Nelkin, 'Whose Body is it Anyway? Disputes over Body Tissue in a Biotechnology Age' (1998) 351(9095) *The Lancet* 53–7; Barbro Björkmann, 'Why We Are Not Allowed'; Cynthia Cohen, 'Selling Bits and Pieces'; Thomas H. Murray, 'On the Human Body as Property: The Meaning of Embodiment, Markets, and the Meaning of Strangers' (1987) 20(4) *University of Michigan Journal of Law Reform* 1055–88; Martin, *Beyond the Market*; Nuffield Council on Bioethics, *Human Bodies*; Singer, 'Altruism and Commerce'; Stephen Wilkinson and Eve Garrard, 'Bodily Integrity and the Sale of Human Organs' (1996) 22(6) *Journal of Medical Ethics* 334–9.

[101] George J. Annas, 'The Prostitute, the Playboy, and the Poet: Rationing Schemes for Organ Transplantation' (1985) 75(2) *American Journal of Public Health* 187–9; Charles Foster, 'Dignity and the Use of Body Parts' (2014) 40(1) *Journal of Medicine and Ethics* 44–7; Jeffrey P. Kahn, 'Three Views of Organ Procurement Policy: Moving Ahead or Giving Up?' (2003) 13 *Kennedy Institute of Ethics Journal* 45–50; Muhammad Nasir, Tehmina Nasir, Hira Ashraf Khan et al., 'Organ Trafficking: Do You Want a Society Where the Destitute Become a Store for the Wealthy?' (2013) 20 *The Professional Medical Journal* 177–81; Ross, 'Saving Lives'.

[102] Along this line of reasoning, it may be argued that the Kantian idea that selling a body part would open the door for slavery does not seem so far-fetched as is generally acknowledged.

respect. In regulated organ markets there is a similar risk that vendors would no longer be regarded primarily as persons with inalienable rights, but instead as sources of body parts that could be bought and sold. Under these circumstances, not only their social status but also their own perception of themselves would be thoroughly corrupted.[103] Moreover, if organs became financial assets and the underprivileged segments of society were expected to be open to selling them, the sense of autonomy of vendors and of the poor in general would also be lost.[104] Consequently, and contrary to what proponents of a regulated organ market proclaim, the opportunities for self-development of the poor would significantly *decrease* instead of increase.

Fifth, and last, an accumulation of these immaterial harms would have a dehumanising and destructive impact of immense proportions on society. An organ market would promote a mindset that regards other individuals in purely instrumental terms, in a domain where this outlook was previously unimaginable. The rich would be invited to capitalise on the desperation of the poor to 'buy' their health, resulting in the creation of an underclass that is considered a reservoir of spare parts for the wealthy.[105]

5.7   Conclusion

As compared to human tissues and genetic material used in research and medicine, organs are currently not the subject of an 'enclosure movement' that is legally sanctioned and reinforced. However, a huge black

[103] Bray, 'Personalizing Personality'; Bob Brecher, 'The Kidney Trade: Or, the Customer Is Always Wrong' (1990) 16(3) *Journal of Medical Ethics* 120–3; Cohen, 'Selling Bits and Pieces'; Karen L. Johnson, 'The Sale of Human Organs: Implicating a Privacy Right' (1987) 21(3) *Valparaiso University Law Review* 741–62; Martin, *Beyond the Market*; Agneta M. Sutton, 'Commodification of Body Parts' (2002) 235 *British Medical Journal* 114; Wilkinson, 'Commodification Arguments'.

[104] Jennifer L. Hurley, 'Cashing in on the Transplant List: An Argument Against Offering Valuable Compensation for the Donation of Organs' (2004) 4(1) *Journal of High Technology Law* 117–37.

[105] Bray, 'Personalizing Personality'; Cohen, 'Selling Bits and Pieces'; Kirpal S. Chugh and Vivekanand Jha, 'Commerce in Transplantation in Third World Countries' (1996) 49(5) *Kidney International* 1181–6; Delmonico and Scheper-Hughes, 'Why We Should Not Pay'; Ross, 'Saving Lives'; Gilbert Hottois, 'Dignity of the Human Body – A Philosophical and Critical Approach' in Peter Kemp, Jacob Rendtorff and Niels Mattsson Johansen (eds.), *Bioethics and Biolaw. Vol. II: Four Ethical Principles* (Copenhagen: Rhodos, 2000), pp. 87–102; Kass, 'Organs for Sale?'; Scheper-Hughes, 'Commodity Fetishism'; Wancata, 'No Value for a Pound'; Wigmore, Lumsdaine and Forsythe, 'Ethical Market in Organs'.

market in organs has come into existence, emerging as soon as transplantation of an organ from an unrelated donor became a feasible procedure, and growing exponentially as organ shortages have increased. As a result of the widening gap between supply and demand, in the most affected countries calls are growing louder to establish a regulated organ market. Despite their admirable aim to help tens of thousands of desperate patients in this way, these proposals are problematic on all levels. Even apart from severe doubts about their feasibility, it is very likely that a regulated organ market would need to rely on exploitation for its proper functioning and that it would result in a net decline in donation rates – the exact opposite of what it would aim to achieve.

Since the labour theory of property that is driving the accelerating commodification of tissues and genetic material is not applicable to organs that are not excised and manipulated, proponents of a regulated organ market are placing their hopes on utilitarian theories of property. However, these theories cannot justify private property rights in organs. More specifically, utilitarian theories of property would not necessarily favour a market approach to organ transplantation. In addition, they might condone the outright exploitation of vendors. Crucially, they also overlook the immense immaterial harms that may arise if a regulated organ market were established. These harms are properly recognised only by personhood theories of property. Precisely because of the enormity of these harms, these theories – relying heavily on insights from both Kantianism and virtue ethics as synthesised by Radin, Dickenson and others – deny that full property rights over the human body and its parts should be granted.

At the most fundamental level, these theories demonstrate that the principle of altruism is essential because organs are too integral to personhood to allow their commodification. Treating organs as articles of commerce would undermine the value of the persons who sell them and, in a broader perspective, would debase humanity in general. Putting a price on an organ would indicate that it has a relative value, inviting a purely instrumental valuation of the person whose organ is considered open to market exchange. Relatedly, altruism in organ donation is important because it allows persons to express and foster communal virtues. Some interpersonal contexts – especially the ones involving lifesaving sacrifices in emergency situations – are essential to a community's understanding of the common good and its sense of solidarity. Therefore, allowing market norms to invade the interpersonal context of organ donation would irreversibly damage the quality of relationships, community identification and notions of shared obligations essential to a flourishing society.

Apart from being rejected on substantive grounds and on grounds of principle, the creation of a regulated organ market would also be reckless, since it is very unlikely that the intrusion of market rhetoric in the transplant context can be rolled back when the problems outlined above do indeed materialise. We cannot risk irreversible harm being done to vendors and to communal values in the name of proposals to increase the organ supply, certainly if their implementation is highly unlikely to be successful in the first place.

6

When There Is No Cure

Challenges for Collective Approaches to Alzheimer's Disease

ROBIN PIERCE

6.1 Introduction

Tremendous scientific and biomedical progress has led to a substantial increase in life expectancy in the Western world. However, one of the great challenges of the twenty-first century has emerged, in part, as a consequence of successful pursuit of increased longevity. As a result of living longer lives, the afflictions of old age have become increasingly prevalent. Alzheimer's disease (AD), a fatal neurodegenerative disease associated with ageing that slowly erodes cognitive capacities as well as underlying brain structures, has come to stand among the most dreaded diseases of an aging population. AD, first described in 1906 by Alois Alzheimer, is characterised by a long period of physical and cognitive degeneration, and the toll that AD takes extends far beyond the debilitation of the individual patient. Globally, the attendant quantifiable demands of dementia – AD in particular – on family, caregivers and society have been estimated in 2015 to come to US$818 billion per year.[1] Nevertheless, the story of biomedical therapeutic approaches to AD has not reached a happy ending or even a promising or short-term resolution. There is no cure and no effective treatment to significantly slow or alter disease progression.

AD is a disease without a cure. Therefore, discussion of medicine (therapeutic interventions) of any kind is necessarily limited to the research phase of the development of therapeutic interventions. While the seeds of collective or individualised medicine are to be found in the research phase, both foundational and translational, characterisation at this stage is complex. Thus, basic research investigating a seemingly

---

[1] World Alzheimer Report, *The Global Impact of Dementia An Analysis of Prevalence, Incidence, Cost & Trends* (London: Alzheimer's Disease International, 2015).

personalised therapeutic approach may subsequently lead to wide population-based strategies while suggested population-based interventions may
eventually prove effective only for a small subsection of AD patients,
perhaps based on genotype. Accordingly, a series of critical questions
must be asked, including when interventions should be located on the
collective–individual spectrum, with what criteria in the research phase,
and when is it appropriate and beneficial to inquire about the collective
versus personalised nature of interventions still in development.

This chapter explores the field of AD research through the lens of
'We Medicine and Me Medicine' (collective and personalised medicine,
respectively) introduced by Donna Dickenson.[2] In this chapter, I explore
the nature and drivers of the research enterprise on AD, and identify
the relatively recent phenomenon of early detection to be at the core.
I conclude that, while the characterisation of personalised versus collective intervention may be of varying significance in the fundamental
research phase, it is essential that the translational phase include one or
more mechanisms that facilitate and prioritise impacts on collective well-
being. While there is still no cure, the personalised and the collective
operate as complementary orientations. Yet, without deliberate consideration throughout the research and development and translational
process, collective approaches to a growing crisis may lose ground to
commercially more profitable individualised approaches.

The AD research community has made great strides in understanding
various aspects of the disease, from identifying highly correlative pre-
symptomatic biomarkers to developing imaging techniques for detecting
process and structural changes that distinguish AD from other neurodegenerative conditions. Next to these advances in understanding stands
a largely unsuccessful effort towards the development of effective therapeutic interventions against AD. At times, the therapeutic prospects
have seemed promising (as judged by news headlines or pharmaceutical
stock prices) and, at other times, they have seemed to be an ever-growing
terrain of disappointing clinical trials and devastated hopes. Over time,
research strategies have shifted and new therapeutic targets have been
identified. One of the most dramatic shifts in AD research is the prioritisation of early detection. As a result, most therapeutic interventions are
now expected to rely on early detection as a key component. A critical
question that must be asked is how the emphasis on early detection will

---

[2] Donna Dickenson, *Me Medicine vs We Medicine: Reclaiming Biotechnology for the
Common Good* (New York: Columbia University Press, 2013).

affect the larger effort to reduce the incidence and prevalence of AD and to effectively treat the growing millions of people who develop the disease. Consequently, a critical question for the research community and its funders is how the prevalence and burden of AD are to be factored into the research strategy. That is, how do we make sense of 'We Medicine versus Me Medicine' when there is as yet no effective medicine and the research effort is very much inconclusive? This chapter explores this question through the lens of AD and, in part, through its focus on early detection, a defining feature of the current AD research strategy, addressing questions regarding 1) the value and cost of early detection as a key feature of AD *treatment*, 2) the effectiveness of this strategy as a response to the nature of the burden of AD, and 3) more fundamentally, whether it is premature to consider collective versus individual therapeutic approaches in the research phase while the search for an effective intervention is still ongoing. When is the optimal time to incorporate a consideration of the collective versus the individual in our quest for optimal healthcare and what should this consideration look like?

6.2 Early Detection

6.2.1 The Holy Grail

A phenomenon that has emerged that cuts across most research strategies is the centrality of 'early detection'. While numerous theories abound regarding the most promising therapeutic approaches, there is general consensus in the AD research community that any success that might come forth in the treatment of AD will involve early detection. The basis for this approach is the belief that the neuropathology associated with AD begins more than a decade before any symptoms appear. The string of disappointing clinical trials prompted researchers to draw the now widely accepted conclusion that the problem was not necessarily one of the wrong target or the wrong pharmaceutical compound, but rather that these experimental therapeutic interventions were being introduced too late in the disease progression. They were missing the 'therapeutic window'.[3] This resulted in robust research efforts to identify AD earlier in the disease progression. The ground-breaking introduction of

---

[3] Robin Pierce, 'Complex calculations: ethical issues in involving at-risk healthy individuals in dementia research' (2010) 36(9) *Journal of Medical Ethics* 553–7.

Pittsburgh Compound B (PIB)[4] that, with the use of PET scans, allows for in vivo detection of amyloid plaques, altered the research landscape in significant ways. With this technology, the presence of amyloid could be detected, quantified and monitored in living patients instead of having to wait for post-mortem confirmation of its presence. Given that amyloid plaques are one of the two primary neuropathologies associated with AD and constitute a necessary, but not sufficient, pathology for a diagnosis of AD, in vivo detection was understandably heralded as a major step forward. Furthermore, many believe that amyloid build-up is an important trigger to the onset of AD[5] and, therefore, has served as a primary target of pharmaceutical research aiming to treat AD. In vivo amyloid detection in living patients also provided an important metric for experimental interventions that sought to measure effectiveness based on a change in the presence and amount of amyloid.

Early detection of AD came to be viewed as a peculiar form of the Holy Grail. Even if researchers were unable to treat the disease, they experienced some success in their efforts to identify elevated risk of it. Careers began to be built not on discovering treatments for AD, but on enhancing the ability to detect it earlier in the disease progression. This led to an avalanche of technological non-fixes that heralded the ability to detect biomarkers for AD before the first symptoms.

The theory behind early detection in AD is not novel. One of the foundational approaches in health policy and public health is that 'early intervention leads to better outcomes'. This rule finds a lot of traction in many disease treatment strategies. Screening programmes for a host of diseases that aim to 'catch' a disease before obvious symptoms manifest have become an accepted and valued component of clinical care, particularly for those diseases that only display symptoms in the middle to late stages, e.g. colon cancer.

Early detection efforts in AD research have led to the identification of several biomarkers. In 2010 discussions of the presence of biochemical changes in cerebral spinal fluid (CSF)[6] led to proposals of possible

---

[4] William Klunk, H. Engler, A. Nordberg, Y. Wang, G. Blomqvist, D. P. Holt et al., 'Imaging brain amyloid in Alzheimer's disease with Pittsburgh Compound-B' (2004) 55(3) *Annals of Neurology* 306–19.

[5] John Hardy and D. J. Selkoe, 'The amyloid hypothesis of Alzheimer's disease: progress and problems on the road to therapeutics' (2002) 297(5580) *Science* 353–6.

[6] Kai Blennow and H. Zetterberg, 'Cerebrospinal fluid biomarkers for Alzheimer's disease' (2009) 18(2) *Journal of Alzheimer's Disease* 413–17.

introduction of spinal taps for AD biomarkers as routine clinical care.[7] This was quite controversial for reasons including cost-effectiveness, challenges in identifying optimal screening populations, possible side effects and the absence of an effective therapy should CSF suggest a diagnosis. Reports of early detection strategies employing novel modalities have emerged with some regularity, including eye tests,[8] nanosensors[9] and blood tests[10]. Nevertheless, even the most compelling methods of asymptomatic detection make no claim to even the slightest therapeutic effect.

Although it is clear that early detection alone, even if achieved, will not deliver effective interventions, it has come to occupy centre stage in the AD research effort. Ironically, it is precisely this development in the research landscape that may lead to greater challenges for collective approaches to effectively combatting AD as the epidemic that it has become. An examination of how early detection is achieved in practice yields insight into some of these challenges.

6.2.2   Early Detection Technology and Its Beneficiaries

The first major breakthrough in the field of early detection was the discovery of Pittsburgh Compound B (PIB), a chemical compound that, with the use of a PET scan, enabled detection of amyloid plaques.[11] Introduced in 2004, PIB was a game-changer in its ability to confirm the presence of amyloid plaques in vivo whereas previously this could only be done post mortem. As both a research and clinical tool, PIB/PET scan served as a major catalyst in the move toward the centrality of early detection.

[7] Manuel Menendez-Gonzalez, 'Routine lumbar puncture for the early diagnosis of Alzheimer's disease. Is it safe?' (2014) 6(65) *Frontiers in Aging Neuroscience* 1–2.

[8] Swati More, J. Beach and R. Vince, 'Early detection of amyloidopathy in alzheimer's mice by hyperspectral endoscopy' (2016) 57 *Investigative Ophthalmology & Visual Science* 3231–8.

[9] Ajeet Kaushik, R. D. Jayant, S. Tiwari, A. Vashist and M. Nair, '80 Nano-biosensors to detect beta-amyloid for Alzheimer's disease management' (2016) *Biosens Bioelectron* 273–87; 'Nanosensors for the diagnosis of Alzheimer's disease', cordis.europa.eu/result/rcn/188315_en.html.

[10] Henrik Zetterberg, D. Wilson, U. Andreasson, L. Minthon, K. Blennow, J. Randall and O. Hansson, 'Plasma tau levels in Alzheimer's disease' (2013) 5 *Alzheimers Research & Therapy* 9.

[11] Klunk, 'Imaging brain amyloid', 306–19.

A second major early detection technology was promoted in early 2010 in the form of cerebral spinal fluid (CSF).[12] This fluid flows through the spine and is obtained through the administration of a 'spinal tap'. This fluid can be analysed for the presence of markers that were highly associated with the onset of AD, and could be detected some time before behavioural and cognitive changes could be detected. However, despite the high concordance of these biochemical changes with the onset of AD, CSF proved to be a very controversial technology. Questions arose about screening and who should get a spinal tap for AD detection and how these people would be identified out of the general population. Discussions of spinal taps as a component of routine clinical care met with substantial resistance.[13] With no effective treatment for incipient AD that might be detected, the value of pre-symptomatic AD pathology screening as routine care was less than compelling. Furthermore, none of these biomarkers for early detection have been validated.[14] So, at best, the most reliable indicators of the presence of incipient AD pathology are risk indicators rather than diagnostic tools. Despite the ever-increasingly sophisticated technologies to detect AD earlier in the disease progression, this is not accompanied by the ability to prevent, treat, delay or cure the onset of AD. Rationally speaking, the fanfare for early detection can only be a muted one.

6.2.3   The Cost and Value of Early Detection

Advantages offered by PIB were that it allowed for differential diagnosis as well as greater diagnostic certainty. From a research perspective, it facilitated quantification of the impact of therapeutic interventions seeking to manipulate the production or presence of amyloid in the living brain as a way of altering disease progression. Not only could the target phenomenon be detected, it could be measured pre- and post- intervention. For early detection research, it also facilitated the identification of patients and potential clinical trial participants who carried an amyloid burden, thus allowing the enrichment of trial participant populations. As a research tool, some value could be shown. The clinical value outside of differential diagnosis is considerably less compelling.

[12] Blennow, 'Cerebrospinal fluid biomarkers', p. 413.
[13] Shima Mehrabian, P. Alexopoulos, M. Ortner, L. Traykov, T. Grimmer, A. Kurz et al., 'Cerebrospinal fluid biomarkers for Alzheimer's disease: The role of apolipoprotein E genotype, age, and sex' (2015) 11 *Neuropsychiatric Disease and Treatment*, 3105–10.
[14] Alzheimers Association, www.alz.org/research/science/earlier_alzheimers_diagnosis.asp

In Western countries, the use of sophisticated technologies for early detection of AD has already met with resistance. This contrast became perhaps most visible in the anxiously awaited decision in the USA by the Center for Medicare and Medicaid (CMMS), the federal agency that determines which medical interventions will be covered by Medicare and Medicaid. This was a particularly critical decision regarding the question of whether social insurance would pay for the use of MRI scans for the clinical care of AD.[15] Given that Medicare is the publicly available medical insurance for persons over 65, this decision was of paramount importance to the AD research community, not least for the financial implications. The centrality that these expensive scans could take on in clinical care for AD and mild cognitive impairment (MCI)[16] from a financial perspective, would not be insubstantial. With nothing else in the AD treatment arsenal, these scans could become standard of care and be seen as a core part of clinical care. Moreover, these scans could become a centrepiece around which all other future interventions must interact, thus entrenching the technology further into the AD 'treatment' paradigm. Of course, many treatment paradigms involve the use of a specific technology, e.g. dialysis. However, the imaging of amyloid is currently of ambiguous value. It is neither a treatment modality nor an assistive technology. So when the CMMS applied their criteria for coverage – the proposed intervention improves health outcomes, proponents of the uptake of the scans by Medicare had an uphill battle.

In 2013, following a proposal for the inclusion of PET scans to detect the presence of amyloid plaques as part of AD diagnosis for Medicare coverage under specified circumstances, the federal agency making such decisions rejected this inclusion. Even though the technology was acknowledged to perform the necessary task competently and reliably, a positive impact on health outcomes could not be shown, as a general matter.[17] The CMMS concluded that there was insufficient evidence of therapeutic benefit or effect on patient outcomes for it to be covered by Medicare. Two exceptions were made: 1) differential diagnosis of fronto-

[15] Centers for Medicaid and Medicare, 'Decision Memo for Beta Amyloid Positron Emission Tomography in Dementia and Neurodegenerative Disease' (CAG-00431 N). (2013) www.cms.gov/medicare-coverage-database/details/nca-decision-memo.aspx?NCAId=265.
[16] Karl Herholz and K. Ebmeier, 'Clinical Amyloid Imaging in Alzheimer's Disease' (2011) 10 The Lancet Neurology 667–70.
[17] Centers for Medicare and Medicaid, 'Decision Memo for Beta Amyloid'.

temporal dementia (FTD) and Alzheimer's disease (AD) under specific requirements; or, 2) use in a CMS approved practical clinical trial focused on the utility of FDG-PET in the diagnosis or treatment of dementing neurodegenerative diseases.[18] This decision is significant for multiple reasons. First, by a focus on the benefit rather than on efficacy alone, the CMMS rejected an almost sacrosanct technological imperative in favour of a more value-based method of evaluation. This was widely regarded as an enormous blow to the AD research community; it probably marked a 'win' for medicine in the public interest. Although Medicare coverage would also have meant wider availability, this would not necessarily have resulted in benefit to patients.

The ambiguity of benefit of early detection of amyloid is further underscored by the fact that while plaques are invariably a feature of AD, the presence of these plaques is not invariably associated with AD. In other words, amyloid plaques are not necessarily indicative of AD in that a not insubstantial percentage of the cognitively healthy population carries amyloid plaques at the time of death.[19] Thus, the value of being able to identify amyloid asymptomatically is somewhat diminished. Moreover, several trials have put this hypothesis to the test with perhaps the biggest blow occurring in the *aducanumab* trial that succeeded in reducing amyloid burden but resulted in no impact on cognitive capacities.[20]

Early detection of AD is a very technology-intensive enterprise. It is expensive and generally inaccessible relative to the size and resources of the patient population. That is, there is no way to accomplish early detection without the use of sophisticated technology. A brief look at the economic costs of early detection shows that many of the technologies required for early detection are quite high. For example, a spinal tap through which cerebral spinal fluid (CSF) is obtained costs roughly between €3,000 and €5,000.[21] The average cost of a Florbetapir F18 PET scan (for in vivo detection of amyloid burden) is approximately $3000.[22] This does not address the initial costs to develop the appropriate

[18] Ibid. [19] Herholz, 'Clinical Amyloid Imaging', p. 668.
[20] Jeff Sevigny, P. Chiao, T. Bussière et al., 'The antibody aducanumab reduces Aβ plaques in Alzheimer's disease' (2016) 537 *Nature* 50–56.
[21] Cristina Valcarcel-Nazco, L. Perestelo-Perez, J. L. Molinuevo, J. Mar, I. Castilla, P. Serrano-Aguilar, 'Cost-effectiveness of the use of biomarkers in cerebrospinal fluid for Alzheimer's disease' (2014) 42(3) *Journal of Alzheimers Disease* 777–88.
[22] Alzheimer's Association, 'For Healthcare Professionals: Frequently asked questions about Amyloid Beta Imaging' (2013), www.alz.org/documents_custom/hps_auc_faq.pdf

expertise and infrastructure necessary to provide access to this technology. This could present substantial barriers to access in low- and middle-income countries (LMIC) or in rural areas. Moreover, in countries without universal health insurance, individual patients would be required to pay the cost of early detection, potentially limiting access further. Healthcare of the elderly may be covered by programmes like Medicare in the USA or national healthcare systems, like the NHS in the UK; these technologies will be limited by eligibility criteria, which inevitably incorporates some degree of cost-effectiveness analysis.

6.2.4 Early Detection and the Right (Not) to Know.

The centrality of early detection must make sense not only scientifically, but also from a social perspective. The Human Genome Project's Ethical Legal and Social Implications (ELSI) project generated a field of literature highlighting the fact that early (risk) detection is not an unqualified benefit.[23] Even if early detection ultimately proves capable of contributing to the development of effective intervention, it is naive to think that this aspect would not come at a cost. The debates occasioned by the Human Genome Project called attention to the complexity of the use of genetic risk information. Even in cases where effective therapies existed, the concept of the 'right not to know' held a certain ground.[24] Moreover, debates unveiled a distinct unspoken belief that knowledge of disease risk may not necessarily be the prevailing value in society. Other things matter.

In the case of AD, the right not to know takes on particular valence given the nature of the disease. Frequently regarded as among the most dreaded diseases, AD erodes multiple aspects of ourselves, including a sense of self, the ability to recall cherished memories and recognise loved ones. Moreover, it robs us of one of our greatest forms of currency in the Western world – our cognitive capabilities. Consequently, early detection of a disease that erodes this currency can ultimately serve to intrude on many aspects of our functional life, depending on how early this early detection takes place. In AD, the estimates of the time before symptoms of the neuropathology associated with AD range from 10 to 20

---

[23] Troy Duster, *Backdoor to Eugenics* (New York: Routledge, 2003).
[24] Roberto Andorno, 'The right not to know: an autonomy-based approach' (2004) 30(5) *Journal of Medical Ethics* 435–9.

years.[25] Thus, as early technology improves and becomes more accurate, integration of early detection also will mean intrusion of a highly compromising disease into our vibrant personal and professional lives. With the incursions on the Genetic Information Non-discrimination Act (GINA) opening up more loopholes that allow for the lawful collection and use of genetic information – for example, the Wellness Program exception[26] – confidence in protections against undesirable use of early detection information not limited to genetic information stands on very little. As such, the question arises regarding the relationship between early detection and collective approaches to AD and healthcare.

6.3   Finding a Place for Early Detection: Collective versus Individual Approaches

6.3.1   Early Detection for Some Things But Not Others

In the absence of a cure, early detection presents challenges to prioritisation of collective or public health approaches. First, early detection generally requires the use of expensive and sometimes invasive technologies inaccessible to the majority of patients. Secondly, there is still no evidence supporting the hypothesis that early detection leads to better outcomes for AD, and so it yields little benefit in exchange for the use of limited resources. However, given the evidence showing incipient AD pathology more than 10 years before symptoms, early detection may serve as a component of some research strategies. It may not be possible to make useful assessments of the value of early detection when it is not altogether clear what role, if any, it will ultimately play. But whatever the relationship between early detection and collective approaches turns out to be, its ability to yield a therapeutic benefit to more than a select few individuals will be required. That this inquiry needs to begin at the research phase seems highly appropriate as a critical question of stewardship and resource allocation.

---

[25] Reisa Sperling, P. S. Aisen, L. A. Beckett, D. A. Bennett, S. Craft, A. M. Fagan et al., 'Toward defining the preclinical stages of Alzheimer's disease: Recommendations from the National Institute on Aging-Alzheimer's Association workgroups on diagnostic guidelines for Alzheimer's disease' (2011) 7(3) *Alzheimers and Dementia*, 280–92.

[26] American Society of Human Genetics, 'ASHG Opposes H.R.1313, the Preserving Employee Wellness Programs Act: Bill Would Undermine Genetic Privacy Protections' (8 March 2017), www.ashg.org/press/201703-HR1313.html

6.3.2   Genetic versus Non-Genetic Basis of AD

Early detection informed by genetic information presents perhaps a clearer case. The distinction between strategies aiming to address the genetic versus non-genetic basis of AD is one widely recognised as essential and important by patients, researchers and policymakers.[27] However, within this distinction sits the basis for several alternative strategies. From an ethical and social justice perspective as well as scientific perspective the specific targeting of the small population of AD sufferers who have or are at risk for the familial form of AD can be justified. This population represents approximately 2 per cent of AD patients who typically develop the disease earlier in life, resulting in the disease designation of Early Onset Alzheimer's Disease (EOAD).[28] The burden of this disease for affected persons justifies a dedicated approach, in part because of the generally greater loss experienced by this AD sub-population in comparison to sporadic AD patients who tend to develop the disease much later in life. Seeking to allocate more resources to a population that suffers a greater loss would be defensible on many grounds, including solidarity.

On the other hand, a different type of focus on genetic involvement in AD would appear to fall in line with the Precision Medicine agenda, propagated by the US and other western governments. This genetic contribution to non-EAOD form of AD suggests for some that the only way to address the heterogeneity of AD aetiology is to personalise treatment strategies.[29] This has two consequences that are likely to prove problematic for collective approaches to AD. First, various degrees of patient stratification can lead to the creation of ever-growing AD patient subsets, each of which generated drug development and pursuit of approval under 'rare disease' status,[30] thereby establishing small patient population, a perverse form of tribalism in direct conflict with collective approaches. The second consequence is more general in that, in order to know the genetic risk of a particular AD patient, some form of

---

[27] Kai Blennow, M. J. de Leon and H. Zetterberg, 'Alzheimer's disease' (2006) 368 *The Lancet* 387–403.

[28] Xing Peng, P. Xing, X. Li et al., 'Towards personalized intervention for Alzheimer's disease" (2016) 14(5) *Genomics, Proteomics & Bioinformatics* 289–97.

[29] Ibid., p. 289.

[30] Aaron Kesselheim, C. L. Treasure and S. Joffe, 'Biomarker-defined subsets of common diseases: policy and economic implications of Orphan Drug Act coverage' (2016) 14(1) *PLoS Medicine* e1002190.

genotyping must occur. This avenue of research carries little promise where the availability of one's genetic information might be limited.

Consequently, an inquiry into the impact on the collective burden of disease of this research arm suggests that research into EOAD, the rarer form of AD, can be justified on social justice grounds. Therefore, measures like the Orphan Drug Act[31] and other types of initiatives aiming to support the health and well-being of 'disease minorities' who would otherwise present as commercially unattractive to 'for-profit' medical innovation – collective approaches rooted in solidarity, in principle – seek to move the entire patient population toward health and well-being. Nevertheless, early detection is a technologically dependent intervention that comes with infrastructural barriers ranging from the availability and logistics of genotyping to reimbursement schemes. This does not mean that it should not be pursued, but rather that it should not be seen as 'the' solution if it operates to exclude a substantial proportion of AD patients from access to effective treatment. Research oriented toward broader access must be promoted and supported.

6.4   Alternatives: Orienting towards the Right Goal

6.4.1   Cure/Treatment versus Care: Debates on Futility

Despite the investment of billions of dollars and years of research, there is no cure or effective treatment. This conundrum demands reflection. Perhaps the most recent indication of such reflection can be found in the announcement in January 2018 by pharmaceutical giant Pfizer that it would discontinue research on pharmaceuticals for Alzheimer's disease. Pfizer explained that 'Alzheimer's has always been a highly challenging area with not much progress being made despite the investment of a lot of funds and resources'.[32] The sense of futility and frustration are not the only bases giving rise to re-evaluation. There are many who think that, given that AD is a disease closely associated with ageing attempts to identify a cure may be futile and that the more realistic and attainable goal is to find ways to slow progression of the disease, particularly in ways

---

[31] Orphan Drug Act of 1983. Pub L. No. 97–414, 96 Stat. 2049.

[32] 'Pfizer halts research into alzheimer's and parkinson's treatments' (2018) NPR, www.npr .org/sections/thetwo-way/2018/01/08/576443442/pfizer-halts-research-efforts-into-alz heimers-and-parkinsons-treatments; 'Alzheimer's takes another hit as Pfizer ends research in this area' Nasdaq (8 January 2018), www.nasdaq.com/article/alzheimers-takes-another-hit-as-pfizer-ends-research-in-this-area-cm901602.

that extend the functional phase and shorten the most severe stages.[33] Thus, one way of distinguishing research strategies is by the goal that is sought, whether cure or treatment (stopping/reversing progression or slowing progression/lessening symptoms).

Despite even this relatively modest goal, some have asserted that the investment in pharmacological interventions to effect a cure is a poor allocation of limited resources. This camp stresses that, because the disease is inextricably tied to ageing, a cure is unlikely.[34] Proponents of this view argue that the money is much better spent on care and social arrangements for persons affected by dementia.

It is difficult to say whether a treatment/cure versus care approach is preferable in terms of propelling a collective approach given that such a characterisation is highly dependent on precisely what kind of treatment/ cure emerges, if any. On the other hand, heavy monetary and time investments in futile or unpromising treatment strategies are unlikely to serve anyone, except perhaps in the form of a fleeting sense of hope. The belief that the disease can be effectively treated if the right target(s) are reached, with the right intervention at the right time, clashes dramatically with ardent care proponents who argue that the billions of dollars invested in cure research is money that would be better spent on learning how to best care for this growing patient population. Among the most vocal in this camp, Peter Whitehouse, author of *The Myth of Alzheimer's*,[35] sees AD as not so much a disease, but a form of the incurable phenomenon of ageing. Whitehouse makes the argument that the spending of vast financial resources searching for a cure to what is essentially part of the ageing process should be redirected to various forms of care and care research. The reasoning goes that we all age differently, partly or largely by virtue of how we have lived – have we exercised regularly, eaten healthy foods, attended to our social needs, and so on? Consequently, this view suggests that acknowledging that this age-related disease is a natural consequence of ageing, sometimes referred to as 'severe ageing', and is not curable, would be a more responsible approach. An emphasis on pharmaceutical intervention for many care proponents raises concerns about a misallocation of limited resources that ultimately serves not the collective but rather pharmaceutical interests.

[33] Margaret Lock, *The Alzheimer Conundrum: Entanglements of Dementia and Aging* (Princeton, NJ: Princeton University Press, 2015).
[34] Ibid., p. 27.
[35] Peter Whitehouse and D. George, *The Myth of Alzheimer's: What You Aren't Being Told About Today's Most Dreaded Diagnosis* (New York: St Martin's Press, 2008).

Any number of reasons could explain the lack of success with early intervention experimental therapies. Some speculate that it could stem from the nature of the disease itself. As a multifactorial disease, AD is known to have different aetiologies, which may, in turn, affect the effectiveness of experimental interventions. Other reasons could include the obvious – wrong target, wrong pharmaceutical compound or influence of undetected comorbidities.

While an emphasis on care over treatment may present as a more promising means of actually delivering something of concrete benefit to the collective, it precludes any possibility of ameliorating the chances to reduce or eliminate affliction. However, should costly pharmaceutical research result in an effective treatment, it could ultimately attend to the collective nature of the burden of AD, *depending on the nature of the intervention*. Consequently, both approaches could present opportunities for collective orientation, one perhaps more immediate and less speculative than the other. But foregoing the long-term vision for the short-term reward also carries certain risks that are, in this instance, probably better avoided in favour of a more diversified research portfolio that concurrently attends to both dimensions of healthcare.

6.4.2 Prevention: What do we know so far?

An alternative strategy to cure or care is prevention. Effective prevention strategies have assumed a place in the AD research agenda, with studies on readily available ingestibles such as Vitamin D.[36] As a potential approach to prevention, it could contribute to collective approaches if proven to be effective in that these are in ready and inexpensive supply and would be more widely accessible.

A number of risk factors have been identified that are highly correlated with the onset of AD. Most of these risk factors are modifiable and can serve as targets for health promotion and public health strategies.[37] These modifiable risk factors are shared with a number of other serious diseases and many are themselves considered morbidities, including hypertension, diabetes, obesity, cardiovascular diseases as well as some lifestyle-

[36] Thomas Littlejohns, W. E. Henley, I. A. Lang, C. Annweiler, O. Beauchet, P. H. Chaves et al., 'Vitamin D and the risk of dementia and Alzheimer disease' (2014) 83(10) *Neurology* 920–8.
[37] Ewilena Maliszewska-Cyna, M. Lynch, J. J. Oore, P. M. Nagy and I. Aubert, 'The benefits of exercise and metabolic interventions for the prevention and early treatment of alzheimer's disease' (2017) 14(1) *Current Alzheimer Research* 47–60.

related risk factors such as excessive alcohol consumption, smoking, cognitive inactivity, physical inactivity, low education and social inactivity.[38] Essentially, what is known about the onset of AD in terms of modifiable risk factors points to lifestyle changes that are generally accessible to everyone regardless of location, income and health infrastructure. Moreover, aerobic exercise has been tentatively shown to have a positive effect on MCI and cognitive decline.[39]

These correlations speak volumes, often echoing public health wisdom long embraced. For example, among the most robust associations are those pertaining to cardiovascular health. Additionally, high blood pressure, stroke and excess weight in midlife have been strongly associated with risk of AD.[40] Consequently, one prevention strategy would be to piggy back on the existing public health strategies. Thus, AD prevention strategies could include such things as reduction of salt intake, regular aerobic exercise and reduced fat and sugar intake.

As well, positive behaviours such as cognitive activity and social engagement have been identified as having a positive effect on the likelihood of cognitive decline.[41] Both these interventions are ripe for collective uptake via health promotion initiatives.

Prevention as a public health strategy is appealing in part because of the collective impact that it could generate in comparison to pharmaceutical and technology-intensive interventions which have hitherto proven unsuccessful. A turn to prevention as a healthcare strategy would seem to make good sense. Prevention holds out few, if any, barriers to a collective approach, including for LMIC. If it is possible to minimise the risk of AD before it starts, and the ways that this can be done are generally accessible, then prevention may serve as the most practical and effective collective approach.

Whether one stands on either end of the 'curable/treatable disease'–'incurable/untreatable severe ageing' spectrum, it is undeniable that the body ages, sometimes badly. Prevention as an alternative to or robust complement to early detection as a strategy to combat AD would seem to stand as a critical and necessary component of any agenda seeking to minimise the

[38] Kimberly Ashby-Mitchell, R. Burns, J. Shaw and K. Anstey, 'Proportion of dementia in Australia explained by common modifiable risk factors' (2017) 9(1) *Alzheimers Research & Therapy* 11.
[39] Maliszewska-Cyna, 'The benefits of exercise', p. 48.
[40] Simone Lista, B. Dubois and H. Hampel, 'Paths to Alzheimer's disease prevention: from modifiable risk factors to biomarker enrichment strategies' (2015) 19(2) *Journal of Nutrition Health & Aging* 154–63.
[41] Maliszewska-Cyna, 'The benefits of exercise', p. 48.

burden of this disease. The overall impact from even minor modifications of disease incidence and progression could bode well for society.

6.5 Timing the Inquiry about Collective Approaches

Although it is probably premature to conclude that the most that really can be done (or should be done) is to promote and administer public health measures aimed at modifiable risk factors, the importance of a collective approach must be kept within view. Any number of reasons could explain the lack of success with early intervention experimental therapies. As a multifactorial disease, AD is known to have different aetiologies, which may, in turn, affect the effectiveness of experimental interventions. Other reasons could include the obvious – wrong target, wrong pharmaceutical compound, influence of undetected comorbidities, and so on.

In some ways, it is reasonable to argue that all AD research has the potential to have a significant impact on the collective burden, regardless of whether its therapeutic target is extremely narrow or aims for broad impact. On this basis, we may be tempted to give a pass to research on prohibitively costly interventions with narrow patient population targets because of the fundamental knowledge that it could yield. This would be a mistake. The pursuit of effective therapeutic interventions for an ultimately fatal disease with increasing incidence which has been characterised as an epidemic, requires that the development of an intervention that may ultimately be introduced into clinical care must consider how it will be administered, when and to whom.

This does not need to tie the hands of researchers conducting research on therapeutic interventions; rather, consideration at this stage requires an honest assessment and articulation of the grounded expectations of how integration into healthcare may ultimately look. The narrative that accompanies the research should reflect this assessment of grounded possibilities for healthcare.

The example of Deep Brain Stimulation (DBS) serves as a good example of therapeutic research on a relatively inaccessible intervention, if it ultimately proves effective. DBS is currently under investigation as a possible intervention for early AD.[42] As a clinical care intervention,

---

[42] Adrian Laxton and A. Lozano, 'Deep brain stimulation for the treatment of Alzheimer disease and dementias' (2013) 80(S28) *World Neurosurgery* e21–S28.

should DBS show therapeutic benefit, the cost and technological sophistication of the contemplated intervention could place DBS outside of the reach of the majority of AD patients. Of course, DBS has taken a prominent role in the treatment of Parkinson's Disease, a disease of considerably lower prevalence and incidence. Thus, a rather individualistic approach to treatment serves a larger percentage of the patient population than would be the case in AD, depending on the indications of successful use. That is, the AD population for whom DBS might be effective is so narrowly circumscribed in the investigational phase that any narrowly defined patient population would be further narrowed by highly selective eligibility criteria.[43]

Characterised as a 'growing epidemic', AD is a great 'leveller'. That is, characterised by having age as its highest predictive association, the non-genetic form of AD appears to strike fairly indiscriminately. It could happen to any one of us and, according to some researchers, *would* happen to everyone if they lived long enough. Consequently, this is a disease that 'belongs' to everyone, either by affliction or the sharing of a familial or community burden. Consequently, the emergence of an effective treatment for AD will have implications for everyone – either as a therapeutic basis for optimism or as a distant treatment that exists but is only for a select few, literally adding insult to injury. Aside from the not insubstantial exclusionary impact of elitist availability is the minimal impact on the general burden of AD that can be had by such a narrowly targeted intervention. This is especially disturbing when one considers that funding devoted to investigation of narrowly targeted interventions may be funds that could have been allocated to research on interventions that, if successful, would be more widely available to AD patients. In terms of collective approaches, DBS presents as a substantially less responsive intervention to the burden presented by this disease.

Low cost–benefit ratio and justice are only two of the reasons why research into narrowly tailored therapeutic interventions is problematic when the burden of disease is so substantial. Yet even these highly compelling reasons do not justify abandoning such research in all instances. These reasons do suggest that if collective impact is to be prioritised in any meaningful way, some scrutiny should attend the

---

[43] Tejas Sankar, M. Chakravarty, A. Bescos, M. Lara, T. Obuchi, A. Laxton et al., 'Deep brain stimulation influences brain structure in Alzheimer's disease' (2015) 6(3) *Brain Stimulation* 645–54.

funding and agenda of such research. The type of scrutiny needed at this phase could pertain to the claims made and the orientation of the research. If we consider the case of DBS as a possible treatment of AD, it is highly unlikely that DBS will ever have a substantial impact on the burden of disease. As a coherent research strategy, relatively little hope can be placed on the use of DBS in the treatment of AD as a way of addressing the burden of this disease. Instead, research on the effect of DBS on AD does have an arguably compelling justification in its potential to yield highly valuable fundamental knowledge, possibly pertaining to the mapping of brain functions, interconnectivity and thresholds for impact and adverse effects. This is knowledge that could serve the entire neurological research community and support the study of multiple neurological diseases. Moreover, the mapping function of DBS research on AD conceivably could, in fact, ultimately contribute to the discovery or development of effective treatment by offering a greater understanding of possible targets, their effects and interactivity. Consequently, despite the highly personalised nature of DBS, it may contribute to fundamental research.

The problem arises when research goals and therapeutic goals are conflated in the presentation of both avenues. DBS, as a technologically intensive treatment modality, flies in the face of collective approaches. As fundamental research, it could yield valuable knowledge. As a neurodegenerative disease in which critical parts of the brain degenerate, the effectiveness of DBS as a treatment for AD can probably be expected to have a limited effect. Even the neurophysiological effect that it has been reported to have has been minimal and variable and its impact on cognitive function even smaller and short-lived.[44]

Buried here is the dilemma arising when research that produces knowledge that can be used in further research on the development of therapies with no clear distinction between a goal of generalisable knowledge versus a therapeutic effect. Each requires a different type of scrutiny. But, of course, this is easier said than done, and is even more so in the context of a disease for which people are desperate for any type of disease-altering effect.

6.6   AD and 'We Medicine'

This chapter points to a few possible strategies for how consideration of collective versus individual approaches could inform the research stage

---

[44] Sankar et al., 'Deep brain stimulation', p. 646.

when there is no cure. In essence, it would require, first, an examination of the burden of disease and an assessment of the effect the contemplated intervention would have if it were to prove effective. This is not merely or even principally a question of how many people suffer from a particular disease, but rather a call to deliberate regard of the overarching policy implications of certain research strategies. Policymakers and regulators have long recognised the importance of protecting research for diseases that afflict a relatively small population. This inquiry is driven by principles of justice and solidarity that translate into shared goals of health and well-being. And, as articulated by Donna Dickenson, this includes a sense of shared burden and address – 'We Medicine'.

A 'We Medicine' approach would scrutinise therapeutic research and would put forth questions regarding availability, accessibility, adequacy of infrastructure and availability of expertise. As the DBS example shows, a conflation of therapeutic with foundational research in some ways is a disservice to funders, society and patients in that a coupling with therapeutic potential holds out a promise that it cannot fulfil for the overwhelming majority of AD patients even if it were to prove effective. A 'We Medicine' approach would find the DBS highly inadequate as a strategy to address the burden of AD, but perhaps permissible as a fundamental research effort conducted on a limited scale.

More difficult to analyse through the lens of collective versus individual approaches is the phenomenon of early detection. With the public health mantra that 'early intervention leads to better outcomes', it is difficult to know how to best understand the role of early detection in potentially addressing AD. In the context of AD, a relatively simple intervention becomes a technologically intensive treatment, again placed out of the reach for many AD patients. A screening programme of some sort would need to become routine for healthy vibrant individuals at the prime of their functional lives. This, of course, raises other concerns. In fact, the concordance of even the most reliable methods using sophisticated technologies, such as fMRI and cerebral spinal fluid, are not 100 per cent accurate in their ability to diagnose or predict the onset of AD and no biomarkers have been validated. Diagnosis is, at best, a complicated endeavour, and prediction even more so.

But if, in the future, the effectiveness of a new drug is proven, but only if taken at a stage in the disease progression detectable by one of the technology-intensive early detection methods currently available, it is difficult to make a case that such an intervention should not be pursued, even if the centrality of early detection makes the treatment unavailable to a majority of patients. This would seem to leave us with little choice but to settle for a largely individualised approach to a widely dispersed burden. If early detection is essential, research should prioritise low cost, low-tech methods of detection that can be widely accessed.

6.7 Conclusion

Alzheimer's disease stands as one of the greatest global challenges in the twenty-first century. A neurodegenerative disease that requires considerable care and that is ultimately fatal exerts a great toll on individual patients and on family and caregivers. Yet, despite billions of dollars invested in research, no treatment or cure has been found. Consequently, the search for anything that might prove effective in arresting this disease garners interest and support. However, research resources are finite and must be handled responsibly. The commitment to widely available interventions that would be accessible to the patient community as broadly as possible must be vigorously pursued. Given the growing incidence of AD in LMIC, ensuring broad accessibility of any therapeutic intervention that may be developed would seem to merit utmost priority. For the research enterprise to emerge with a narrowly tailored and inaccessible intervention would be a modest success, at best, in the face of the millions suffering from this dreaded affliction.

Undoubtedly, what a commitment to 'We Medicine' looks like when there is no cure is complex. Such phenomena as technologically intensive early detection or with highly individualised treatments, such as DBS, may be valuable in the research phase, yielding valuable knowledge that can later be used to develop more accessible therapies. In a landscape barren of effective treatment options, a certain degree of patience and flexibility seems to be required. Nevertheless, regard for the collective burden would advise some priority for interventions that can be 'up-scaled' to meet the challenge that faces communities worldwide. Admittedly, there is little profit in the promotion of modifiable lifestyle risk behaviours. Our permissible acceptance, even celebration, of small victories for a handful of AD patients even at great cost, should not blind us to our long-term goals and foundational regard for health and well-being for everyone, including when there is no cure.

7

Lost and Found

Relocating the Individual in the Age of Intensified Data Sourcing in European Healthcare

KLAUS HOEYER

7.1 Introduction

Places with intense human traffic, such as train stations and airports, often have an office for the lost and found. Ideally, a lost and found office reconnects people with the objects they might lose in the course of their journey. To achieve the purpose somebody has to find the lost object – it must be handed in at the office, catalogued, and thus be made available for retrieval. Lost and found offices can be fascinating places. Like Simmel's famous figure of 'the stranger',[1] they are products of modernity's complex forms of social organisation and mobility. Simmel notes that a 'stranger' unites what is far away in a social sense with that which is near in a physical sense, and that the 'stranger' is both an outsider to a social group, while concomitantly being granted a social position – that of *stranger* – thanks to the group. In lost and found offices, things act as strangers, and strange things happen. Sometimes what is 'lost' was never meant to be retrieved; it was lost on purpose, and sometimes it is retrieved by others than the original owner. The passage from being lost to being found can redefine an object and make it into something else for somebody else.[2] Even when returned to the original owner, an object can acquire a new meaning and significance after having been lost.

This chapter is about being lost and found in new places of intense traffic: the digital infrastructure for health data. It is about the passage from individual data to population data, where the interests of individuals are lost, as it were, and how these data can be used to create

---

[1] G. Simmel, 'The Stranger' in K. Wolff (ed.) *The Sociology of Georg Simmel* (New York, NY: Free Press, 1950), pp. 402–8.

[2] K. Hetherington, 'Secondhandedness: consumption, disposal, and absent presence' (2004) 22 *Environment and Planning D: Society and Spaces* 157–73.

personalised advice which is applied to individuals. A new 'owner' is found. Health data can operate as 'strangers' in the sense that users of data can experience physical nearness to data subjects despite social distance. Sometimes a researcher will know things about an individual that not even close relatives would know, but still not know the individual as an actual person. As data change hands, they potentially change meaning and function, much like the stuff in the lost and found office. Health data always relate in some way to individuals and, in the end, the various uses of this data are supposed to benefit individuals, one way or another. Benefits are never guaranteed, however, and the routes to potential benefit are many and not always easily understood. As data uses multiply, data come to live more promiscuous lives.

As laid out in the introduction to this book, Dickenson suggests a distinction between We Medicine and Me Medicine to interrogate contemporary developments in healthcare.[3] With We Medicine, Dickenson refers to the publicly organised delivery of healthcare that takes solidarity as its primary starting point, while Me Medicine begins in the individual and transforms collective challenges to individual opportunities and risks. Using this distinction, this chapter explores how the ongoing data intensification relates to this spectrum of Me Medicine and We Medicine. How do public and commercial forms of data sourcing operate? What counts as collective and individual risk and benefit? How do the public and the private forms of data sourcing compare? What are the stakes for individuals in those processes? What are the interests of society? How do the two relate? Who are lost and what is found? What is lost, and who are found?

7.2   Data Sourcing and Use in Denmark

Health data are collected, stored and exchanged all over the world, but the ways in which this happens differ according to place and the political, economic and social norms and material infrastructures of different healthcare systems. The Nordic healthcare systems deliver universal access and they are primarily financed through taxes. In the following discussion of infrastructures for data, I will take most of my examples from one Nordic country, Denmark, where public collection and use of

---

[3]   D. Dickenson, 'A reality check for personalized medicine' in D. Dickenson, *Me Medicine vs We Medicine: Reclaiming Biotechnology for the Common Good* (New York, NY: Columbia University Press, 2013), pp. 1–6.

health data is pervasive.[4] Thanks to the use of personal identity numbers in all encounters with public services, Danish health data can be combined with data on socio-economic and educational status from employers and tax authorities.[5] The other Nordic countries have similar elaborate register infrastructures[6], but Denmark has taken what can be seen as a more radical approach to research facilitation than the other Nordic countries by allowing data to be used without consent.[7]

The remarkable opportunities for population-based research in Denmark have regularly been discussed in, for example, the journal *Science*, describing the whole country as a 'cohort study'.[8] To retain this

[4] M. K. Saunders, 'In Denmark, Big Data Goes To Work' (2014) 33(7) *Health Affairs* 1245.

[5] L. C. Thygesen and A. K. Ersbøll, 'Danish population-based registers for public health and health-related welfare research: Introduction to the supplement' (2011) 39 (Suppl 7) *Scandinavian Journal of Public Health* 8–10; L. C. Thygesen and A. K. Ersbøll, 'When the entire population is the sample: strengths and limitations in register-based epidemiology' (2014) 29(8) *European Journal of Epidemiology* 551–8. The registers are regularly validated (M. Schmidt, S. A. Schmidt, J. L. Sandegaard et al., 'The Danish National Patient Registry: a review of content, data quality, and research potential' (2015) 7 *Clinical Epidemiology* 449–89 and they are primarily used for epidemiological research designs where the ability to control how the diseased compare to a background population implies that many of the criticisms raised against new Big Data methodologies (e.g. D. Boyd and K. Crawford, 'Critical questions for big data: Provocations for a cultural, technological, and scholarly phenomenon' (2012) 15(5) *Information, Communication & Society* 662–79 and poor administrative and clinical data systems in other countries are not particularly relevant (e.g. M. S. Lauer, E. H. Blackstone, J. B. Young and E. J. Topol, 'Cause of Death in Clinical Research' (1999) 34(3) *Journal of the American College of Cardiology* 618–20; L. Li and P. M. Rothwell, 'Biases in detection of apparent "weekend effect" on outcome with administrative coding data: population based study of stroke' (2016) 353 *British Medical Journal* 1–9; D. M. Maslove, J. A. Dubin, A. Shrivats and J. Lee, 'Errors, omissions, and outliers in hourly vital signs measurements in intensive care' (2016) 44 *Critical Care Medicine* e1021–e1030). The special status of the Nordic health data can be illustrated for example with the fact that when the (public) American Food and Drug Administration approved the (private) company Merck's vaccine for human papillomavirus, it was on the condition that they would use the (publicly sanctioned but privately run) Nordic registers to follow up on long-term vaccine outcomes (Food and Drug Administration). *8 June 2006 Approval Letter – Human Papillomavirus Quadrivalent (Types 6, 11, 16, 18) Vaccine, Recombinant* (Rockville, MD: Department of Health and Human Services, 2006).

[6] A. Cool, 'Detaching data from the state: Biobanking and building Big Data in Sweden' (2015) 11(3) *BioSocieties* 277–95.

[7] K. Hoeyer, 'Denmark at a crossroad? Intensified data sourcing in a research radical country' (2016) 29 *The Ethics of Biomedical Big Data* 73–93. Cohort studies and other research initiated data collections typically use informed consent, and some databases do too, not least if they are sponsored by or work closely with industry – but for public registers and clinical databases consent is not legally required.

[8] J. Couzin-Frankel, 'Science gold mine, ethical minefield' (2009) 324 *Science* 166–8; L. Frank, 'When an entire country is a cohort' (2000) 287(5462) *Science* 2398–9; L. Frank, 'The epidemiologist's dream: Denmark' (2003) 301(5630) *Science* 163.

position, the Danish parliament in 2014 deleted an opt-out register in which 16 per cent of the population featured.[9] People could not opt out of register-based research,[10] but with the registration they could avoid being contacted by researchers wanting further information from them. It will come as a surprise to many outside observers that nothing about the abolition of the opt-out register was communicated to the people who were now again eligible for invitation to active participation in research, but in Denmark the abolition gave rise to little public comment. Lately, the government has proposed the use of the publicly gathered health data to attract international investment in the Danish pharmaceutical industry. In the 'national lost and found office' of health data, data can not only change custodianship, but also purpose and beneficiary.

Taking the metaphor of the lost and found office and Donna Dickenson's notion of We versus Me Medicine[11] as the points of departure for my analysis, this chapter presents some reflections on changing meanings and uses of health data in an ever more data-intensive healthcare system. I first clarify my conceptual approach to data intensification and then outline some trends in, and outcomes of, data sourcing practices in the public sector followed by some examples from private-sector initiatives. Though using 'public' and 'private' casually as descriptive concepts, it will be clear that the public–private distinction is itself in need of critical scrutiny,[12] but it is beyond the scope of this chapter to discuss this. Subsequently, I discuss how We and Me Medicine as a conceptual pair work in relation to an assessment of what is lost and what is gained through intensified data sourcing in its various manifestations.

7.3   The Data Circle and Intensified Data Sourcing

During the past decade, health services have undergone significant changes as they have sought to take advantage of new information and

---

[9] F. Nordfalk and K. Hoeyer, 'The rise and fall of an opt out system' (2018) *Scandinavian Journal of Public Health*, Published online.

[10] It is still the case that register data can be used for research without consent. Denmark and a few other countries lobbied hard to ensure exemption for the general consent rules of the EU Data Protection Regulation and succeeded in ensuring opportunities for continuation of the old system. This is also discussed by Sterckx, Dheensa and Cockbain in this volume.

[11] Dickenson, *Me Medicine vs We Medicine*.

[12] S. Gal, 'A semiotics of the public/private distinction' (2002) 13(1) *A Journal of Feminist Cultural Studies* 77–95.

communication technologies in an intense process of digitalisation and integration of information platforms.[13] Everyday healthcare activities also generate numerous tissue samples taken for diagnostic purposes. Such samples, when stored, can be retrieved for quality assurance and research purposes.[14] A blood sample can be used for whole genome or exome sequencing or be used to identify new biomarkers. As a result, patients today give rise to increasing amounts of traceable healthcare data every time they use health services.

Accelerated data intensiveness has paved the way for a much hyped 'revolution' in science towards what is often framed as Big Data mining.[15] However, healthcare data are typically produced in conjunction with routine *care*, hence data intensification is not just a matter of facilitating *research*. Therefore, I have suggested supplementing the focus on Big Data with an interest in what I call *intensified data sourcing*,[16] by which I mean attempts to get more data, of better quality, on more people in a dynamic process of creating, collecting, curating and storing data while simultaneously making it available for multiple purposes. Big Data debates are strongly focused on research,[17] but scientific research is only one of many purposes for which health data are used. Also, I think 'sourcing' is a better concept than 'data mining' because 'mining' suggests that data are found, extracted and consumed. Yet data are not 'found', but *made* to exist, and unlike raw metals and other mining products, there is no such thing as 'raw data'.[18] Furthermore, metals are finite resources, while data can be

[13] L. Olsen, D. Aisner and J. M. McGinnis, *The Learning Healthcare System: Workshop Summary* (Washington, DC: The National Academies Press, 2007).
[14] M. Richards, R. Anderson, S. Hinde et al., *The Collection, Linking and Use of Data in Biomedical Research and Health Care: Ethical Issues* (London: Nuffield Council on Bioethics, 2015).
[15] V. Mayer-Schönberger and K. Cukier, *Big Data: A Revolution that Will Transform How We Live, Work and Think* (London: John Murray, 2013).
[16] K. Hoeyer, 'Denmark at a crossroad? Intensified data sourcing in a research radical country' (2016) 29 *The Ethics of Biomedical Big Data*, p. 74.
[17] D. Boyd and K. Crawford, 'Critical questions for big data: Provocations for a cultural, technological, and scholarly phenomenon' (2012) 15(5) *Information, Communication & Society* 662-79; M. Hildebrandt, 'Who needs stories if you can get the data? ISPs in the era of big number crunching' (2011) 24(4) *Philosophy & Technology* 371-90; J. P. Ioannidis, 'Informed consent, big data, and the oxymoron of research that is not research' (2013) 13(4) *The American Journal of Bioethics* 40-2; B. D. Mittelstadt and L. Floridi, 'The ethics of Big Data: Current and foreseeable issues in biomedical contexts' (2015) *Science and Engineering Ethics* 1-39.
[18] L. Gitelman and V. Jackson, 'Introduction' in L. Gitelman (ed.), *'Raw Data' Is an Oxymoron* (Cambridge & London: The MIT Press, 2013), pp. 1-14.

sold again and again, re-used and retained while forwarded.[19] Finally, metal retains essential material properties irrespective of its users, while data as semiotic products modulate when entering new networks with new users: data are epistemologically and ontologically unstable.[20]

Partly, the new data opportunities reflect rapidly lowering cost of genetic sequencing technologies and electronic data storage,[21] partly new real-time processing opportunities facilitating ever more uses.[22] Scientific research is only one of many drivers of data production. Data are produced to increase accountability, to ensure proper remuneration, to feed into performance measurement, quality development and because of changed clinical needs.[23] In consequence, the health services are likely to increase their data intensity irrespective of research uses. Interestingly, this emphasis on reuse of data often leads policymakers and data users to ignore well-established social science insights into how secondary uses impede data validity.[24] Data are conceptualised as if immune to the social processes bringing them about.[25]

One of the medical research areas thriving on (and stimulating) the data surge is personalised medicine.[26] Though it is termed 'personalised medicine', it is of course still a matter of creating sub-populations with particular characteristics and directing health guidance based on

---

[19] M. T. Mayrhofer, 'About the new significance and the contingent meaning of biological material and data in biobanks' (2013) 35(3) *History and Philosophy of the Life Sciences* 449–67.

[20] J. van Dijck, 'Datafication, dataism and dataveillance: Big Data between scientific paradigm and ideology' (2014) 12(2) *Surveillance and Society* 197–208.

[21] M. Richards, R. Anderson, S. Hinde et al., *The Collection, Linking and Use of Data in Biomedical Research and Health Care: Ethical Issues* (London: Nuffield Council on Bioethics, 2015); The Expert Group on Dealing with Ethical and Regulatory Challenges of International Biobank Research, *Biobanks for Europe: A Challenge for Governance* (Brussels: European Comission, 2012).

[22] J. Roski, G. W. Bo-Linn and T. A. Andrews, 'Creating value in health care through big data: Opportunities and policy implications' (2014) 33(7) *Health Affairs* 1115–22.

[23] T. Hey, S. Tansley and K. Tolle, *The Fourth Paradigm* (Redmond, WA: Microsoft Research, 2009); P. C. Smith, 'Reflecting on "Analytical perspectives on performance-based management: an outline of theoretical assumptions in the existing literature"' (2015) *Health Economics, Policy and Law* 1–5.

[24] M. L. Markus, 'Toward a theory of knowledge reuse: Types of knowledge reuse situations and factors in reuse success' (2001) 18(1) *Journal of Management Information Systems* 57–93.

[25] O. Halpern, *Beautiful Data: A History of Vision and Reason since 1945* (Durham and London: Duke University Press, 2014).

[26] L. Hood and M. Flores, 'A personal view on systems medicine and the emergence of proactive P4 medicine: predictive, preventive, personalized and participatory' (2012) 29 (6) *New Biotechnology* 613–24.

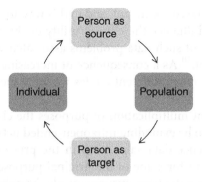

Figure 1 The Data Circle

population characteristics to individual members of that population.[27] Therefore, personalised medicine necessitates a flow of data that can be described as following a classic public health data circle (see figure 1).

With the data circle I mean the way in which individuals, named and known, serve as sources of data in the construction of population data. As data become accumulated at a group level in a smaller or larger 'population', the individual is *lost*, so to speak (in the sense of information being disentangled and anonymised). But when knowledge from population data is put to use, it is again applied to named and known persons, who are *found* and targeted with preventive advice or treatment options expected to suit their case.

The image of a data circle might simplify the data journeys involved a little too much when we consider some of the intricate features of intensified data sourcing. Data travel in many directions, and some of the data uses influence the data values and thereby affect the goals of the idealised public health data circle. For example, some of the administrative uses of data, such as remuneration, are known to influence data quality.[28] When diagnostic codes are used to differentiate between prices for services, it is well known that more 'expensive' diagnoses become more prevalent, irrespective of the distribution of the disease burden in society.[29] The diagnostic coding system is used differently depending on

---

[27] C. Holmberg, C. Bischof and S. Bauer, 'Making predictions: Computing populations' (2013) 38(3) *Science, Technology & Human Values* 398–420.

[28] See also M. L. Markus, 'Toward a theory of knowledge reuse: Types of knowledge reuse situations and factors in reuse success' (2001) 18(1) *Journal of Management Information Systems* 57–93.

[29] E. Silverman and J. Skinner, 'Medicare upcoding and hospital ownership' (2004) 23 *Journal of Health Economics* 369–89.

the uses to which the codes are put, and in this way administrative uses of medical data can influence the clinical utility of the same data. In fact, there is a long list of such data problems associated with performance-based management.[30] As a consequence of increasing uses of data, they come to feed into many different circles whereby their valences potentially change.

With the current multiplication of purposes the classic public health data circle seems to be exploding into open-ended networks. Competing uses of data influence data values and in the process the information might lose its worth for some of the original purposes. If uses of diagnostic codes for remuneration purposes erode their clinical accuracy, the information loses both clinical and scientific value. As a lost-and-found office, data infrastructures can make simple pieces of information such as diagnostic codes change meaning and value as they are put to use by new 'owners' for new purposes. Even when publicly financed, collected and used, data might work through mechanisms that contain elements of both solidarity (We Medicine) and individualised gain (Me Medicine). To understand the value tensions in data sourcing better, I now discuss in a bit more detail how data is created, collected, curated, stored and used for multiple purposes, first in public and then private settings. Today, digital data dependency is engrained in most clinical work practices, including record keeping, communication between units and the construction of treatment plans: it is not an option to return to an analogue mode of narrative record keeping in a closed closet. But does it bring more Me or more We Medicine to the table (or the bedside)? Both, I think, as I shall seek to illustrate in the following section.

7.4   Public Data Intensification

To assess the collective and individual values of public data sourcing and use, I present some trends and examples – but for obvious reasons I cannot claim that these provide a comprehensive picture. Nevertheless, in Denmark, data intensification in public healthcare institutions can be said to revolve around, and contribute to: 1) governance; 2) clinical care; and 3) research.

[30]   S. Wadmann, S. Johansen, A. Lind, H. O. Birk and K. Hoeyer, 'Analytical perspectives on performance-based management: an outline of theoretical assumptions in the existing literature' (2013) *Health Economics, Policy and Law* 1–17.

I have already described the multiple purposes of public *governance*. Data are seen as essential in the creation of transparency, accountability and predictability.[31] Without data there are fewer options for financial control, quality control and planning – at least, that is a common perception among policymakers.[32] This can be seen as a matter of We Medicine, because it is about the efficiency of a shared public system. Ironically, however, data are used to model tax-financed services on market ideals, for example, by enhancing competition between the different units in the healthcare sector (reflecting methods of governance emphasising self-interest more in line with Me Medicine). Also, data intensification gives rise to new initiatives to facilitate cross-sector data sharing with potentially detrimental effects for distributive justice and access to care,[33] as for example when health data are increasingly becoming part of decisions concerning the allocation of benefits in the social sector. The Director of the Danish National Board of Health, Søren Brostrøm, has suggested that the social sector puts such pressure on the health sector for diagnostic codes that the meaning of the diagnostic codes is gradually changing.[34] When health data are used to allocate social benefits it also means that the notion of 'sharing information' changes, because of the differences between the interests of the individuals and the systems involved in the sharing.

When it comes to data intensification in the *clinical* setting, it is important to notice that it is co-produced with technologies of care that necessitate large datasets to find the right treatment for individuals.[35] Clinical guidelines and other support tools are now part of everyday care, and interaction with them depends on support software that guides both diagnosis and follow-up care. This type of software depends on translation of narratives about symptoms into data and diagnostic codes. A new data trend is to also facilitate patient-generated

---

[31] L. Olsen, D. Aisner and J. M. McGinnis, *The Learning Healthcare System: Workshop Summary* (Washington, DC: The National Academies Press, 2007).

[32] P. C. Smith, 'Reflecting on "Analytical perspectives on performance-based management: an outline of theoretical assumptions in the existing literature"' (2015) *Health Economics Policy and Law* 1–5.

[33] Dickenson, *Me Medicine vs We Medicine*, pp. 72–7.

[34] Rasmussen, L. I. (2016), 'Danmark er et diagnosesamfund', *Politiken*, March 27, (pp. 4–6).

[35] A. Hedgecoe, *The Politics of Personalised Medicine: Pharmacogenetics in the Clinic* (Cambridge: Cambridge University Press, 2004); R. Tutton, 'Personalizing medicine: Futures present and past' (2012) 75(10) *Social Science & Medicine* 1721–8; R. Tutton, *Genomics and the Reimagining of Personalized Medicine* (Farnham: Ashgate Publishing, 2014).

data.[36] It adds to the number of expectations, stakeholders and data types, as well as the potential uses: physicians might need to contemplate data in new formats produced by new data suppliers, and patients might acquire new responsibilities they had not foreseen.[37]

It is often the *research* uses of public health data that are most hotly debated at the expense of the *governance* and *clinical* implications of data intensification.[38] This emphasis easily creates the impression that data intensification calls for well-known measures from medical ethics, such as informed consent, irrespective of whether it speaks to the collective (We) or individual (Me) challenges that come along with data intensification.[39] In the international perspective, Denmark has taken a radical route to promote research uses of health data by insisting on consent exemption rules and by deleting the opt-out register. In Denmark, everyone is included and this is defended with reference to public interest.[40] While this is not what Dickenson means by We Medicine, it is indeed a route providing little emphasis on the rights of the individual in order to protect what the state defines as the interests of the collective. In the Danish context, researchers, policy workers and politicians use arguments of solidarity and the common good when justifying the system, though in the international literature it has been argued that solidarity presupposes awareness (e.g. through informed consent) of the purposes to which you as a citizen contribute.[41] This is

[36] P. J. van der Wees, M. W. G. Nijhuis-Van der Sanden, J. Z. Ayanian et al., 'Integrating the use of patient–reported outcomes for both clinical practice and performance measurement: Views of experts from 3 countries' (2014) 92(4) *The Milbank Quarterly* 754–75.

[37] C. Dedding, R. van Doorn, L. Winkler and R. Reis, 'How will e-health affect patient participation in the clinic? A review of e-health studies and the current evidence for changes in the relationship between medical professionals and patients' (2011) 72(1) *Social Science & Medicine* 49–53. See also Huijer and Detweiler in this volume.

[38] L. F. Hogle, 'The ethics and politics of infrastructures: Creating the conditions of possibility for big data in medicine' in L. Floridi and B. Mittelstadt (eds.), *The Ethics of Biomedical Big Data* (Switzerland: Springer, 2016), pp. 1–32.

[39] B. D. Mittelstadt and L. Floridi, 'The ethics of Big Data: Current and foreseeable issues in biomedical contexts' (2015) *Science and Engineering Ethics* 1–39.

[40] Danske Regioner, *Handleplan for bedre brug af sundhedsdata i regionerne* (Copenhagen: Danske Regioner, 2015), pp. 1–19; Danske Regioner, *Sundhedsdata i spil* (Copenhagen: Danske Regioner, 2015); Ministeriet for Sundhed og Forebyggelse, *National Strategi for Adgang til Sundhedsdata* (Copenhagen: Ministeriet for Sundhed og Forebyggelse, 2014), pp. 1–2.

[41] B. Prainsack and A. Buyx, *Solidarity in Biomedicine and Beyond* (Cambridge: Cambridge University Press, 2017).

not the case with respect to register-based research for the wider Danish population.

What type of research has been used to justify the consent exemption? What are the public registers used for? The best way of addressing these questions is to look at the examples that the official committee coordinating register-based research itself brings forward – that is, how it justifies register-based research. These justifications have been gathered in a document summarising key research results achieved using Danish health data,[42] and I use that document as a reference for the examples below.

The document presents 29 examples of research with international impact. Thousands of studies use the registers, but these examples were selected to show how data representative of a whole population can give rise to many different types of knowledge that probably could not be gained in any other way.[43] Through comprehensive registers, the healthcare system becomes an in vivo experiment with long-term follow up. I convey the results as the researchers present them though some readers might doubt their validity. Indeed, what counts as true today can always be questioned tomorrow, but the examples have been chosen by the committee because of their high current standing in the scientific establishment. Civic groups, social scientists and ethicists typically continue to oppose medical findings, e.g. when it is stated that a treatment is 'safe',[44] but here I merely present the findings used by the medical establishment to justify national register-based research.

It is striking that the examples chosen demonstrate how registers have been used to document side effects of drugs that could not be identified in short-term trials (e.g. risks associated with new types of contraceptive pills), but also erased doubts about potential side effects and dangers associated with particular treatments. They thereby serve to create a better understanding of safety, at least from a medical perspective. For example, for years it was assumed that heavy use of pain relief medication increased the risk of recurrence among breast cancer

---

[42] Strategisk Alliance for Register- og Sundhedsdata, *Eksempelsamling. Brug af sundhedsdata i forskning til gavn for patient og borger* (Copenhagen: Strategisk Alliance for Register- og Sundhedsdata, 2016), pp. 1–55.

[43] The document itself groups the examples somewhat arbitrarily, seemingly according to the research groups producing them: 'quality of treatment', 'biological data', 'children', 'pregnancy', 'cancer', 'medicine', 'vaccine' and 'prevention'.

[44] See also C. L. Decoteau and K. Underman, 'Adjudicating non-knowledge in the Omnibus Autism Proceedings' (2015) 45(4) *Social Studies of Science* 471–500.

patients. The comprehensive Danish registers allowed researchers to compare the medication schemes and cancer prevalence in the whole population and thereby debunk the hypothesis and facilitate more effective pain relief without fears of negative impact on cancer risk. In another example, American researchers claimed that abortion was associated with a higher risk of developing breast cancer, while the Danish registers were used to debunk this claim, because all abortions in Denmark can be linked to all registered cancers in the whole population and show there was absolutely no correlation. Another example of suggested dangers that comprehensive registers suggest are non-existent, is the idea that it would be dangerous to live close to high-voltage lines. For many years it was assumed it could be dangerous, but Danish registers made it possible to combine data of residence and workplace (and their proximity to high-voltage lines) with rates of mortality, morbidity and use of medication, and found no such correlation. One day the medical consensus might change again, of course, but for now this is regarded as the best available evidence. Similarly, expecting parents have for years feared the effects on babies of particular diseases during pregnancy, and the registers suggest that many of these fears were unfounded. The Danish registers were also used to investigate the effects of some vaccines accused of having serious side effects, showing that there was no reason to assume they could cause, for example, autism, as some researchers had hypothesised. Registers have also been used to debunk claims with potentially stigmatising effects, such as the one that cancer patients commit suicide more often. Furthermore, the registers have been used to document inequality in health (here, examples are numerous because inequality in health has been a key interest of Nordic epidemiologists – see, for example, the lifetime contributions of Finn Diderichsen, which inform WHO work in this area). Note that many of these research results constitute knowledge that can underpin new guidelines or policies. They do not need to be translated into commercially sold products to have an impact on public health. In this sense, they form part of We Medicine.

   The research value of Danish registers depends on the full inclusion of an unbiased population (through universal access to healthcare) and the absence of opt-out opportunities. While Dickenson emphasises a right to informed consent even in We Medicine, I suggest that this Danish model could be seen as We Medicine in a double sense; the benefits of research are shared with the public and depend on shared access to services and shared obligations to deliver data. There are, however, trends that undermine this 'mandatory-solidarity' approach. The World Medical

Association, the European Union and the National Council of Ethics have all discussed the introduction of informed consent in register-based research. Probably many women who have had an abortion would opt out of research on abortion, not because they do not like the results described above, but because they would consider the past event sensitive and, given the option, that it is more appealing to ask for less attention, rather than more. Few of the Danish women who have had an abortion, however, will know that they have contributed to the research results mentioned above, or even think about it when reading about the results in the newspaper. They have been connected with a stranger, the data analyst, in the lost-and-found office, but never experienced any consequences. Their intimate knowledge of an abortion has been able to travel as data without returning to them as individuals. Informed consent, however, operates in a different way. It creates an emotional and personalised relation to data: it becomes 'My Data', even when researchers only work on population statistics, 'Our Data'. Informed consent makes the individual feel 'found', and thereby some of the opportunities for the population are lost. Furthermore, opt-out registers literally are registers and thereby a new source of knowledge about people and the research types from which they wish to opt out. As long as people feature as part of a population only, their identities can be better protected than when singled out as autonomous decision-makers. The data are gathered irrespective of research uses, so opting out of data-intensive medicine is never an option.

Another trend toward Me Medicine that affects the uses of population data for research is the recent rise in private healthcare delivery. Private hospitals are supposed by law to deliver data to the national registers, but here well-known problems from the USA pop up: there is a lack of incentives for proper reporting and no effective sanctions when data are not sent as agreed. It causes problems not only for the utility of population data, but also in some cases for the patients opting for private healthcare because they still depend on public healthcare in other instances, but now their medical records have gaps and omissions. Hence, Me Medicine also involves risks for the individual who cannot be found in the data jungle when having left the collective grid.

Finally, the We Medicine approach in data use is under pressure as a result of public authorities seeking to attract private investments into the Danish pharmaceutical industry by making the publicly collected data available for commercial partners.[45] There are similarities here to the *care.data* case in the UK[46] and the collaboration between Google's DeepMind project and the National Health Service in the UK.[47] As noted by Cool[48] in a discussion of big data practices in Sweden, the state-centred notion of 'sharing' in relation to health issues is under pressure in an increasingly globalised world economy.[49]

7.5   Private Data Intensification

Data are created, collected, curated, stored and made available for multiple purposes also – and perhaps chiefly – outside the public sector. Commercial data intensification is less transparent, however, and because data here equals competitive edge and monetary potential, it is difficult to gain any clear understanding of who accumulates which types of data, and how they do it. Huge amounts of data are gathered passively as people accept terms of use for their phone or cookies on homepages, and thereby allow companies to gather and sell data about their mobility patterns or interests.[50] Data is also gathered from people who opt for so-called 'free services' (apps or Internet searches such as Google, Gmail or other presumably 'free' platforms). As Andrew Lewis has put it: 'If you're not paying for something, you're not the customer; you're the product being sold.'[51] Data can also be acquired as people purchase direct-to-consumer health services, such as various tests.[52] Here they might

---

[45] See e.g. Danske Regioner, *Handleplan for bedre brug af sundhedsdata i regionerne* (Copenhagen: Danske Regioner, 2015), pp. 1–19; Danske Regioner, *Handlingsplan for personlig medicin* (Copenhagen: Danske Regioner, 2015); Danske Regioner, *Sundhedsdata i spil* (Copenhagen: Danske Regioner, 2015); Ministeriet for Sundhed og Forebyggelse, *National Strategi for Adgang til Sundhedsdata* (Copenhagen: Ministeriet for Sundhed og Forebyggelse, 2014), pp. 1–2.

[46] S. Sterckx, V. Rakic, J. Cockbain and P. Borry, '"You hoped we would sleep walk into accepting the collection of our data": controversies surrounding the UK care.data scheme and their wider relevance for biomedical research' (2015) *Medicine, Health Care and Philosophy* 1–14; P. Vezyridis and S. Timmons, 'Understanding the care.data conondrum: New information flows for economic growth' (2017) *Big Data & Society* 1–12.

[47] J. Wakefield, 'Google Deepmind: Should patients trust the company with their data?' BBC, September 2016.

[48] A. Cool, 'Detaching data from the state: Biobanking and building Big Data in Sweden' (2015) 11(3) *BioSocieties* 277–95.

[49] See also the chapter by Sterckx, Dheensa and Cockbain in this volume.

[50] See, for example, Huijer and Detweiler in this volume.

[51] E. Pariser, *The Filter Bubble* (London: Penguin, 2011), p. 21.

[52] See, for example, S. Sterckx, J. Cockbain, H. Howard et al., '"Trust is not something you can reclaim easily" – Patenting in the field of direct to consumer genetic testing' (2013) 15 (5) *Genetics in Medicine* 382–7.

opt for a discount by way of giving the company access to their data (this is typically presented as a matter of allowing 'research' on it). In principle, private data sourcing is mediated by some form of contractual acceptance as people have to accept cookies and agree to data policies to use the services through which their data are being sourced. It might look very much like Me Medicine with its praise of individual choice, but companies like 23andMe actively promote themselves as working for the common good. In this realm 'informed consent' serves to establish commercial rights for those who accumulate the data, and some participants were horrified when 23andMe took out a patent on a gene for Parkinson's Disease though the consent form mentioned that 'intellectual property' would belong to the company.[53] Still, the notion of autonomous choice often lacks substance; in fact, the practices of accepting 'cookies', 'terms of conditions', etc., seem no less constricted than the public data sourcing initiatives described above because the terms of agreement often change, the agreements are obscure, or people are forced by other factors to use the services and thereby accept (even unreasonable) agreements.

If public data sourcing contributes to the development of public governance, clinical care and research, what are privately created and collected health data used for? Basically, commercially gathered data are sold to those who can afford it. Uses of data therefore develop continuously and cannot be predicted. There is limited knowledge about the concrete data market flows because this type of information (data about data) constitutes a commodity in its own right, beyond the reach of academic research. Ethical analysis in this way becomes restricted through the new modes of organising health data markets. Commercial competition thus redirects the ethical analysis away from commercial data sourcing and back to national tax-financed initiatives, at least those that are (hopefully accurately) disclosed to the public, simply because this is what ethicists can analyse. Still, it seems safe to say that privately organised data collections contribute to, or are at least expected to contribute to three areas: 1) development of new health products; 2) 'personalised' pricing structures; and 3) personalised marketing.

Big Pharma has always used commercially gathered data to develop *new health products*, but some of the Big Data methodologies involved today are new. New types of products include also the devices and software used for data collection and handling. Furthermore, software with algorithms that allow development of personalised risk profiles, lifestyle

---

[53] E. C. Hayden, 'A broken contract' (2012) 486 *Nature* 312–4.

guidance and clinical decision-support tools also constitute important product innovations with a potentially big impact on healthcare.[54] Most of these products are sold direct to the consumer as tools for self-improvement.[55] Some of these new self-monitoring apps are installed on people's mobile phones and thereby deliver the data circle – full circle – right in people's pockets: it is possible to generate data and to measure yourself against others and get your feedback right away.[56] You are never lost, so to speak; but a new question emerges: how many companies and other actors may find you?[57] The Veteran's

[54] L. F. Hogle, 'The ethics and politics of infrastructures: Creating the conditions of possibility for big data in medicine' in L. Floridi & B. Mittelstadt (eds.), *The Ethics of Biomedical Big Data* (Switzerland: Springer, 2016), pp. 1–32.

[55] M. Bode and D. B. Kristensen, 'The digital doppelgänger within: A study on self-tracking and the quantified self-movement' in D. Bajde and R. Canniford (eds.), *Assembling Consumption* (Oxford/New York, NY: Routledge, 2015), pp. 119–34.

[56] T. Sharon and D. Zandbergen, 'From data fetishism to quantifying selves: Self-tracking practices and the other values of data' (2016) 19(11) *New Media & Society* 1695–1709. doi:10.1177/1461444816636090. See also Huijer and Detweiler in this volume.

[57] According to some observers, it is a general feature of the self-monitoring device industry that the start-ups begin selling devices and then acquire their real value based on the data they gather: the data becomes a selling point for the companies (H. K. Holst, 'Forsikringsselskaber vil tjekke dig døgnet rundt med smartwatch og skridttæller', *Berlingske Business* September 2016). Another, more publicised example, is Facebook's takeover of the message service app *WhatsApp*. Facebook wanted to data source although WhatsApp had promised not to do so. Nevertheless, WhatsApp had gained value through accumulation of the enormous amounts of data on people who had opted out of more easily accessible data (e.g. from Gmail accounts), and Facebook did not consider itself bound by the previous owners' assurances. Facebook's intentions were questioned by authorities in the USA (Federal Trade Commission, 'FTC Notifies Facebook, WhatsApp of Privacy Obligations in Light of Proposed Acquisition', Federal Trade Commission, April 2014), and in the UK the Information Officer is also looking into the legality (E. Denham. *Statement on Changes to WhatsApp and Facebook's Handling of Personal Data*. United Kingdom Information Comissioner's Office, 2016), though revelations of terrorists using WhatsApp have stimulated the British Government also to pursue access to the data for investigative purposes. Most recently, the Hamburg commissioner for data protection has started proceedings to stop the data sourcing (Hamburg Commissioner for Data Protection and Freedom of Information, *Administrative Order Against the Mass Synchronization of Data Between Facebook and WhatsApp*. Hamburg, Germany: Commissioner for Data Protection and Freedom of Information, 2016), which comes as a continuation of the attempts by the German *Bundeskartellamt* to prevent Facebook from using its privileged market position to impose 'unreasonable' terms of agreement on its costumers (Bundeskartellamt, *Bundeskartellamt Initiates Proceeding against Facebook on Suspicion of Having Abused its Market Power by Infringing Data Protection Rules*. Bonn, Germany: Bundeskartellamt, 2016). Furthermore, data live promiscuous lives also due to problems with data security. Basically everything can be hacked, and many of the new self-monitoring technologies (especially those dependent on Bluetooth technology) have serious security flaws according to some studies (R. Goyal,

Administration (VA) in the USA, that Dickenson[58] mentions as an example of classic We Medicine, has tested tools for the identification of people at risk of suicide based on changes in their typing speed and the vocabulary they use on social media.[59] Keeping track of the data gathered on the many new devices can be extremely difficult. Some of the new data products can become engrained in classic We Medicine healthcare systems, while others circumvent ideas about shared responsibility and allocate benefits and risks to individuals.

Another avenue opened by private data collection and use of health data is *personalisation of prices*. In countries with private insurance coverage, data profiles of potentially expensive health service users (e.g. those at risk of low compliance) can be a valuable commodity for insurance companies.[60] According to Hogle,[61] the data market in the USA is now taking over the insurance market. In Denmark, it was recently proposed to make it illegal to use genetic information to differentiate insurance prices (the insurance industry does not agree with this proposal),[62] yet at the same time insurance companies experiment with pricing models where those who are willing to provide access to apps and mobile devices that demonstrate high levels of physical activity can get discounts on their insurance.[63] It might look like a matter of free choice (Me Medicine), but it does remove other choices; e.g. not to share your data without paying extra, or to enjoy a run in the forest without bringing your devices along to prove your good health. Moreover, those who, for various reasons, cannot comply with the standards of healthy behaviour will have to pay a higher price if those who can comply get cheaper insurance.

According to some observers, this whole personalisation of the pricing structure is still only in its infancy, at least when compared to the

N. Dragoni and A. Spognardi, 'Mind the tracker you wear: A security analysis of wearable health trackers' (2016) *31st ACM Symposium on Applied Computing (SAC'16)* 131–6).

[58] Dickenson, *Me Medicine vs We Medicine*, p. vii.

[59] L. F. Hogle, 'The ethics and politics of infrastructures: Creating the conditions of possibility for big data in medicine' in L. Floridi and B. Mittelstadt (eds.), *The Ethics of Biomedical Big Data* (Switzerland: Springer, 2016), pp. 1–32.

[60] See also examples mentioned by Sterckx, Dheensa and Cockbain in this volume.

[61] L. F. Hogle, 'Data-intensive resourcing in healthcare' (2016) 11(3) *BioSocieties* 372–93.

[62] Lov (L 157) Om ændring af lov om forsikringsaftaler og lov om tilsyn med firmapensioner, www.retsinfo.dk.

[63] H. K. Holst, Forsikringsselskaber vil tjekke dig døgnet rundt med smartwatch og skridttæller, *Berlingske Business*, September 2016.

personalisation taking place through the use of data-intensive methodologies in other sectors.[64] In the area of Internet-based commodity trade, differentiated pricing furthermore goes hand-in-hand with *personalised marketing*. Algorithms and models are constructed in order to adequately describe and predict patterns of behaviour and interest. Based on predictions, individuals are targeted with offers using customised price-setting and other features aimed at optimising the chances of a deal with maximum profit. Amazon pioneered this mode of personalisation, but today this type of data market is converging with health, as insurance companies and healthcare suppliers learn about the value of 'knowing their customer', as noted also by investigative journalist Eli Pariser.[65] This constitutes an arena of Me Medicine, and some customers are bound to love the effects of an online sphere that knows them so well that they 'coincidentally' come across the very health products they are most likely to buy.

There is, however, a darker side to the personalised modes of marketing. According to researcher and data analyst Henrik Legind Larsen,[66] the market in health data is intertwined with illegal trade in sensitive information, which gains its value because the people with the most desperate health needs can be targeted with offers of treatment with little or no evidence of efficacy at very high costs.[67] Marketing here typically interacts with medical tourism, although tourism is a flawed metaphor when we consider the nature of the travel undertaken by people desperately seeking a cure when there are no medically sanctioned opportunities left.[68] Others can be targeted for their potential interest in treatments that are either illegal or extremely expensive in their home countries. Still others can be targeted with treatments that involve materials in short supply within medical systems dependent on free donations

---

[64] H. M. Krumholz, 'Big data and new knowledge in medicine: the thinking, training, and tools needed for a learning health system' (2014) 33(7) *Health Affairs* 1163–70; J. Roski, G. W. Bo-Linn and T. A. Andrews, 'Creating value in health care through big data: Opportunities and policy implications' (2014) 33(7) *Health Affairs* 1115–22.

[65] E. Pariser, *The Filter Bubble* (London: Penguin, 2011).

[66] Larsen, personal communication, 5 September 2016.

[67] A recent episode revealed that IT criminals do target emails from Danish health authorities to harvest health data (O. N. M. Toft, 'Blixt kræver samråds-svar i data-sag', Altinget, September 2016).

[68] A. Wahlberg and T. Streitfellner, 'Stem cell tourism, desperation and the governing of new therapies' in A. Leibing and V. Tournay (eds.), *Technologies de l'espoir. Les débats publics autour de l'innovation médicale* (Montreal: Université de Montréal, 2009).

of organs, gametes and tissues.[69] Here again, Me Medicine takes over from We Medicine, but it is not simply a matter of granting new opportunities to wealthy individuals who can purchase treatment – it can easily put the wealthy at risk too, as they chase treatment options with no guarantees and little legal (and scientific) backing.

Just as we saw with public data sourcing, data sourcing is ubiquitous in the private sector. It cuts across sectors, and even if the research uses of data were to be more legally restricted, the data practices are not likely to become less intense or more aimed at the common good. Though primarily operating in the realm of Me Medicine, many of the privately mediated data practices are in practice no less inescapable than the ones in the Danish public sector.

7.6   Concluding Reflections

In the current age of intensified data sourcing, data creation, collection, storage and use have become ubiquitous. Collective and individual interest in the new data practices can be difficult to pinpoint. Data can serve individuals and collectives, but can also expose them to potential harm. Public data intensification is intertwined with attempts to ensure key values of public administration – transparency, efficiency, evidence – but it also feeds into new forms of obscuration, increased expenditure and initiatives based on unfounded promises of prediction. In practice, data gathered in the public and the private sector may cross over and be used for new purposes irrespective of their mode of production. Unless carefully regulated, data infrastructures easily acquire traits of the lost-and-found office. Like Simmel's 'stranger', they can give people who are far away from data sources in a social sense a physical presence to information that is highly intimate. Moreover, data infrastructures can – by way of the outside position of the data analyst (the stranger) – create new social groupings, ideas about disease and notions of the self.

Because ethicists typically have access to more information about data flows in the *public* sector, and because medical ethics has a long tradition of discussing the terms of *research* participation, there is a tendency to focus criticism of data intensive methods on *public* data used for *research*

---

[69] D. A. Budiani-Saberi and F. L. Delmonico, 'Organ trafficking and transplant tourism: A commentary on the global realities' (2008) 8(5) *American Journal of Transplantation* 925–9; J. P. Pirnay, E. Baudoux, C. Olivier et al., 'Access to human tissues for research and product development: From EU regulation to alarming legal developments in Belgium' (2015) 16(5) *EMBO Reports* 557–62.

purposes. In particular, critique tends to focus on study methods that violate norms from clinical ethics associated with the right to give an informed consent.[70] It is problematic, however, to nail the analysis to the notion of informed consent as a 'solution' developed to address a different set of problems.[71] The private sector thrives on forms of data sourcing that are no less inescapable than those of register-based public research, though in principle relying on 'consent', and commercial data practices are furthermore combined with less transparency. 'Acceptance of cookies' and similar clicks do little to care for consumer rights and interests. Do we expect that quick 'click' options would do much good in the public health sector? Also, informed consent for data usage for *research* purposes leaves all the other uses of data unexamined, and might in fact expose the individual more (not less) because it involves creating a tighter connection between the individual and the data which will be gathered anyway. If individuals are to access and administer research access to their personal data then the digital networks will need to have more entry points and become easier to hack. It will not necessarily protect individuals better.

So are Danish health data practices part of We Medicine or Me Medicine? I think there are elements of both. When publicly sourced data are used to attract commercial investments and generate profit, it looks more like Me Medicine thriving on the illusion of We Medicine. When data are used for identifying individuals based on algorithmic profiling and this identification individualises risks and benefits it similarly comes across more like Me Medicine using We Medicine as a veil. Nevertheless, if we believe at all in the value of medical consensus, the common goods derived from research uses can also be significant. Without the Nordic registers and consent exemption rules, there would

---

[70] K. Hoeyer and N. Lynöe, 'Is informed consent a solution to contractual problems? A comment on the article "'Icelandic Inc.'? On the ethics of commercial population genomics" by Jon F. Merz, Glen E. McGee and Pamala Sankar' (2004) 58(6) *Social Science and Medicine* 1211–13; J. F. Merz, G. E. McGee and P. Sankar, '"Iceland Inc."?: On the ethics of commercial population genomics' (2004) 58(6) *Social Science & Medicine* 1201–9.

[71] D. Grande, N. Mitra, A. Shah, F. Wan and D.A. Asch, 'The importance of purpose: Moving beyond consent in the societal use of personal health information' (2014) 161(12) *Annals of Internal Medicine* 855–62; L. F. Hogle, 'The ethics and politics of infrastructures: Creating the conditions of possibility for big data in medicine' in L. Floridi & B. Mittelstadt (eds.), *The Ethics of Biomedical Big Data* (Switzerland: Springer, 2016), pp. 1–32; B. D. Mittelstadt and L. Floridi, 'The ethics of Big Data: Current and foreseeable issues in biomedical contexts' (2015) *Science and Engineering Ethics* 1–39.

be fewer options for checking and challenging the claims made by the pharmaceutical companies based on short-term randomised controlled trials (RCTs). The registers have been used to identify unknown side effects, to stimulate a better understanding of poly-pharmacy effects, and have also shown that certain fears were probably unfounded. Many of these research results arising from public Danish health registers are now freely available and implementable in a non-rivalrous manner and to the benefit of the people delivering the data in the first place. In this sense, the data circle works and it works as We Medicine. If research uses were to be restricted through the use of informed consent, the risks would be differently distributed and the benefits of unbiased information disappear.

Rather than insisting on informed consent, would it not be more adequate to focus on the responsibilities that authorities and companies incur through mandatory data sourcing? Responsibilities for insuring safety, communal purposes and fair use? For compensating those harmed by data leaks or hacking? For ensuring that secondary purposes with data sourcing do not overrule primary purposes so that clinical utility is hampered in the pursuit of administrative or research utility? Responsibilities to think through carefully how data usage can avoid undermining the entitlement to healthcare for vulnerable individuals? Furthermore, there is a need to complement the current focus on the privacy and autonomy interests of those from whom data derive and to take into account also the group privacy interests of those at the receiving end of the new data tools developed with the big datasets to ensure they are put to use for the common good and not just as profiling tools that individualise risks and benefits.[72] Will it be possible to be lost and stay lost? Is there a right to be forgotten as well as a right not to be tagged as a particular profile? There is a need to find ways of countering the risks associated in particular with private data sourcing, and to help individuals manoeuvre the landscapes of personalised pricing, marketing and services that might make the user into the product. Data intensification involves many challenges, but they are hardly solved with rules about informed consent. They demand communal approaches setting rules for collectives rather than distributing responsibilities to individuals. Those scholars who continue to insist on informed consent as an obligatory

---

[72] L. Taylor, 'Safety in numbers? Group privacy and big data analytics in the developing world' in L. Taylor et al. (eds.), *Group Privacy. New Challenges of Data Technologies* (Dordrecht: Springer, 2017).

passage point for data sourcing will have to address these challenges too, lest they simply aim at individualising responsibilities in a complex data-intensive age.

Intensified data sourcing changes medicine as we know it. It reflects and affects epistemological issues (what we can know), issues of citizenship (the rights and duties of individuals), economic issues (costs of healthcare and accumulation of capital), as well as issues of societal morality (public values and the distribution of goods and risks). In many ways, it looks as if data intensification tends to take healthcare in the direction of Me Medicine. Still, if we think of the common good not as 'accumulated goods' (akin to accumulated data), but as goods that derive from the collective,[73] intensified data sourcing could also be a prime example of We Medicine when only directed towards common good goals. It is, however, a key task to ensure that the collective goods do not become redirected into private pockets – and that collectives help each other to counter individual risks. I believe it is possible to bring some of the old values of We Medicine to the table of a data-intensive healthcare system and work for communal use, shared risk and collective benefits. It is well worth a try, considering that there is little reason to assume that healthcare will become any less data-intensive in the future.

Acknowledgements

This chapter is based on a project that has received funding from the European Research Council (ERC) under the European Union's Horizon 2020 research and innovation programme (grant agreement number 682110). I would like to thank also Francisca Nordfalk and the participants at the workshop ('Me Medicine versus We Medicine') on which this book is based for their comments and suggestions, as well as the organisers Sigrid Sterckx, Britta van Beers and Donna Dickenson for the invitation and for comments on earlier versions of this chapter.

[73] H. Widdows and S. Cordell, 'Why communities and their goods matter: Illustrated with the example of Biobanks' (2011) 4(1) *Public Health Ethics* 14–25.

Presuming the Promotion of the Common Good by Large-Scale Health Research

The Cases of care.data 2.0 and the 100,000 Genomes Project in the UK

SIGRID STERCKX, SANDI DHEENSA AND JULIAN
COCKBAIN

8.1 Introduction[1]

8.1.1 Background

Before World War One (WWI), levels of financial inequality world-wide had reached previously unknown magnitudes,[2] despite forms of democracy having been introduced into many Western countries. WWI was, however, to yield a world 'fit for heroes',[3] one in which the common person had a fair share. Between WWI and World War Two (WWII), little was done to reduce inequality. With WWII's outbreak, the problem of inequality was set to one side. However, after Germany had capitulated, the UK general elections brought in a socialist government whose stated promise was to establish a 'Welfare State', to provide education, health, unemployment benefits and pensions for all, and to nationalise utilities and key infrastructures.

UK citizens and residents are not required to have identity cards or record their domicile with the local authorities. However, the UK government and its agents keep extensive data records, e.g. of births, marriages, deaths, passports, driver's licences, entries into and departures

---

[1] All information in this chapter is up to date as of 6 November 2017.

[2] Thomas Piketty, *Capital in the Twenty-First Century* (Cambridge, MA: Harvard University Press, 2014).

[3] Politician David Lloyd George promised the British public to undertake major reforms to address education, health, housing and transport inadequacies and to create a land 'fit for heroes to live in'.

from the UK, (un)employment, tax, crime and, not least, healthcare.[4] To some, it may be obvious that it is in the interest of the state to collate these records to give a clearer picture of the population and to improve the allocation of state resources. The records are of particular value in optimising healthcare, crime prevention and education, three of the primary tasks of the UK government. To others, the spectre of Big Brother comes to the fore with fears of a totalitarian state such as those well-known from the last century.

8.1.2   Health Data Collection in the UK

In this chapter, we are concerned with the collection of health-related data in the UK, in particular those deriving from *institutional care* (e.g. care in hospitals – the majority of which are still public institutions), *personal care* (e.g. data held by family physicians, known in the UK as General Practitioners, or GPs, who are not state employees but contractors) and from *specific government initiatives* such as UK Biobank (which holds material and data from about half a million citizens) and the 100,000 Genomes Project (which is to hold information from about 70,000 people with cancers and rare diseases and their relatives, as discussed further in this chapter).

   The collation of such health data clearly could improve the efficiency of the UK's National Health Service (NHS),[5] for example, by identifying treatments that are more effective and improving regional allocation of resources. Research using the collated data may help the development of new diagnostic and treatment methods and drugs. This may well fall under the label of 'We Medicine',[6] understood as accessible and publicly funded healthcare aiming to benefit all. However, where commercial players become involved as potential vendors of new products, rather than simply as contractors for the NHS, the benefits may flow to more limited sets of individuals.

---

[4] Digital Economy Act 2017, www.legislation.gov.uk/ukpga/2017/30/contents/enacted, accessed 6 November 2017.

[5] As Vezyridis and Timmons explain, health data has also become a valuable source of income for the NHS. Paraskevas Vezyridis and Stephen Timmons, 'Understanding the care.data conundrum: New information flows for economic growth' (2017) *Big Data and Society*. Published online.

[6] Donna L. Dickenson, *Me Medicine vs We Medicine – Reclaiming Biotechnology for the Common Good* (New York, NY: Columbia University Press, 2013).

In April 2005, the UK government set up a (publicly owned) company, the 'Health and Social Care Information Centre', which acquired institutional personal health data with at least the aim of making it available for research where the researcher was neither within nor a contracted agent of the NHS. This company (HSCIC-1) went under the names of 'The Information Centre' and the 'NHS Information Centre'. Following the enactment of the Health and Social Care Act 2012,[7] HSCIC-1 was dissolved in March 2013 and its functions were transferred to a new publicly owned company, also called the Health and Social Care Information Centre, which was created on the following day. This new company, which we will refer to as *HSCIC-2*, was empowered to integrate into its health database the *personal health records held by GPs*. The scheme for harvesting GP data was referred to as 'care.data', and, although due to begin in 2014, was suspended that same year. In April 2016, the government announced that, from July 2016, HSCIC-2 would change its name to NHS Digital, and in July 2016 the care.data scheme was officially scrapped.[8] However, although the name has been dropped and the 'consent' model underlying it has been changed, the scheme continues, as we will explain.

In the same year as the Health and Social Care Act 2012, the UK government announced the launch of 'The 100,000 Genomes Project' (hereinafter 100kGP) to 'bring the benefits of personalised medicine to the NHS'.[9] The project involves sequencing the whole genomes of NHS patients with either a rare disease or cancer. Genomics England, a company owned by the Department of Health (DoH), is delivering the project through thirteen Genomic Medicine Centres (GMC) in NHS trusts.

This project has been developing the infrastructure for a national genomic medicine service in which whole-genome sequencing will become a routine and frontline test in cross-cutting areas of medicine. There are plans to 'concentrate all NHS genomic testing into the same

---

[7] Health and Social Care Act 2012, www.legislation.gov.uk/ukpga/2012/7/contents, accessed 6 November 2017. This Act epitomised the privatisation of the NHS by facilitating the contracting of NHS services to private providers. Allyson M. Pollock, Alison Macfarlane and Sylvia Godden, 'Dismantling the signposts to public health? NHS data under the Health and Social Care Act' (2012) 344 *British Medical Journal* e2364.

[8] George Freeman, 'Written statement to Parliament: Review of health and care data security and consent' (2016), www.gov.uk/government/speeches/review-of-health-and-care-data-security-and-consent, accessed 6 November 2017.

[9] NHS England, 'Genomics' (2012), www.england.nhs.uk/ourwork/qual-clin-lead/personalisedmedicine/genomics, accessed 6 November 2017.

data centre' with 'access to . . . industry for the purpose of developing new knowledge, methods of analysis, medicines, diagnostics and devices'.[10]

8.1.3   Concerns

The collection of residents' health-related data undoubtedly has the potential for public benefit, but is surrounded by concerns regarding privacy, autonomy and justice. While the UK government's schemes do, at least superficially, take these concerns into account, we address in this chapter what we see as a gap – indeed a gaping chasm – between the government's rhetoric and the governance structures they put in place. By taking a closer look at both in the cases of care.data and the 100kGP, we demonstrate that what is presented as 'We Medicine' in fact falls far short. We begin our review with care.data before turning to the 100kGP and the ethical issues we consider to be most pressing.

8.2   Care.data

8.2.1   Current Sharing of Health Data

As David Springate, a biostatistician who works on electronic data base research at the University of Manchester, has noted:

> For a sizeable proportion of the UK population, the sharing of their electronic medical records . . . is already a reality and has been for decades. About a third of UK patients already have their electronic medical records held on the main current UK primary care databases . . . and many have their pseudoanonymised data accessible (for a fee) to both medical researchers . . . [and] private companies, including drug companies . . . In the majority of cases now, patients will not even be aware that their data are being collected, let alone be offered the opportunity to consent.[11]

Physician and science writer Ben Goldacre commented:

> [A] government body handed over parts of my medical records to people I've never met, outside the NHS and medical research community, but it is

---

[10] Sally Davies, 'Generation Genome. Annual Report of the Chief Medical Officer' (2016) www.gov.uk/government/uploads/system/uploads/attachment_data/file/631043/ CMO_annual_report_generation_genome.pdf, accessed 6 November 2017 (chapters 14 and 2).

[11] David Springate, 'Health database could help avoid another pharma scandal' (2014) *The Conversation*, www.theconversation.com/health-database-could-help-avoid-another-pharma-scandal-23730, accessed 6 November 2017.

refusing to tell me what it handed over, or who it gave it to, and the minister is now incorrectly claiming that it never happened anyway. There are people in my profession who think they can ignore this problem. Some are murmuring that this mess is . . . a public misunderstanding to be corrected with better PR. They are wrong: it's like nuclear power. Medical data, rarefied and condensed, presents huge power to do good, but it also presents huge risks. When leaked, it cannot be unleaked; when lost, public trust will take decades to regain.[12]

Survey results show that only 54 per cent of the public support commercial access to their health data for health research. However, there is a clear desire for the NHS to seek permission before allowing access to companies. Some participants think data access is unacceptable if it is solely for private benefit and do 'not want anyone . . . to be able to co-opt health data for political ends'.[13]

8.2.2   Concerns Regarding the (Im)Possibility of Opting Out from Care. data

In April 2013, nine months before care.data launched, Jeremy Hunt, the UK Secretary of State for Health, gave the public a reassurance that any patient who did not want personal data in their GP records to be shared with HSCIC-2 'would have their objection respected'.[14] On 12 September 2013, he added that 'All they have to do in that case is speak to their GP and their information won't leave the GP surgery'.[15] Objections to information leaving the GP surgery became known as a 'Type 1' objection. At the same time, for objections to information leaving the HSCIC-2, a 'Type 2' objection, was proposed.[16]

The option to opt out of care.data is not overseen by the Information Commissioner's Office (the ICO), and is *not* guaranteed by law. Moreover, the Health and Social Care Act 2012 (HSCA), the law that

[12] Ben Goldacre, 'Care.data is in chaos. It breaks my heart' (2014) *The Guardian*, 28 February.
[13] Wellcome Trust/IPSOS Mori, 'The one-way mirror: Public attitudes to commercial access to health data' (2016), www.ipsos.com/sites/default/files/publication/5200–03/sri-wellcome-trust-commercial-access-to-health-data.pdf, accessed 6 November 2017.
[14] Fiona Caldicott, 'Review of data security, consent and opt-outs' (2016), www.gov.uk/government/uploads/system/uploads/attachment_data/file/535024/data-security-review.PDF, accessed 6 November 2017.
[15] Department of Health (DoH), 'Jeremy Hunt confirms commitment to balance patient safety and privacy' (2013), www.gov.uk/government/news/jeremy-hunt-confirms-commitment-to-balance-patient-safety-and-privacy–2, accessed 6 November 2017.
[16] Caldicott, 'Review of data security, consent and opt-outs'.

provided the basis for the care.data scheme, 'trumps' key provisions of the Data Protection Act 1998.[17] Specifically, the HSCA allows all patient data to be used for purposes that extend beyond patient care without consultation, i.e. without the patients' knowledge. Indeed, the HSCA *makes it impossible for patients to prevent their data from being used for research.*

In autumn 2013, NHS England set up a care.data website where citizens could record their views and in January 2014 an information leaflet on care.data was sent to all English households.[18] However, public concern rose, as did concern among General Practitioners. Many patients began to take advantage of the opportunity to opt out that Hunt had offered. Hunt had effectively promised that the data for those who opted out would *not* be harvested from the GPs' records. In reality, the intent was to harvest that data anyway and then 'de-identify' their records.[19]

Amendments to the HSCA in the Care Act 2014[20] went some way towards addressing public concerns regarding confidentiality and inappropriate use of patient health data, not least by allowing data releases only 'for the purposes of the provision of healthcare or adult social care, or the promotion of health'. However, this amendment clearly does not prevent data being made available to drug researchers, pharmaceutical firms and tech giants like Google.

Care.data was not just problematic for patients. As Vezyridis and Timmons[21] observe, the new obligation on GPs to share data with HSCIC-2 created pressure on GPs who are responsible for telling patients about a scheme that they know little about themselves. As data controllers with legal liability for their patients' information, they face conflicting statutory obligations to process patient data fairly and yet disclose

---

[17] Jamie Grace and Mark J. Taylor, 'Disclosure of confidential patient information and the duty to consult: The role of the health and social care information centre' (2013) 21(3) *Medical Law Review* 415–47; Data Protection Act 1998, www.legislation.gov.uk/ukpga/1998/29/contents, accessed 6 November 2017.

[18] Vezyridis and Timmons point out that the leaflet was sent out without checks, was biased towards the programme's benefits and had little information about the so-called opt-outs. It was later deemed 'unfit for purpose'. (Vezyridis and Timmons, 'Understanding the care.data conundrum').

[19] NHS England, 'Privacy impact assessment: care.data' (2014), www.england.nhs.uk/wp-content/uploads/2014/04/cd-pia.pdf, accessed 6 November 2017.

[20] Care Act 2014, www.legislation.gov.uk/ukpga/2014/23/contents, accessed 6 November 2017.

[21] Paraskevas Vezyridis and Stephen Timmons, 'Dissenting from care.data: an analysis of opt-out forms' (2016) 42(12) *Journal of Medical Ethics* 792–6.

data. Many GP practices provided patients with opt-out forms, but they provided extremely variable information and could have been confusing and unintentionally misleading.

With many GPs showing concern, in February 2014 the government decided to delay GP data harvesting to allow NHS England the opportunity to persuade GPs, healthcare professionals and patients that care.data was necessary and that sufficient safeguards had been put in place. Key elements of the discussions included: appropriate consent mechanisms for data collection and use; the right to object to processing of personal data; the extent of the data collected; and the uses of the data by the NHS or third parties. Citizens also raised several of these concerns.[22]

In September 2015, Hunt bought more time for care.data by commissioning the National Data Guardian, Fiona Caldicott, to review the protection of personal health data and the provision of appropriate opt-outs. The Caldicott Review could then be held out as legitimately dealing with the public's concerns. Shortly thereafter, in November 2015, one concerned GP, Dr Neil Bhatia, made a request under the Freedom of Information Act asking whether the extraction of GP data would still be the same care.data scheme, albeit with an 'updated' dataset, or whether it would be an additional, parallel, extraction for a different project. The following month, NHS England confirmed that 'There will be a single national GP dataset which would therefore replace the dataset as currently defined for the care.data pathfinder stage.'[23]

8.2.3   The Caldicott Review

In July 2016, the UK government issued the long-awaited report on the initiation of the Iraq War, the Chilcot Report. Astonishingly, on the same day, the Caldicott Review[24] was issued, and the UK government announced that the care.data scheme had been scrapped. However, it stated that it remained '*absolutely committed to realising the benefits of sharing information*

---

[22] Sigrid Sterckx, Vojin Rakic, Julian Cockbain et al., '"You hoped we would sleep walk into accepting the collection of our data": Controversies surrounding the UK care.data scheme and their wider relevance for biomedical research' (2016) 19(2) *Medicine, Health Care and Philosophy* 177–90; Rebecca Hays and Gavin Daker-White, 'The care.data consensus? A qualitative analysis of opinions expressed on Twitter' (2015) 15 *BMC Public Health* 838.

[23] NHS England, Letter dated 10 December 2015, responding to a Freedom of Information Request by Dr Neil Bhatia, www.whatdotheyknow.com/request/single_national_gp_data set_2, accessed 6 November 2017.

[24] Caldicott, 'Review of data security, consent and opt-outs'.

... Therefore, *this work will now be taken forward* ... in order to retain public confidence and to drive better care for patients' (emphasis added).[25]

The Caldicott Review was clear that it had been an exercise in generating public trust in the use of their health data:

> This has been a report about trust. ... Because of the importance of earning public trust, the Review concluded that people should be able to opt out of their *personal confidential data* being used for purposes beyond their direct care unless there is a mandatory legal requirement or an overriding public interest.[26] (emphasis added)

However, Caldicott recommended that: confidential patient information should nonetheless be collected by HSCIC-2, *irrespective* of any opt-out by individual patients; and that 'data that has been de-identified [by HSCIC-2] according to the [Information Commissioner's Office's] anonymisation code should *not* be subject to the opt-out' (emphasis added).[27] Interestingly, Caldicott noted the government's decision to re-brand HSCIC-2 as NHS Digital saying that '[t]his will provide [HSCIC-2] with a good opportunity to use the NHS brand to make it clear to everyone that it is part of the NHS "family"'.[28]

Since the effects of the opt-outs proposed by Caldicott would conflict with the Type 1 opt-out promised by Hunt in relation to care.data, Caldicott recommended that 'the Government should consider the future of the care.data programme'.[29] More particularly, Caldicott noted that applying the Type 1 opt-out 'to all HSCIC[-2] data collections, including existing data collections from hospitals, would degrade the quality of data currently available to ... researchers'.[30] It is thus abundantly clear that the function of the Caldicott Review was to advise the government *how to restart the care.data scheme for the same purposes, but without the risk of public outcry* and without Hunt's misleading promise that opting-out would prevent data being harvested from the GP records. We refer to the 'new' scheme as care.data 2.0.

Rhetoric aside, Caldicott proposed that NHS England consider two approaches to opt-outs, and present these to patients on forms with tickboxes. One approach offers two alternatives (which we will label, for clarity, 'broad' – the default option – and 'narrow'), while the other also adds a third (which we will label 'limited'):

25 Freeman, 'Written statement to Parliament: Review of health and care data security and consent'.
26 Caldicott, 'Review of data security, consent and opt-outs'.   27 Ibid., p. 8.
28 Ibid., p. 7.   29 Ibid., p. 8.   30 Ibid., p. 34.

Broad: *'Information about me can be used to run the NHS and social care system and to support research to improve treatment and care for everyone.'*
Limited: *'Information about me can be used to run the NHS and social care system, but not for research.'*
Narrow: *'Information about me can only be used by the people directly providing my care.'*

This way of representing the opt-outs is problematic for at least three reasons. First, in the wording of each of the options, the patient is told that this relates to 'information about me', while the opt-out applies to 'confidential patient information'. The patient is given no indication that the latter is a term with a specific and narrow legal definition (see below) and that the HSCIC-2 is *free to share de-identified, pseudonymised or anonymised data* (which patients think is also 'information about me'[31]) *with anyone* as long as it is 'for the purposes of the provision of healthcare or adult social care, or the promotion of health'. The information provided also fails to make clear the technical limitations of pseudonymisation as a de-identification technique.[32] Second, in the Limited option, the patient is not offered the choice between research by or for the NHS and research by and for commercial organisations,[33] and hence is 'nudged' away from this option. Third, in the Narrow option, the patient is not advised that persons directly providing their care are not just the physicians and other healthcare professionals with whom they interact.

This misleading nature of the Caldicott opt-outs is also shown in the language used in introducing the proposed opt-outs:

> You are protected by the law. Your *personal confidential information* will only ever be used where allowed by law ... [Y]ou can ask your health care professional not to pass on particular information *to others involved in providing your care. You have the right to opt out.* You have the right to opt out of your *personal confidential information* being used for these other purposes beyond your *direct care* ... *This opt-out will be respected by all*

---

[31] Wellcome Trust/IPSOS Mori, 'The one-way mirror'.
[32] Kieron O'Hara, *Transparent Government, Not Transparent Citizens: A Report on Privacy and Transparency for the Cabinet Office* (Southampton: University of Southampton, 2011).
[33] Caldicott noted that 'people hold contrasting views about information being used for purposes beyond direct care and some people became concerned when data is shared outside the NHS "family"'. Nevertheless, she took the view that the opt-out model 'should be set around the purpose to which data is put ... and that dividing up NHS and "non-NHS organisations" without reference to purpose can be artificial and misleading'. This decision is highly problematic, as we will explain in the section on ethical questions. Caldicott, 'Review of data security, consent and opt-outs', p. 23.

organisations that use health and social care information ... You can
change your mind ...[34] (emphasis added)

In sum, the Caldicott Review makes it clear that the opt-out *only*
applies to data from which the patient may be directly identified, and
even then *only* to data supplied to those not involved directly with the
patient's care, with 'direct care' being defined more broadly than the
normal person would understand this term. This is problematic, as a
Wellcome Trust/IPSOS Mori[35] report shows that people are already
unclear about who can access their data. The obfuscatory language in
the Caldicott Review will only exacerbate the confusion.

8.2.4 Has the GDPR Any Effect?

In 2016, the EU enacted the *General Data Protection Regulation*
(Regulation (EU) 2016/679, GDPR), a law that came into force in EU
member states in May 2018. Under Article 18(1)(d) GDPR, people are
given 'the right to obtain ... *restriction* of processing ... [of data relating
to them] pending the verification whether the legitimate grounds of the
[data] controller override those of the data subject' (emphasis added).
Article 21(1) GDPR, moreover, states that 'The data subject shall have the
right to *object* ... to processing of personal data ... unless the [data]
controller demonstrates compelling legitimate grounds for the processing which override the interests, rights and freedoms of the data subject. ... ' (emphasis added).

However, Article 6(1) GDPR reads, in relevant part, as follows:

> Processing shall be lawful only if and to the extent that [it is necessary]: for
> *compliance with a legal obligation* to which the [data] controller is subject ...
> [or] for the performance of a task *carried out in the public interest* or *in the
> exercise of official authority* vested in the [data] controller. (emphasis added)

Perhaps not surprisingly, the GDPR thus allows EU member states to
override the data subject's rights in certain (if not most) circumstances
concerning state use. Until at least March 2019 the UK is covered by EU
regulations. Thus it will come as no surprise that the UK government has
introduced in the House of Lords the Data Protection Bill,[36] which, when
accepted, will be UK law.

---

[34] Ibid., p. 39.   [35] Wellcome Trust/IPSOS Mori, 'The one-way mirror'.
[36] Data Protection Bill [HL], www.publications.parliament.uk/pa/bills/lbill/2017–2019/
0066/18066.pdf, accessed 6 November 2017.

In Section 15 of the Data Protection Bill, the relevant government minister is to be given the right to override the GDPR *without* Parliament approval, by issuance of a Rule:

> – to adapt the application of rules of the GDPR . . . *for compliance with a legal obligation*, for the performance of a task *in the public interest* or *in the exercise of official authority*;
> – [under Article 23(1) GDPR to restrict] the scope of the obligations [to] and rights [of the data subject] . . . *to safeguard certain objectives of general public interest*; [and]
> – [under Article 89 GDPR] to provide for derogations from the rights mentioned in paragraphs (2) and (3) of that Article . . . *for scientific . . . research [or] statistical purposes* (emphasis added)[37]

In other words, the Data Protection Bill, when passed, will allow free use of *de-identified* personal health data.

8.2.5   Post-Caldicott: The 'National Data Lake'

Following the issue of the Caldicott Review, but before releasing its response, in July 2017 the government undertook a consultation exercise[38] and in August 2017 a document setting out the proposals for a 'Target Architecture' for care.data 2.0 was leaked to the press.[39]

---

[37] Article 23(1) GDPR, in relevant part, reads: 'Member State law . . . may restrict . . . the obligations and rights provided for in Articles [18 and 21 GDPR] when such a restriction . . . is a necessary and proportionate measure in a democratic society to safeguard . . . important *objectives of general public interest* of . . . a Member State, in particular . . . an important economic or financial interest of the . . . Member State, including . . . public health' (emphasis added). Likewise, Article 89 GDPR, in relevant part, reads: 'Processing . . . . *in the public interest* [or for] *scientific . . . research* purposes or statistical purposes, shall be subject to appropriate safeguards . . . Where those purposes can be fulfilled by further processing which does not permit or no longer permits the identification of data subjects, those purposes shall be fulfilled in that manner.' (emphasis added). Regulation (EU) 2016/679 of the European Parliament and of the Council of 27 April 2016 on the protection of natural persons with regard to the processing of personal data and on the free movement of such data, and repealing Directive 95/46/EC (General Data Protection Regulation), *Official Journal* L 119/1, 4 May 2016.

[38] Department of Health, 'Your data – Better security, better choice, better care. Government response to the National Data Guardian for Health Care's Review of data security. Consent and opt-outs and the Care Quality Commission's Review "Safe data, safe care"' (2017), www .gov.uk/government/uploads/system/uploads/attachment_data/file/627493/ Your_data_better_security_better_choice_better_care_government_response.pdf, accessed 6 November 2017.

[39] NHS England, 'Enabling evidence-based continuous improvement. The Target Architecture. Connecting care settings and improving patient experience' (2017),

The consultation exercise showed the importance of public trust but had also indicated that, while a need for a national data collection existed, the public is 'less willing to share their data when the direct benefit for them and their local population is unclear'.[40] The proposal is thus to harvest data into local pools, each representing the maximum size for which a high degree of public trust can be predicted: about 2–5 million people. With a common architecture in the format of each pool, and with a national spine making the pools interconnectable, a 'National Data Lake' will be created which merely appears to be a set of local pools for local people.

NHS England effectively admits this in the target architecture plan:

> Sensitive personal and confidential data (which is fully identifiable) will almost certainly be required to achieve interoperability and to facilitate precision medicine and case finding. The [Caldicott] Review opt-out will not apply.[41]

Such data, however, obviously remains sensitive. It is 'confidential patient information', a term which is *precisely defined by law and does not mean personal health records in general*, as most people would think. It refers to information[42] which, without a court order, generally cannot be released to parties outside the NHS and its contracted agents without the patient's consent, distinguishing it from information that the NHS *is* permitted to release without the patient's consent, *even if the patient has opted out.*

Care.data 2.0 thus involves NHS Digital collecting confidential patient information, and, by de-identifying it, creating a database of

---

https://medconfidential.org/wp-content/uploads/2017/09/2017-07-13-Target-Architecture.pdf, accessed 6 November 2017.

[40] NHS England, 'Enabling evidence-based continuous improvement', p. 35.
[41] Ibid., p. 31.
[42] National Health Service Act 2006, www.legislation.gov.uk/ukpga/2006/41/contents, accessed 6 November 2017. Section 251(10) defines 'patient information' as follows: '(a) information (however recorded) which relates to the physical or mental health or condition of an individual, to the diagnosis of his condition or to his care or treatment, and (b) information (however recorded) which is to any extent derived, directly or indirectly, from such information, whether or not the identity of the individual in question is ascertainable from the information.' However, Section 251(11) goes on to make clear that patient information is 'confidential patient information' where: '(a) the identity of the individual in question is ascertainable—(i) from that information, or (ii) from that information and other information which is in the possession of, or is likely to come into the possession of, the person processing that information, and (b) that information was obtained or generated by a person who, in the circumstances, owed an obligation of confidence to that individual.'

'non-confidential' information. The new Caldicott opt-outs have *no effect whatsoever* on the release to *any* party of personal health data which has been 'de-identified', to whatever extent the government sees fit.

The government warmly welcomed and supported Caldicott's recommendations, and HSCIC was duly rebranded as NHS Digital. A national data opt-out is being prepared, i.e. a single opt-out to replace the Type 1 and Type 2 opt-outs (to prevent uploading of GP data to HSCIC-2's database, and to prevent release of identifiable data by HSCIC-2, respectively). This national opt-out is to be available from March 2018. In effect, the only thing the national opt-out will provide is the right to prevent fully identifiable data from being used for research and 'planning'.

The timeline set out in the government's response to the Caldicott Review sets a date of September 2019 for NHS Digital to implement a new mechanism to de-identify data on collection from GP practices, so we can presume that this is likely to be the new start date for care.data 2.0.

8.3   The UK 100,000 Genomes Project

8.3.1   Background, Focus and Patient Recruitment

The 100kGP is a hybrid of a biobank for research (including by industry and commercial actors) and clinical practice (in that participating in the project might lead to a diagnosis or to the identification of a treatment for that patient's presenting condition).

The 100kGP is being delivered and implemented using existing NHS resources. NHS clinicians treating potentially eligible patients identify and refer them to the project. Those who want to take part have a preliminary discussion with a healthcare worker and are sent information documents to read. Genomics England has designed these documents via piloting with public/patient involvement groups and discussion with different advisory committees. Notably, research showed that some patients found the documents too lengthy and complex and they have been revised.[43]

At least 24 hours after receiving the information, patients and family members are seen in a face-to-face consent appointment with NHS staff at a Genomic Medicine Centre. There, they give samples of blood, tissue and saliva which are sent to the sequencing hub. The sequence data are sent for storage to Genomics England's data centre. Genome data

---

[43] Caroline Benjamin, 'Findings from the National Consent Evaluation' (2016) www.geno micsengland.co.uk/consent-evaluation-findings, accessed 6 November 2017.

are then combined with data about the patient from their hospital or clinic, their GP records, national disease registries, social care records and Public Health England. The data is to be extracted over the patient's whole life into a database built in partnership with NHS Digital. In a bid to protect privacy, the linked dataset is 'de-identified'. The samples are also stored for future research. These sample and data banks are controlled by Genomics England (although what will happen to them once the project is over will be left to the Secretary of State for Health to decide).

The project shares some similarities with the 500,000-participant strong UK Biobank,[44] which also collected biomaterial and detailed health-related information linked to GP and hospital data. The key differences are that UK Biobank had broad recruitment criteria and offered test results such as blood pressure readings and body mass index, while 100kGP recruitment is more tightly linked to the NHS patient 'family' and provides results from tests otherwise unavailable through the NHS (whole-genome sequencing and, eventually, other 'omics'). Many patients and families in the rare diseases arm will be those who have had earlier tests which failed to achieve a diagnosis. Whole genome sequencing is a last hope after a long 'diagnostic odyssey'. Although patients and family members are told that diagnoses are not guaranteed, they *are* told they are possible. In fact, newspaper coverage of the project's pilot phase has shown that several patients in the rare disease arm have been diagnosed.

Tested people can also opt to have their genomes searched against a constantly updated predefined list of 'additional findings' for potentially serious but actionable risks, e.g. familial hypercholesterolemia and familial cancer syndromes. This offer – as Genomics England's Chief Scientific Officer Mark Caulfield suggests – is made on the basis of increasing fairness and trustworthiness: '[patients] have entrusted us with their genomic information, it seems only fair that we can offer ... options ... [that] may benefit their future health'.[45] Genomics England sends reports to physicians about their patients, and so any feedback about results is offered as part of clinical consultations.

[44] UK Biobank, 'Participants' (2016) www.ukbiobank.ac.uk/participants, accessed 6 November 2017.

[45] Genomics England, '100,000 Genomes Project gains ethical approval to offer NHS patients further information about their genomic results' (2015) www.genomicseng land.co.uk/100k-genomes-projectp-gains-ethical-approval-to-offer-nhs-patients-further-information-about-their-genomic-results, accessed 6 November 2017.

The focus is on rare diseases since, in 80 per cent of cases, these diseases have a genomic basis. Although individually uncommon, the diseases affect 6–7 per cent of the UK population. Finding the genetic cause can shed light on the nature of the disease, its prognosis and potential treatments, and areas for further research. Half of new cases of such disease are found in children. The list of eligible rare diseases consists of: diseases for which there is a clinical diagnosis but no molecular diagnosis and no readily detectable genetic mutation in known disease-related genes; diseases for which there is a *suspected* clinical diagnosis; and diseases that are 'ultra-rare'. Since comparing sequences can aid interpretation, multiple family members are invited to participate in the project.

In the cancer arm, patients' germline genomes and the genomes of their cancers will be sequenced, because mutations in tumours are a central factor in determining the progression of the cancer and its likely response to therapy. The project's focus on cancer is unsurprising: in the UK, cancer killed 160,000 people in 2014 and over 350,000 new cases were reported that same year. Given that cancer is extremely heterogeneous, even among people with the 'same' diagnosis, the stated aim of the project here is to make diagnoses that are more precise, as well as to find better, more 'personalised', treatment choices – i.e. those that have a better balance of response rate to toxic side effects. Genomics research has already led to success in this respect, showing that HER2 positive breast cancers respond to the drug Herceptin (trastuzumab).

8.3.2   Research and Development

One of the project's aims – enabling new scientific discovery and insight – is said to be possible only through research on the genomic and clinical information. Thus for patients, having their clinical tests and any chance of a diagnosis is presented as being contingent upon giving broad consent to future, unspecified research on their data. Some of this research is to be done by industry and commercial companies. This is said to be because: 'if any new diagnostic tests and treatments are to come from this project, they will need to be developed, as they always have been, by the private sector and not within government or the NHS'.[46]

[46] Chelsea and Westminster Hospital, 'West London Genomic Medicine Centre', www .chelwest.nhs.uk/about-us/research-development/west-london-genomic-medicine-cen tre, accessed 6 November 2017. This is of course misleading. Many diagnostic tests and pharmaceuticals have been discovered and developed, if not commercially marketed, by

There are strict restrictions about who can access the data for research. Insurers, marketers and other government agencies, such as the police, are disallowed automatic access, although the police and Home Office can seek a court order for access. Researchers can access only de-identified subsets of the data for research purposes approved by the 'access review committee', in a monitored, secure data environment. Priority and royalty-free access to data is given to members of the Genomics England Clinical Interpretation Partnerships (GeCIPs) which are domains of over 2000 researchers, clinicians, trainees and funders from academia, charitable organisations, government or healthcare. GeCIPs will carry out research into particular disease-types or cross-cutting issues (e.g. health economics) and get free access because their research will aid the interpretation of data. Researchers who do not meet the eligibility criteria to join a GeCIP (e.g. private healthcare institutions or commercial companies) will be able to access the dataset for a fee.

Regarding intellectual property and patenting, Genomics England has adopted a relatively standard approach to inventions made by public bodies carrying out research on its data: patents may be sought and may be licensed to commercial entities and academic institutions on favourable terms. Genomics England also states that there may be cases where it decides not to patent an invention for public policy reasons, e.g. if it would serve the public interest to make the invention freely available for use. The key question, of course, is the extent to which patent rights may vest in commercial entities carrying out research on its data.

8.3.3 Funders and Commercial Actors Involved

Genomics England is largely government funded: the UK government committed £250 million as part of its 2016 spending review after an initial investment of £300 million. The Medical Research Council contributed £24 million towards computing power for the analysis and interpretation of data. NHS England agreed to underwrite an NHS contribution of up to £20 million over the duration of the project. The Wellcome Trust contributed £27 million towards a sequencing facility near Cambridge, UK. Illumina, the US biotechnology company carrying out the genome sequencing, is investing £162 million in return for its £78 million sequencing contract.

the public sector. One has only to think of the antibiotic penicillin and the anti-cancer drug paclitaxel.

In 2015, Genomics England granted access to a subset of aggregated data to twelve pharmaceutical, biotechnology and diagnostic companies from the UK and abroad, including GSK, Roche and AstraZeneca, as part of an industry trial. They asked each company to identify areas of improvement in data collection and to invest money (a fee of £250,000) and staff (scientists and bioinformaticians) to aid the storage, security and analysis of data. These companies have been obliged to publish all research from the industry trial 'at the point at which intellectual property for any product is protected, in common with best practice in the pharmaceutical industry'.[47] Notably, intellectual property is only 'protected' once all the relevant patents are granted: something that will normally occur only 5–15 years after the initial invention. Thus this is by no means a promise of rapid publication. As Samuel and Farsides[48] comment, 'little is known about the outcome of this trial ... [and] how the ethical issues associated with partnering with commercial entities might unfold'. Several other commercial companies, including Illumina, have access to the data centre or data pipelines because they are providing technical services, such as computing infrastructure, data storage or genome analysis.

At its core, 100kGP is a vehicle through which the government can build a database and capabilities to analyse the data that can lead to health benefits and stimulate economic growth. Indeed, when launching the project in 2012, then-Prime Minister David Cameron stated his government's desire 'to see the emergence of genomic platforms in the UK that ... support the emergence of new companies and innovations' leading to the developments of 'valuable new products that are sold around the world'.[49]

8.4   Ethical Questions

The developments regarding care.data 2.0 and 100kGP validate Donna Dickenson's concern that: '*Me Medicine* is eclipsing what I call *We*

---

[47] Genomics England, 'FAQs about how we are working with industry' (2014), www.genomicsengland.co.uk/working-with-industry/working-with-industry-faqs, accessed 6 November 2017.

[48] Gabrielle Natalie Samuel and Bobbie Farsides, 'The UK's 100,000 Genomes Project: manifesting policymakers' expectations' (2017) 36(4) *New Genetics and Society* 336–53.

[49] Department of Business, Innovation and Skills (DBIS), 'Industrial strategy: government and industry in partnership. Strategy for UK life sciences. One year on' (2013), www.gov.uk/government/collections/industrial-strategy-government-and-industry-in-partnership, accessed 6 November 2017.

Medicine, so that we're losing sight of the notion that biotechnology can and should serve the common good'.[50] Without pretending to be exhaustive, in this section we will discuss three ethical issues that these schemes highlight.

8.4.1 Obfuscatory Language and Promissory Discourse

NHS England and Genomics England use the contentious terms 'personalised care' and 'personalised medicine'. The terms are often used interchangeably with 'precision medicine' and 'stratified medicine'[51]. Donna Dickenson has observed that:

> [O]ne meaning of personalized medicine that does seem genuinely beneficial [is] drug treatment tailored to the patient on an evidence-based model for better clinical care. Whether that's really personalized in the sense of *individualized*, however, is arguable ... individuals are classified into *groups* according to which allele (variant) of the relevant gene they have ... Even the biotechnology industry-linked Personalized Medicine Coalition concedes that pharmacogenetics is about population subgroup response to particular drugs.[52]

However, she also rightly remarks that 'Patients' enthusiasm for pharmacogenetics would take quite a hit if they saw it as a rationale for denying them therapy, but in an era of cost cutting, that's exactly what could happen.'[53]

Indeed, highly targeted 'personalised' drugs (i.e. 'Me Medicine' – helping me and people like me), available at huge mark-ups over the production costs, could reduce the strength of the population-wide 'safety net' ('We Medicine') that is the NHS. What's more, personalised care could lead to an even more fragmented NHS. In an ethnographic study exploring the translation of stratified medicine into a London cancer centre, Day and colleagues found that:

> [S]tratified medicine placed additional strains on the service through its requirement for a highly-skilled workforce and a meticulously integrated patient pathway that, in the context of budget constraints, were difficult to deliver. Highly-skilled staff have moved increasingly to back-office functions such as laboratory analysis [and] replaced in frontline functions by

---

[50] Dickenson, *Me Medicine vs We Medicine*, p. 2.
[51] Sara Day, R. Charles Coombes and Louise McGrath-Lone, 'Stratified, precision or personalised medicine? Cancer services in the "real world" of a London hospital' (2017) 39 *Sociology of Health and Illness* 143–58.
[52] Dickenson, *Me Medicine vs We Medicine*, p. 8. [53] Ibid., p. 75.

less qualified staff following the protocols of the new medicine ... [T]his recalibration of staff roles has enabled hospitals to trim budgets and carry on, but staff and patients alike reported increasing fragmentation and particular difficulties in coordinating the steps along a pathway ... [M]easures to improve coordination and navigation ... do not always work, with the result that some patients describe care that is far from personalised.[54]

Echoing Day's findings, Samuel and Farsides highlight 'the pitfalls of unfulfilled promissory genohype' around the 100kGP. They found that staff at, or working with, Genomics England, felt that policymakers driving the project had 'grandiose expectations': implementation brought several organisational tensions, for example, about whether the 'cash-strapped busy' NHS and 'stressed and busy' staff not trained in genomics would be capable of delivering the project. Other participants felt that the political rhetoric surrounding the project, and the fact that an 'entrepreneurial company' was responsible for the project, was a positive force – mobilising the project and overcoming so-called clinical inertia. As one participant said, 'The objective was ... to drive this fast ... and not to give people time to downgrade it'.[55] Along similar, but less positive, lines, a *Lancet* editorial from 2017 about the UK Chief Medical Officer's report cites research that whole-genome sequencing is unlikely to benefit day-to-day care and argues that the NHS might not be the right place to mainstream genomic medicine because it is struggling to deliver even basic services.[56]

The promissory discourse that is so prevalent in relation to both care. data and 100kGP is particularly problematic in view of the multiple unanswered questions and epistemological challenges that surround Big Data projects in biomedicine. These challenges imply fundamental questions regarding the scientific utility and validity of these types of projects, and each of the epistemological problems also has ethical implications.[57] All these problems simply remain unmentioned, so as not to threaten the hype, it would seem.

[54] Day, Coombes and McGrath-Lone, 'Stratified, precision or personalised medicine?', p. 154.
[55] Samuel and Farsides, 'The UK's 100,000 Genomes Project'.
[56] Editorial, 'Public genomes: the future of the NHS?' (2017) 390 *The Lancet* 203.
[57] We do not have the space here to elaborate on this, but for particularly interesting discussions of the problems involved, see, for example, John Ioannidis, 'Informed consent, big data, and the oxymoron of research that is not research' (2013) 13(4) *American Journal of Bioethics* 40–2; Wendy Lipworth, Paul Mason, Ian Kerridge et al., 'Ethics and epistemology in big data research' (2017) 14(4) *Journal of Bioethical Inquiry* 489–500;

8.4.2   The Ethical (In)Defensibility of the Consent Models

As we have hinted at above, the 'consent' model for care.data 2.0 is hugely problematic. The consent model in 100kGP has some shortcomings, but the project is much more limited in scope.

8.4.2.1   The Opt-Out Model Recommended by the Caldicott Review

The Privacy Impact Assessment of care.data undertaken by NHS England (NHS England 2014) made it clear that the GP data of those registering an opt-out *would* be passed to the HSCIC and would most likely be used in research to which those patients have not consented:

> Where patients have objected to the flow of their personal confidential data from the general practice record, the HSCIC will receive clinical data without any identifiers attached ... If a patient is (a) content for personal confidential data from their GP record to be extracted into the secure environment of the HSCIC but (b) objects to flows of personal confidential data from the HSCIC ... then the HSCIC will extract the fact of the objection, the date of the objection and the individual's NHS number. The NHS number will be used internally within the HSCIC to match these data to other data held for that patient *so that the data can be anonymised before release.*[58] (emphasis added)

In this context, 'anonymisation' actually meant 'pseudonymisation', a 'technique that replaces identifiers with a pseudonym that uniquely identifies a person', i.e. what is frequently called 'coding' of health data. Astoundingly, what is being said here is that a patient's wish that their confidential information is *not* extracted or used, is respected by extracting and using the data anyway, but in pseudonymised form. This is not what the average person understands by 'opting out' – arguably, people understand this as meaning that their data *will not be used in any way.* Little has changed in the wake of the Caldicott Report since the recommended opt-outs relate only to 'confidential patient information', and, as mentioned in Section 8.2.4 ('Has the GDPR Any Effect?'), data collected by NHS Digital and de-identified is not considered to be confidential patient information. In other words, the opt-out is not actually an opt-out. This scheme is simply care.data 2.0.

This is ethically problematic. As argued by bioethicist Julian Savulescu:

> Each [mature] person has values, plans, aspirations, and feelings about how that life should go. People have values which may collide with research goals ... To ask a person's permission to do something to that person is to involve her actively and to give her the opportunity to make the project a part of her plans. When we involve people in our projects without their consent we use them as a means to our own ends.[59]

This illustrates why the care.data consent model amounts to a violation of people's autonomy. The principle of respect for autonomy is based on the principle of respect for persons.[60] Respecting people implies that they should be offered ethically appropriate and clearly understandable ways to consent (or not) to have their health records included in central databases. Except for purely privacy-related concerns, de-identification of health data *cannot* overcome any of the important ethical concerns that many people have about the creation and use of databases and/or tissue banks for research purposes.[61] For example, various studies indicate that people may consider commercial uses to be at odds with their original motivation to participate in research *even* when they explicitly agreed to take part in research.[62]

---

[59] Julian Savulescu, 'For and Against: No consent should be needed for using leftover body material for scientific purposes. Against' (2000) 325 *British Medical Journal* 648–9, p. 649.

[60] National Commission for the Protection of Human Subjects of Biomedical and Behavioral Research, *The Belmont Report – Ethical Principles and Guidelines for the Protection of Human Subjects of Research* (1979) www.hhs.gov/ohrp/regulations-and-policy/belmont-report/index.html, accessed 6 November 2017.

[61] NBAC, 'Research Involving Human Biological Materials: Ethical Issues and Policy Guidance (Executive Summary)' (1999) https://bioethicsarchive.georgetown.edu/nbac/hbm_exec.pdf, accessed 6 November 2017; Kristof Van Assche, Serge Gutwirth and Sigrid Sterckx, 'Protecting dignitary interests of biobank research participants: lessons from *Havasupai Tribe* v. *Arizona Board of Regents*' (2013) 5 (1) *Law, Innovation and Technology* 54–84. At most, anonymisation might offer protection with regard to privacy, although various studies suggest that even this cannot be guaranteed. Genome data pose a high risk of re-identification. This is doubly problematic since genome data have implications for the patient *and* her family members. Melissa Gymrek, Amy L. McGuire, David Golan et al., 'Identifying personal genomes by surname inference' (2013) 6117 *Science* 321–4.

[62] Tore Nilstun and Göran Hermerén, 'Human tissue samples and ethics–attitudes of the general public in Sweden to biobank research' (2006) 9(1) *Medicine Health Care and Philosophy* 81–6; John Arne Skolbekken, Lars Ø. Ursin, Berge Solberg et al., 'Not worth the paper it's written on? Informed consent and biobank research in a Norwegian context' (2005) 15 *Critical Public Health* 335–47.

8.4.2.2 The Consent Model Underlying 100kGP

Policymakers are using the 100kGP model as a starting point to design an appropriate approach to consent for NHS genomic medicine services. At the time of writing, this approach was still in development.[63] It remains to be seen whether broad consent, i.e. consent for unspecified and unknown research, and the entwinement of consent for the clinical aspect (e.g. a primary diagnosis) and research will be carried forward. Broad consent could be argued to be morally justified in the name of 'We Medicine': seeking consent for individual studies could slow down research of potential social value. However, the question arises as to how the potential for benefit to the common good of any research project can be assessed. Without an answer to this question, it is difficult to justify the use of broad consent on the grounds of the common good. Further questions arise, such as how public and individual interests can be balanced and who should carry out these balancing exercises. In 100kGP, Genomics England's Access Review Committee[64] takes on this role. It is up to NHS England to decide whether such a committee should continue to exist post-100kGP.

As we will discuss next, notions of altruism and solidarity are sometimes invoked in arguments supporting broad consent. Caulfield and Kaye have pointed out that there is a danger of conflating the idea that people want to participate in a project 'altruistically' – in the name of the common good – with the idea that the ethical and legal norm (i.e. consent) should be altered in its service.[65] Interestingly, some research suggests that the public and patients *do not* see broad consent as acceptable. A systematic review of studies from the USA showed that participants preferred tiered or specific forms of consent, and were less supportive when data could be shared with pharmaceutical companies.[66] Moreover, one survey of over 1000 participants found that initial support for broad consent diminished once specific types of controversial research (e.g. including research into safer abortion methods,

[63] Becki Bennett, 'What does consent mean for Generation Genome?' (2017) *BioNews*, 18 September, www.bionews.org.uk/page_886840.asp, accessed 6 November 2017.

[64] Chaired by Professor Jonathan Knowles, who is also chairman of the board of Adappimunne Ltd and Immunocore Ltd, two UK-based biotechnology companies.

[65] Tim Caulfield and Jane Kaye, 'Broad consent in biobanking: reflections on seemingly insurmountable dilemmas' (2009) 10 *Medical Law International* 85–100.

[66] Nanibaa' A. Garrison, Nila A. Sathe, Armand H. Matheny Antommaria et al., 'A systematic literature review of individuals' perspectives on broad consent and data sharing in the United States' (2016) 18(7) *Genetics in Medicine* 663–71.

xenotransplantation and, notably, research that would lead to patents) were raised as a possibility.[67]

Other research has shown that the general public is generally positive towards medical research and is usually willing to participate without expecting any personal benefit.[68] However, the willingness to participate decreases if the benefits to society are unclear or if private profits might be derived.[69]

8.4.3   Appealing to Altruism: Furthering a Neoliberal Political Agenda?

Donna Dickenson identifies corporate interests and political neoliberalism as one of the key drivers of 'Me Medicine'. Neoliberalism includes making significant cuts in public spending while at the same time increasing the involvement of private corporations in areas such as healthcare, education and scientific research (and outsourcing from the public to the private sector of an increasing number of services).[70] With regard to biomedicine and healthcare, the neoliberal nature of the political agenda is very clear.

For health services, the agenda translates into the following stratification:

(a) to keep the voters happy, a basic, low-level service should be paid for by the state;

(b) a higher-level service should be available to those who pay, directly or via insurance;

---

[67] Raymond G. De Vries, Tom Tomlinson, H. Myra Kim et al., 'The moral concerns of biobank donors: the effect of non-welfare interests on willingness to donate' (2016) 12 *Life Sciences, Society and Policy* 3.

[68] Dianne Nicol and Christine R. Critchley, 'Benefit sharing and biobanking in Australia' (2012) 21(5) *Public Understanding of Science* 534–55.

[69] Christine R. Critchley, Dianne Nichol, Margaret F. A. Otlowski et al., 'Predicting intention to biobank: a national survey' (2012) 22 *European Journal of Public Health* 139–44; Åsa Kettis-Lindblad, Lena Ring, Eva Viberth et al., 'Genetic research and donation of tissue samples to biobanks. What do potential sample donors in the Swedish general public think?' (2006) 16(4) *European Journal of Public Health* 433–40; Saskia C. Sanderson, Michael A. Diefenbach, Randi Zinberg et al., 'Willingness to participate in genomics research and desire for personal results among underrepresented minority patients: a structured interview study' (2013) 4(4) *Journal of community genetics* 469–82; Wellcome Trust/IPSOS Mori, 'The One-Way Mirror'.

[70] Damien Cahill and Martijn Konings, *Neoliberalism* (Cambridge: Polity Press, 2017); Owen Jones, *The Establishment: And How They Get Away With It* (London: Allan Lane, 2014).

(c) extremely expensive services should be paid for by the state, but on a rationed basis;

(d) expensive infrastructure, for whatever purpose, should be paid for by the state; and

(e) value from the services provided by and infrastructure generated by the state should, as far as is possible, be channelled into the private arena.

Indeed, as Donna Dickenson observes, 'at the highest governmental levels, public backing has been solicited to underpin private-sector profit making from biotechnology'.[71] Moreover, '[the] public sector, as the entrepreneurial state, is being asked to sponsor the growth and shoulder the risks for the private sector'.[72]

Interestingly, two simultaneous trends can be observed in the UK: while healthcare and social care data are *centralised* for research purposes, the provision of healthcare itself is being *decentralised*. Indeed, accompanied by a narrative about building healthcare services 'around the needs of local populations', the UK government has announced the 'restructuring' of the NHS through so-called 'Sustainability and Transformation Plans' (STPs). A total of 44 geographical areas ('footprints') are created that need to develop strategic plans to rationalise services. This is arguably a further step in the process of dismantling the NHS as a *national* health service. The STPs, like care.data, suggest that 'sustainability' and economic growth have become the de facto social values. Moreover, 'Individuals, rather than organisations or public institutions, are forced to deal with the healthcare, social and financial consequences of ever-increasing and ambiguous data dissemination practices among entities they are not always aware of'.[73]

Yet, as we have hinted at in our discussion about broad consent, the neoliberal political agenda is veiled with references to benefits for all and altruism. For example, care.data was promoted by the UK government as a scheme that would 'improve the quality of care for all'.[74] In the case of the 100kGP, the message is that the project enhances altruism and that people who take part are altruistic. As Woods[75] has pointed out,

---

[71] Dickenson, *Me Medicine vs We Medicine*, p. 21.   [72] Ibid., p. 180.

[73] Vezyridis and Timmons, 'Dissenting from care.data'.

[74] NHS England webpage previously available at: www.england.nhs.uk/ourwork/tsd/care-data/better-care.

[75] Simon Woods, 'Big Data governance: solidarity and the patient voice' in Brent Mittelstadt and Luciano Floridi (eds.), *The Ethics of Biomedical Big Data* (Springer International, 2016), pp. 221–38.

Genomics England has used this rhetoric to rally the public to a common cause and to implicitly call upon their civic duty to endorse the project. In this way, 100kGP appeals to the best of 'We Medicine' (i.e. the production of wide social goods through the coming together of rare disease and cancer communities), and 'Me Medicine' (i.e. the chance of a precise diagnosis and treatments). It draws on the language of 'We Medicine', with the ultimate promise of (and hopes for immediate) 'Me Medicine'.

The frequent invoking of the principle of altruism echoes the discourses that have surrounded older healthcare and research ventures, such as National Blood Donation and UK Biobank. The form of altruism applied in such discourses was Richard Titmuss's (1970) 'gift relationship'. An altruistic act within a gift relationship is one that is voluntary and that has no expectation of return. 100kGP is purported to promote altruism and the people taking part are doing so because, at least in part, they are altruistic. Speaking to the *Financial Times*, Professor Mark Caulfield (Chief Scientific Officer) has assumed that the participants are well aware that few will see pharmaceutical benefits themselves: '[T]hey've enrolled on the principle that this is altruistic, and they don't expect any personal benefit. They're doing it because they want someone else to have a better chance than they did.'[76]

However, as we have said, the 100kGP does offer (although does not promise) clinical benefit. So is it accurate to say that people are participating to benefit others? It is likely that at least some are participating to get a diagnosis. Caulfield's assumption, and the references to altruism, thus seem inappropriate.

What function is this rhetoric about common good, civic duty and altruism serving? As others have argued with regard to the biobanks that came before 100kGP, it detracts from the role of industry and from concerns that participants might have about injustice in the research enterprise.[77] It also deflects from the glimmer of hope that there *will* be a diagnosis or a treatment (the 'Me Medicine' aspect). It masks the question as to whether, if new drugs come out of the project, the NHS will even be able to afford them if it is privatised further. This would be a clear

---

[76] Richard Hodson and Clive Cookson, 'NHS launches genetic sequencing centres to develop treatments' (2014) *Financial Times*, 22 December.

[77] Richard Tutton and Barbara Prainsack, 'Enterprising or altruistic selves? Making up research subjects in genetics research' (2011) 33(7) *Sociology of Health and Illness* 1081–95; Lars Ø. Ursin, 'Biobank research and the welfare state project: the HUNT story' (2010) 20(4) *Critical Public Health* 453–63.

loss for 'We Medicine' as a whole, and a win for 'Me Medicine' but only for those who can afford expensive treatments.

While the two schemes we discuss in this chapter purport to promote the common good, we would submit that fairness requires real benefit-sharing and not just rhetoric. The HSCIC reassures people that it will not make a profit from providing data to other organisations, but will only charge an access fee to cover its costs. While this may look unproblematic, what it means is that commercial companies are provided access to assets they have not themselves bought or created and are thus being given a quasi-free commercial boost by the UK government. However, to put NHS databases at the disposal of industry, without requiring a 'kickback' to enhance the service that the NHS is set up to provide, is inappropriate. The mere fact that a new drug might reach the market is not sufficient to count as benefit-sharing with UK citizens, since this benefit (the new drugs) is then also available for citizens in other countries, whose health data has not been mined by the companies in question. Instead, the companies seeking access should be required to provide the NHS with reduced access costs for the resulting drugs or other health-related products. With data being collected from the UK population at the expense of the UK state, we are talking about a concealed Public Private Initiative: something which should not be entered into unless the benefits to the private party are at least balanced by the benefits to the public as a whole.

8.5   Concluding Remarks: Trust versus Trustworthiness

The huge controversy surrounding the care.data scheme clearly showed that the various misleading elements of the scheme undermined citizens' trust. The Caldicott Review[78] and the UK Chief Medical Officer's report[79] rightly mention repeatedly that trust is essential for making any such scheme work. However, we should emphasise that there is a difference between *being trusted* and *meriting trust (i.e. being trustworthy)*. In order to merit any trust, those who acquire health data ought to make sure that they respect the autonomy of individuals whom they expect to *entrust* them with their health data.

Does the 'architecture' proposed by the Caldicott Review and the Chief Medical Officer's report represent a scheme that is trustworthy?

---

[78] Caldicott, 'Review of Data Security, Consent and Opt-outs'.
[79] Davies, 'Generation Genome'.

Transparency is a crucial prerequisite, both for trust and trustworthiness. Regarding care.data 2.0, unfortunately, the misleading and obfuscation continue. In spite of all the Caldicott Review's talk about opt-outs, it is clear that the scheme *is not in fact based on an opt-out regime*, since, as explained above, a patient's wish that their confidential information is *not* extracted or used, is met by extracting and using the data in de-identified form. This makes a mockery of the claim that people can opt out. If somebody opts out, that should mean that their data are simply *not extracted and used*, i.e. HSCIC should receive no data, not even in 'de-identified' form.

It is clear from NHS England's response to Caldicott and from NHS Digital's draft target architecture from July 2017 that NHS England is intent on pressing ahead with care.data 2.0 with a fig-leaf of a national opt-out and the illusory regional fragmentation of the National Data Lake it so desperately wants to create. Health data is to be conscripted regardless.

The consent model underlying the 100kGP arguably might be ethically defensible, on the grounds that the research might promote the common good. However, it is not clear how 'common good' will be defined by policymakers and how the involvement of industry will affect the nature and the extent of any benefits to society. As we have discussed, appeals to altruism can be a thin veil for the neoliberal drive behind 'Me Medicine' schemes and the drastic impact they could have for the NHS and its users. As Dickenson points out, there is a danger that, eventually, people will 'perceive that their altruism is being exploited by commercialisation'.[80] Those who feel exploited will have little recourse, as a commenter on *The Times* newspaper's coverage of the NHS 'National Data Lake' has pointed out:

> [O]nly the very wealthy have a choice as to whether they want a relationship with the NHS . . . however much someone may dislike or distrust the NHS, they cannot seek medical treatment elsewhere. The NHS may want to appear to encourage people to be altruistic . . . but they come very close to compelling rather than promoting the altruism. We are being asked to sign up to the rules of a club that most of us cannot leave.[81]

---

[80] Dickenson, *Me Medicine vs We Medicine*, p. 199.

[81] R. Moss, Comment on article by Kat Lay, 'NHS to share opt-out patients' data' (2017) *The Times*, 19 September.

Clearly, care.data 2.0 and the 100kGP are using the NHS 'brand' to generate trust in a health service that looks very different to the one set up after WWII. However, trust should be merited and not manufactured for the sake of generating support for whatever projects the government wishes to implement.

9

My Genome, My Right

STUART HOGARTH, JULIAN COCKBAIN AND SIGRID
STERCKX

'Everyone has the right to access and understand their personal genetic
information ... It's amazing to me it's so controversial that you should be
able to get your genetic information.'[1]

'The imaginary of rights is gradually replacing social justice. The decolo-
nization struggles, the civil rights and counter-cultural movements fought for
an ideal society based on justice and equality. In the human rights age, the
pursuit of collective material welfare has given way to individual gratification
and the avoidance of evil.'[2]

9.1 Introduction

The growing number of firms offering direct-to-consumer genetic testing
(DTCGT) has prompted commentary from scientists, clinicians, bioethi-
cists and ELSI scholars. Those critical of this nascent consumer industry
have expressed concerns about, inter alia, the absence of evidence supporting the utility of DTCGT, the vulnerability of the public to misleading advertising claims and the appropriateness of marketing tests direct
to the consumer.

But even amongst those sceptics who believe that the business models
of consumer genetics firms are as shaky as their scientific claims, there
can be little doubt that one notable success they have enjoyed has been to
shift the terms of public debate about genetic testing. In the face of a
variety of efforts to regulate the consumer genetics industry, some firms
(and some of their customers and supporters) have asserted the principle
that individuals have a right to 'their genome'. This assertion has proved

---

[1] Anne Wojcicki quoted in Jason Madara, 'The extraction process: meet 23andMe's Anne
Wojcicki', *Wired* (6 March 2017), www.wired.co.uk/article/the-extraction-process,
accessed 28 January 2018.

[2] Costas Douzinas, 'The paradoxes of human rights' (2013) 20(1) *Constellations* 51–67.

extremely powerful, and its broad appeal requires us to pay it careful attention. What assumptions underpin the assertion of this genomic right? What might be its consequences? Should this putative right be seen as a legal right or a fundamental human right? What would be the implication of such a right for regulatory initiatives? What implications would it have for other forms of diagnostic testing? What other rights are invoked (implicitly or explicitly) in the policy debate about consumer genetics and what bearing do they have on any putative right to one's genome?

To understand what it is stake, it is necessary to provide some brief background on the DTCGT industry: the range of services it offers and its business models, the variety of regulatory responses the nascent sector has generated and the commentary such initiatives have provoked.

Given this book's focus on medicine and public health, we shall focus on firms that offer health-related testing, but the industry is broader, encompassing paternity testing, ancestry testing and lifestyle testing, such as genes related to athletic ability. Before 2005, the first wave of health-related DTCGT firms largely focused on nutrigenetics, testing for genes linked to nutrient metabolism and providing tailored dietary recommendations or selling nutritional supplements; a second wave of firms launched around 2007 focused on offering polygenic risk tests for a range of common diseases such as asthma, diabetes and stroke. A recent survey[3] found 246 firms, but the industry comprises mostly small start-up firms with a high failure rate. Even 23andMe, the largest firm offering health-related testing, is still not profitable a decade after launch. 23andMe is notable for experimenting with multiple business models: in particular, it has tried to supplement income from test sales by leveraging its growing DNA database as a research platform for the pharmaceutical industry.

There have been two types of regulatory initiatives that have impacted on the DTCGT market. Legislation in a number of European countries has either banned or limited the availability of genetic tests that can be purchased without the involvement of a medical professional – such legislation is generally not focused solely on the issue of the DTCGT market but has aimed to provide a more general governance framework for genetic testing. Meanwhile in the USA, the Food and Drug

---

[3] Andelka M. Phillips, 'Only a click away – DTC Genetics for ancestry, health, love . . . and more: A view of the business and regulatory landscape' (2016) 8 *Applied & Translational Genomics* 16–22.

Administration (FDA) has policed the sector through a series of warning letters that culminated in November 2013 in action against 23andMe, the most high-profile firm, when the FDA shut down the health-related portion of its testing service.

The FDA's intervention in the DTCGT market was characterised by some commentators as premature,[4] an overreaction[5] or even an infringement of the constitutional right of freedom of speech.[6] The most impassioned responses to the FDA's 2013 action against 23andMe invoked the language of genomic rights and framed the issue as a Manichean conflict between the state and market, with the latter as the guarantor of individual freedom. This position was articulated in *Forbes* magazine by Harry Binswanger, a director of the Ayn Rand Institute: 'The real issue is not the reliability of these tests. The real issue is the right of an individual to act on his own judgment, free of government coercion.'[7]

9.2 The Right to One's Genome

Just what might the widely claimed right to one's genome actually mean? A human right or a legal right? A right in relation to the information carried by the genome or a right to the chemical material itself? A right to own, to access, to exclude, or to use and provide to others?

The claim that people have a right to their genomes is only clear if one establishes which right is being claimed, and particularly whether the subject matter of the claim is material or information. Several commentators making the general claim of a right to one's genome simply conflate the material and the information.[8]

The material is a rivalrous good, one that cannot be shared, and thus potentially the basis for and covered by a claim to 'self-ownership'.

---

[4] Barbara Prainsack, Jenny Reardon, Richard Hindmarsh et al., 'Personal genomes: misdirected precaution' (2008) 456 *Nature* 34–5.

[5] Caroline F. Wright, Alison Hall and Ron L. Zimmern, 'Regulating direct-to-consumer genetic testing: what is the fuss about?' (2011) 13(4) *Genetic Medicine* 295–300.

[6] Robert C. Green and Nita A. Farahany, 'Regulation: the FDA is overcautious on consumer genomics' (2014) 505 *Nature* 286–7.

[7] Harry Binswanger, 'FDA says, "No gene test for you: You can't handle the truth"', *Forbes* (26 November 2013), www.forbes.com/sites/harrybinswanger/2013/11/26/fda-says-no-gene-test-for-you-you-cant-handle-the-truth/#221c75d74156, accessed 28 January 2018.

[8] Michele Loi, 'Nobody's DNA but mine' (2017) *Journal of Medical Ethics*. doi:10.1136/medethics-2017-104188.

The information is a non-rivalrous good, i.e. one that can be and is shared, and one therefore that requires very special reasons for permitting ownership and control rights. Thus, for example, society does occasionally permit short-term ownership and control rights of some non-rivalrous goods (e.g. inventions and unpublished data). Since the information may be shared by more than one person, there can be no question of an ownership right. Equally, since sharing that information with others, e.g. by publishing it, may harm the interests of those having the same genetic sequences, we consider that the 'right to your genome' cannot be an unrestricted right to use the information. For the purposes of this chapter we will therefore consider the 'right' at maximum to be a human right to access your genetic information.

The idea of an inviolable right to access information regarding your genome plays on the concept that your DNA is the key to your personal identity, the genetic blueprint that defines your essential individuality. However, in the post-genomic age, attention has moved beyond the genome to the epigenome, the metabolome, the proteome and the microbiome. Are these new 'omic' sciences creating new rights? In this chapter we suggest that genomes constitute collectives as well as individuals; that genomics is a field replete with tensions between individual rights and collective rights; and that an individual's exercise of her rights needs to be constrained by regulators (rather than self-regulation) to protect those rights of others which trump the individual's rights.

What can an individual be allowed to do with their genetic information once they have received it? Can access to parts of it be denied when there is concern that the individual might suffer from or abuse that information? These questions stem particularly from the right of others to privacy, since genomic information, unlike genetic material (i.e. the physical thing), is not unique to the person. Admittedly, the entirety of your genomic information is unique to you, but relevant and concerning parts of it are shared with others, in particular your relatives and your community.

We thus need to distinguish between:[9]

– A: an individual who wishes to order a DTC test
– 'not A': everybody else (including regulators and the state)
– 'B': individuals who are not A, but who are sufficiently closely related to A that they share a greater degree of (presumable) informational

---

[9] See Wendy Elizabeth Bonython and Bruce Baer Arnold, 'Direct to consumer genetic testing and the libertarian right to test' (2017) *Journal of Medical Ethics*. doi: 10.1136/medethics-2017-104188.

commonality between their genome and the genome of A due to genetic or geographic relatedness than the degree of commonality in the general population.

The interests of 'B' are crucial yet seem to be overlooked by many commentators.

9.3 Human Rights

How might the idea of a right to access or own one's genomic data fit within our existing systems of rights? We might begin by considering this putative right in relation to the Universal Declaration of Human Rights (UDHR),[10] and here we consider two rights: the right to healthcare and the right to access scientific knowledge.

9.3.1 The Right to Healthcare

If we address first the health-related aspects of DTCGT, then the relevant provision would seem to be Article 25 UDHR:

> Everyone has the right to a standard of living adequate for the health and well-being of himself and of his family, including food, clothing, housing and medical care and necessary social services.[11]

To what extent would this right be relevant to DTCGT? Many firms have sought to distance themselves from the world of medical care, arguing that what they offer is 'recreational genomics' or 'lifestyle genomics'. This rhetorical strategy is primarily a form of regulatory arbitrage, intended to provide cover from regulatory agencies like the US Food and Drug Administration (FDA), but if taken at face value, it would appear to exclude the DTCGT firms that adopt such terminology from any consideration that their services might fall under Article 25 UDHR. Further, since many firms offer polygenic risk assessment for common diseases, and this type of testing has not been shown to be clinically useful, let alone medically necessary, it is not clear that even if such tests are marketed as medical care, that they meet the test of something necessary to ensuring health and well-being. Failing such a test would make it

---

[10] Universal Declaration of Human Rights (1948), www.un.org/en/universal-declaration-human-rights, accessed 29 January 2018.
[11] Universal Declaration of Human Rights.

difficult to envisage this portion of DTCGT as part of a right to healthcare.

Article 25 UHDR seems to be more relevant for genetic tests that are deemed clinically useful, such as the carrier testing that 23andMe offers for a range of singe-gene diseases. However, even medically necessary products may not be available direct-to-consumer. For instance, in many jurisdictions essential medicines such as antibiotics and powerful pain-killers are only available via prescription. There is no public outcry about this situation, and this tacit acceptance of the intermediary role played by healthcare professionals in the provision of essential medicines suggests that people understand the distinction between the principle that access to a public good, such as clean drinking water, should be considered a universal human right, and the question of how that right is delivered. Further, many would defend the principle that equitable access to such public goods is best guaranteed by giving the state a monopoly on provision, rather than by relying on the private sector. The UK Human Genetics Commission's (HGC) report Genes Direct supported the prin-ciple of state provision:

> We feel strongly that there should be a well-funded NHS genetics service supported by a genetically literate primary care work force, which can properly manage and allow access to new predictive genetic tests that are being developed. This could involve the NHS providing ready access to testing services provided by commercial testing laboratories. It would enable predictive genetic testing to be retained within a well-respected model of continuing healthcare.[12]

State provision, it should be made clear, is not only a model for ensuring access but also for evaluating what is medically necessary. In the context of the UK, for instance, new genetic tests are evaluated by the UK Genetic Testing Network in order to decide whether they should be available on the NHS and to which patients. This evaluative process is a first level of gatekeeping, but even if the test becomes available, then a clinician must be persuaded that you meet the relevant clinical criteria before she will order the test. In the clinical context of a public healthcare system, access to technological resources must be rationed, and diagnostic tests, of any sort, cannot be ordered simply to satisfy scientific curiosity.

Nevertheless, the HGC's view that medically necessary genetic testing should be available on the UK's National Health Service (NHS), delivered through a publicly funded health service open to all citizens, offers a

---

[12] Human Genetics Commission, Genes Direct (London: Department of Health, 2003).

model of how to ensure the human right enshrined in Article 25 UDHR within an equitable framework founded on the principle of social solidarity rather than relying on market-based satisfaction of human rights through costly consumer services.

As noted earlier, much of the rhetoric of FDA critics suggests a Manichean conflict between the market and the state. It is no surprise then, to discover that Anne Wojcicki, 23andMe's CEO and the most high-profile advocate of genomic rights, is a sceptic about public healthcare systems and believes that consumers should pay directly for medical services. A 2012 article in the UK newspaper *The Times* reported that Wojcicki does not believe in free public healthcare systems like the UK National Health Service: 'I support a monetised system, but one that emphasises prevention and more freedom to choose'.[13] Thus we can see how the assertion of an individual's right to access her genome is predicated on a neoliberal philosophy that disconnects negative rights (to be free from state interference) from positive rights (such as access to publicly funded healthcare). As Jane Mummery characterises the neoliberal refashioning of democracy:

> Having disconnected freedom from social justice, neoliberalism must also reject all ideas and practices of social or distributive justice ... in framing democracy merely as a mechanism for the attainment of individual freedom, neoliberalism can have no understanding of the political and social ends that democracy might serve.[14]

It is in this context that we have to understand how the term 'democracy' is being operationalised when 23andMe claims that it is 'democratizing genomics' (and the hostility of many DTCGT advocates to FDA regulation). However, in response to Wojcicki's neoliberal vision of how to guarantee genomic rights, we might suggest that a right becomes a privilege when it is dependent on a certain level of disposable income – clean drinking water is a political right; bottled mineral water is a consumer luxury. Viewed in this way, it becomes clear that DTCGT could lead to the denial, rather than the protection, of human rights and that state-funded healthcare provision can act as a guarantor of the human right to necessary medical care.

[13] Anne Wojcicki in Tim Teeman, 'Married to Mr Google', *The Times* (4 February 2012), www.thetimes.co.uk/article/married-to-mr-google-nc6qc5znkwt, accessed 20 February 2018.

[14] Jane Mummery, *Radicalising Democracy for the 21st Century* (Abingdon: Routledge, 2017), p. 153.

9.3.2 The Right to Scientific Knowledge

Shifting from the realm of medical necessity and returning to the realm of 'informational' or 'recreational' genomics, a claim frequently made by firms like 23andMe is that they are providing consumers with an opportunity to become familiar with genomic science. In this regard, we might consider the relevance of Article 27 UDHR, which states:

> Everyone has the right freely to participate in the ... cultural life of the community, to enjoy the arts and to share in scientific advancement and its benefits.[15]

For many, the rhetorical allure of the assertion of an individual's right to access her genome lies in the emotional appeal of its underlying assumptions: the Baconian belief that knowledge is power, and the idea that the free circulation of knowledge is fundamental to democratic societies. One immediate line of argument in response to this reasoning would be the one outlined above – that a premium-priced consumer service is not the optimal means to ensure equitable access to something that is a universal human right. A second approach is to critically evaluate the pedagogic role played by DTCGT firms. Notwithstanding Balzer's argument[16] that the contemporary overuse of the term 'curation' has rendered it meaningless, we might suggest that the principal role of DTCGT firms is curatorial – they select from amongst the plethora of novel genotype/phenotype associations those that they deem worthy of reporting to their consumers. This was certainly the model of firms like 23andMe and Navigenics, which launched around 2007: these firms mined the data emerging from the new wave of genome wide association studies (GWAS) to identify genetic risk markers that could be combined together to create polygenic risk scores for a range of diseases like asthma, diabetes and stroke.

However, polygenic risk scores have been subject to considerable scientific critique that brings into question the legitimacy of the pedagogic claims advanced by DTCGT firms. The DTCGT sector has been the target of considerable criticism and has become a lightning rod for broader concerns about the regulation of genetic testing. There are three broad areas of concern about the DTCGT market:

---

[15] Universal Declaration of Human Rights.

[16] David Balzer, *Curationism: How Curating Took Over the World and Everything Else* (London: Pluto Press, 2015).

1) **information provision:** information asymmetries are a classic justification for regulation and the challenges of consumer understanding
in a fast-moving and complex area of science are exacerbated by
failures in information provision by firms. For instance, in 2008 the
European Technology Assessment Group undertook a review of 38
companies offering genetic tests DTC. Using an evaluative framework
comprising a checklist of 12 criteria devised by Datta et al.,[17] it
assessed the quality of information provision and found that 55 per
cent of companies (21 out of 38) complied with four or fewer of the 12
criteria, and concluded that such 'fundamental information deficits
[had] ... possibly far-reaching consequences for consumers'.[18]

2) **test quality and marketing claims:** a series of academic papers argued
that: i) there was insufficient evidence to support the claims made by
many of the companies;[19] and ii) even amongst those firms which only
reported well-validated gene-disease associations there were major dis-
crepancies, with the same individual receiving different risk information
depending on which genetic markers are being tested for.[20]
Furthermore, the field was moving so quickly that a person's risk profile
could change repeatedly as new gene-disease associations were discovered.[21] A 2010 report by the US Government Accountability Office
(GAO) presented at a Congressional hearing summarised these concerns and quoted experts who argued that the genetics of common,
complex diseases was still a science in the making and that therefore
polygenic risk assessment lacked clinical utility.[22] The report concluded

[17] Adrija K. Datta, Tara J. Selman, Tony Kwok et al., 'Quality of information accompanying online marketing of home diagnostic tests' (2008) 101(1) *Journal of the Royal Society of
Medicine* 34–8.

[18] Leonhard Hennen, Arnold Sauter and Els van den Cruyce, *Direct to Consumer Genetic
Testing: Final Report* (Bonn: European Technology Assessment Group, 2009), p. 38.

[19] A. Cecile J. W. Janssens, Marta Gwinn, Linda A. Bradley et al., 'A critical appraisal of the
scientific basis of commercial genomic profiles used to assess health risks and personalize
health interventions' (2008) 82(3) *American Journal of Human Genetics* 593–9.

[20] Raluca Mihaescu, Mandy van Hoek, Eric J. G. Sijbrands et al., 'Evaluation of risk
prediction updates from commercial genome-wide scans' (2009) 11(6) *Genetic
Medicine.* 588–94; Pauline C. Ng, Sarah S. Murray, Samuel Levy et al., 'An agenda for
personalised medicine' (2009) 461 *Nature* 724–6.

[21] Mihaescu, van Hoek, Sijbrands et al., 'Evaluation of risk prediction updates from commercial genome-wide scans'.

[22] Government Accountability Office, *Direct-To-Consumer Genetic Tests: Misleading Test
Results Are Further Complicated by Deceptive Marketing and Other Questionable Practices*
(Washington, DC: Government Accountability Office, 2010), pp. 8–9.

that DTCGT firms were misleading a public that lacked the scientific expertise to assess the veracity of companies' claims.

3) **service quality**: although tests for susceptibility to common diseases have been the mainstay of the DTCGT market, some companies offer more traditional clinical genetic tests to consumers, reporting on a range of monogenic disorders. Here the concern is not the lack of clinical validation, but the lack of medical supervision and pre- and post-test counselling.

Translated into the language of rights, the first two concerns are couched in terms that appeal to statutory consumer rights long established in most, if not all, jurisdictions with mature mass-consumer markets: the right to adequate disclosure of information before the purchase of a service, and the right to expect that goods and services will meet certain pre-established standards. The third of the regulatory concerns outlined above speaks to issues of professional monopoly and the demarcation of certain services as the preserve of appropriately qualified professionals. We will address these issues in turn, dealing with the first two together, before moving on to the third.

9.4 Regulation of Information

The widespread misgivings about whether DTCGT firms could be relied upon as curators of genomic science impelled the FDA to take regulatory action, even as the agency expressed support for the principle that consumers have a right to access their genomic data:

> We don't have an issue with people getting their own DNA data ... We just have concerns with how it's being interpreted ... People have every right to get their data ... We want to make sure they can trust what they're being told about it, too.[23]

After the FDA shut down 23andMe's health-related testing service in 2013, Robert Green and Nita Farahany questioned whether the type of information that the firm offered consumers could really be classed as medical and whether the FDA might be in breach of the First Amendment of the US Constitution, which protects both 'the rights of

---

[23] Alberto Gutierrez quoted in Diane Brady, 'Do genetic tests need doctors? FDA defends its challenge to 23andMe', *Bloomberg Businessweek* (27 November 2013), www.bloomberg .com/news/articles/2013–11–27/do-genetic-tests-need-doctors-fda-defends-its-chal lenge-to-23andme, accessed 29 January 2018.

individuals to receive information, and of "commercial speech".[24] Academic commentators like the lawyer Barbara Evans and the social scientist Jennie Reardon have invoked historical parallels to illustrate the importance of the principles at stake in the free flow of genetic information. Equating the completion of the Human Genome Project to the invention of the printing press, Evans compares contemporary disputes about access to the genomic 'Book of Life' to the debate about whether to translate the Bible into English so that it could be read by ordinary people.[25] Reardon connects the FDA's reaction to 23andMe's attempt to create a mass consumer market for genomic data to historic fears of mob rule undermining democracy.[26] Rather more pragmatically, Anne Wojcicki utilises the idea of information flows to question the very feasibility of regulation:

> If you get your genome done, you can ship it off to Canada or China or other places in the world and get an interpretation. So how do you regulate information? That's one of the issues. I'm not sure you can hold it back.[27]

The need to protect the free circulation of information is not a new argument against the FDA's role in regulating biomedical innovation. It is, moreover, an idea that is closely related to a fundamental tenet of neoliberal philosophy – the superiority of the market as a processor of information – and that links in turn to historic efforts by US neoliberals to undermine the legitimacy of FDA's authority. As Edward Nik-Khah has recently revealed,[28] the Chicago School of Economics has, since 1972, worked with the pharmaceutical industry to challenge the regulatory regime established by the 1962 Kefauver Amendment[29] to the US

---

[24] Robert C. Green and Nita A. Farahany, 'Regulation: the FDA is overcautious on consumer genomics' (2014) 505 *Nature* 286–7.

[25] Barbara J. Evans, 'The First Amendment right to speak about the human genome' (2014) 16(3) *University of Pennsylvania Journal of Constitutional Law* 549–63.

[26] Jenny Reardon, 'The "persons" and "genomics" of personal genomics' (2011) 8(1) *Personalized Medicine* 95–107.

[27] Robert Hof, '"We are going for change": A conversation with 23andMe CEO Anne Wojcicki', *Forbes* (15 August 2014), www.forbes.com/sites/roberthof/2014/08/15/we-are-going-for-change-a-conversation-with-23andme-ceo-anne-wojcicki/#5af96b275477, accessed 29 January 2018.

[28] Edward Nik-Khah, 'Neoliberal pharmaceutical science and the Chicago School of Economics' (2014) 44(4) *Social Studies of Science* 489–517.

[29] Drug Efficacy Amendment ('Kefauver Harris Amendment') PL 87–781 (10 October 1962).

Federal Food, Drug and Cosmetic Act (FD&C),[30] as what can be seen as part of a mobilisation by US industry against the broader rise of consumer protection regulations. In his contribution to the 1972 conference that inaugurated this assault on the FDA, Sam Peltzman, a leading member of the Chicago School of Economics, followed the classic neoliberal line in arguing that it was the marketplace that was most capable of generating new data on pharmaceuticals:

> His primary complaint about the 1962 Amendments was that they had in fact decreased the value of information available to consumers: FDA restrictions on pharmaceutical companies' claims would decrease the amount of information on non-sanctioned uses of drugs, while any reduction in marketing for a drug of a particular brand would reduce information about the drug type in general.[31]

Thus, in the absence of measured discussion of what regulation of the DTCGT market might look like in practice, the FDA's critics frequently simply conflated regulation with proscription and presented a stark choice between rights and regulation. However, to return to our analogy with the state's role in ensuring clean water supply as a human right, even those who advocate privatisation of water services might concede the need for state regulation to create a framework within which firms can operate (indeed the privatisation of public utilities has generally been accompanied by the establishment of state agencies to regulate the newly created markets). Regulators play a variety of functions in such markets, but two fundamental regulatory functions that are relevant here are the setting and enforcement of standards; it is precisely these functions that FDA has now performed in the DTCGT market in the course of approving two submissions from 23andMe. The first approval in 2015 covered carrier testing for a number of genetic diseases and the second was for a number of genetic risk tests (although not any polygenic risk scores). Each approval was accompanied by a special controls document, a regulatory guidance that established a new standard for validating this specific class of tests. These standards encompassed not only the scientific approach to validation of diagnostic accuracy, but also the evidentiary requirements for firms to

[30] Federal Food, Drug, and Cosmetic Act (FD&C).
[31] Sam Pelzman cited in Edward Nik-Khah, 'Neoliberal pharmaceutical science and the Chicago School of Economics' (2014) 44(4) *Social Studies of Science* 489–517.

demonstrate that consumers can understand the information they receive.[32]

9.5   Regulation through Professional Monopoly

Nonetheless, these recent approvals notwithstanding, FDA continues to restrict what 23andMe can offer. In relation to genetic risk assessment, the agency has not approved BRCA1/2 testing for breast cancer risk and has publicly stated that the potential consequences of positive BRCA results, in particular prophylactic mastectomy, are so serious that the test requires the involvement of healthcare professionals.[33] Again, to return to the analogy with the sale of medicines, what has been created is a mixed market in which some tests are available DTC and others can only be accessed via a clinician. This approach might seem like an appropriate balance of freedoms and protections to some, and has been implicit in the approach of most DTCGT firms, which have been highly selective in the types of genetic data they report to customers.

The prescription-only approach speaks to the issue of the quality of service provided, which was the third of the regulatory concerns outlined above, and in particular to issues of professional monopoly and the demarcation of certain services as the preserve of appropriately qualified professionals. Professional standard-setting is another a way to guarantee standards for consumers, but the recourse to professional monopoly as a means to ensure those standards has been attacked by DTCGT advocates as the protection of producer rights at the expense of consumer choice. In the neoliberal era, producer rights have increasingly been eclipsed by consumer rights; however, even Adam Smith, who was first to crown the consumer sovereign, stated that: 'Consumption is the sole end and purpose of all production and the welfare of the producer ought to be attended to, only so far as it may be necessary for promoting that of the consumer.'[34] Smith's assertion leaves open the possibility that producer

---

[32] Margaret Curnutte, 'Regulatory controls for direct-to-consumer genetic tests: A case study on how the FDA exercised its authority' (2017) 36(3) *New Genetics and Society* 209–26.

[33] Alberto Gutierrez in Diane Brady, 'Do genetic tests need doctors? FDA defends its challenge to 23andMe', *Bloomberg Businessweek* (27 November 2013), www.bloomberg .com/news/articles/2013-11-27/do-genetic-tests-need-doctors-fda-defends-its-chal lenge-to-23andme, accessed 29 January 2018.

[34] Adam Smith, *Wealth of Nations* (Oxford: Oxford University Press, 2008), p. 376.

rights may in some instances be a necessary guarantor of consumer rights.

Aside from the FDA's regulatory intervention in the US market, there are other legal restrictions that address the consumer diagnostics market and/or genetic testing in particular. Some states have limits on the legal right to purchase diagnostic tests without the involvement of a healthcare professional or have specific restrictions relating to genetic testing. A succession of policy reports in the last two decades has established a broad consensus on the standard of care for clinical genetic testing, including the need for informed decision-making, supported by appropriately qualified healthcare professionals (often encompassing genetic counselling), and the need to ensure rigorous, independent evaluation of tests before they enter routine clinical use. These ideas have been enshrined in transnational standards such as the Council of Europe's 2008 Additional Protocol to the Convention on Human Rights and Biomedicine, concerning Genetic Testing for Health Purposes, and the Organisation for Economic Cooperation and Development's 2007 Best Practice Guidelines for Quality Assurance in Molecular Genetic Testing.[35] However, both these documents state that not all genetic tests require the same standard of care. The need for the involvement of a healthcare professional in genetic testing is also enshrined in legislation in some EU member states, including France, Germany and Portugal, although there is no evidence of active enforcement[36] (it is also unclear how many states have implemented the standards set out in the OECD guidelines).

In the USA, state law also dictates whether healthcare provider authorisation is required to obtain a laboratory test, including a genetic test. Some states explicitly permit labs to deal directly with patients without authorisation from a healthcare provider for specific tests (such

---

[35] Council of Europe, Additional Protocol to the Convention on Human Rights and Biomedicine, concerning Genetic Testing for Health Purposes (2008) (CETS No. 203); OECD, Best Practice Guidelines for Quality Assurance in Molecular Genetic Testing (2007); Dolores Ibarreta and Stuart Hogarth, 'Quality issues in clinical genetic services: regulatory issues and international conventions' in Ulf Kristoffersson, Jörg Schmidtke and Jean-Jacques Cassiman (eds.), Quality Issues in Clinical Genetic Services (Dordrecht: Springer, 2010).

[36] Pascal Borry, Rachel E. van Hellemondt, Dominique Sprumont et al., 'Legislation in direct-to-consumer genetic testing in seven European countries' (2012) 20(7) European Journal of Human Genetics 715–21.

as cholesterol or pregnancy tests).[37] Other states, such as New York, explicitly proscribe all DTC testing, and still other states have no relevant legislation. Currently, 25 states and the District of Columbia permit DTC laboratory testing without restriction, whereas 13 categorically prohibit it. DTC testing for certain specified categories of tests is allowed in 12 states but it is not clear whether these laws would extend to genetic tests. In 2014, the Clinical Laboratories Amendments Act was amended to let patients request that test reports be sent to them, instead of or as well as to their physician. This amendment only applies to laboratories covered by the Health Insurance Portability and Accountability Act Privacy Rule and is designed to give patients 'control of their personal health information'.

> Upon request by a patient (or the patient's personal representative), the laboratory may provide patients, their personal representatives, and those persons specified under 45 CFR 164.524(c)(3)(ii), as applicable, with access to completed test reports that, using the laboratory's authentication process, can be identified as belonging to that patient.[38]

9.6 Conclusion

This chapter has addressed two fundamental aspects of the debate about genomic rights: the assumption that a right to one's genome trumps other rights and the framing of regulatory intervention as a Manichean conflict between state and market. Much of the preceding discussion might be considered as an exploration of conflicting genomic rights – the right to unfettered access to information regarding one's genome conflicts with legislation and regulations designed to safeguard other rights. The FDA's regulation of DTCGT firms has sought to ensure that consumers rights have access to clear and comprehensive information in the testing process. Documents such as the OECD Guidelines and the Council of Europe's Additional Protocol that emphasise the need for the involvement of a healthcare professional with genetic expertise in the pre- and post-test processes of deciding to order a test and then

---

[37] Genetics and Public Policy Center, *Survey of Direct-to-Consumer Testing Statutes and Regulations* (Washington, DC: Genetics and Policy Center, 2007), https://repository .library.georgetown.edu/bitstream/handle/10822/511162/DTCStateLawChart.pdf? sequence=1&isAllowed=y, accessed 29 January 2018.
[38] 42 CFR 493.1291(l).

interpreting, and acting upon the test results, can be seen as establishing the individual's right to a certain standard of care.

Thus, there is the question of whether the right to access information regarding one's genome is absolute and inalienable or whether it must take its place somewhere within a field of overlapping and sometimes conflicting rights, taking precedence over some but outranked by others. Furthermore, in practical terms, the ability to exercise this right is limited by the availability of genetic testing. As noted above, in public healthcare systems, access to genetic testing must be balanced against other clinical priorities. The individual's right to access to information regarding their genome might be outranked by the collective right to prioritise healthcare spending.

But what if the individual is willing to spend their own money on buying a genetic test from a private provider? Here we return to the issue of the conflict between the right to exercise autonomy as a consumer in a market and the right of consumers/patients to enjoy a collectively defined standard of care (and of course such standards are always collectively defined). Absent the collective enforcement of this standard of care, then consumers are vulnerable to those wishing to offer cheaper testing services which may not be of the same quality. Would it be an unacceptable breach of autonomy to regulate the commercial genetics market to ensure certain standards, keeping out companies which do not meet those standards? We would submit that the assertion of the autonomous individual's right to access their genomic information does not preclude the possibility of legitimate forms of state intervention in the consumer genetics market.

In sum, we would suggest that, given its relevance to healthcare, an individual has a human right to access to their genomic information, but that this is a negative rather than a positive right and is subject to reasonable state regulation. The right extends to a right to control access to and use of genomic information derived from the individual, and to limit publication of genomic information from close relatives. However, the right does not equate to *ownership* of data. In view of the corresponding rights of others, the individual's right cannot extend to an unlimited right to publish their genomic information.

The complex interplay of individual and collective rights and the question of the state's role in establishing and enforcing such rights illustrates the inadequacy of the state/market dichotomy that underpins much criticism of regulatory initiatives in this field. Such rhetoric is not uncommon amongst DTCGT firms like 23andMe, which are part of a

Silicon Valley culture of disruptive innovation and operate with a business model predicated on regulatory arbitrage and a hostility to government fuelled by the libertarian anti-statism of Ayn Rand, a key intellectual inspiration for many leading figures in the West Coast technology sector.[39] Such anti-statism, redolent of an older tradition of Jeffersonian democracy, not only fails to translate well to Europe, but it perpetuates a misconception of American success as predicated on a weak federal government, a myth that is nowhere more apparent than in Silicon Valley, where industrial success has been heavily reliant on state funding for R&D.

In fact, public and private sector institutions are densely intertwined in the field of genomics. Much attention is focused at the moment on standards for genomic data and the respective roles of public and private actors in establishing standards and platforms for the sharing of scientific data. In the USA, the Obama administration's Precision Medicine initiative linked academic science, industrial R&D and the FDA together to pursue new standard-setting initiatives. The language of pipelines and flows draws us back to our analogy with the water supply. In contemporary society, we accept that some fundamental forms of physical infrastructure are best provided by the state, but in the nineteenth century there was considerable resistance to the right of the state to compel individual households to connect to a communal system for the supply of water and the disposal of human waste.

Consumer genomics companies already benefit from the free flow of scientific data from publicly funded research. The second wave of DTCGT firms including Navigenics and 23andMe that launched in 2007 did so on the back of the new wave of scientific data emerging from large, transnational genome wide association studies (GWAS) such as the Wellcome Trust Case Control Consortium.

The interpenetration and mutual dependence of state and market indicate the limitations of rights-based rhetoric that pits one against the other. As this chapter has demonstrated, the invocation of genomic rights is not a short cut to closure on deliberation about the complex trade-offs between different needs and interests. Instead it opens up a complex terrain on which can be mapped out a variety of positions and interests.

[39] Stuart Hogarth, 'Valley of the unicorns: Consumer genomics, venture capital and digital disruption' (2017) 36(3) *New Genetics and Society* 250–72.

10

'The Best Me I Can Possibly Be'

Legal Subjectivity, Self-Authorship and Wrongful Life
Actions in an Age of 'Genomic Torts'

BRITTA VAN BEERS

10.1 Introduction: 'Persons' in Personalised Medicine and 'Persons' in Law

Who is the person in personalised medicine? Terms such as 'personal genomics', 'personalised medicine' and 'Me Medicine'[1] each raise the question as to which concept of the person and of the self is at the root of these emerging medical-technological practices. Somewhat predictably, enthusiasts and sceptics of personalised medicine answer the question differently.

According to the 'believers', personalised medicine is able to do justice to the patient's biogenetic uniqueness and individuality. They point out that the abandonment of the traditional 'one size fits all' model of healthcare may result in new forms of patient empowerment and self-authorship. Their hope is not only that personalised medicine will enable targeted and more 'customised' types of medical treatment (e.g. pharmacogenetics), but also allow patients to make better informed health and lifestyle decisions, manage their own health data (e.g. personalised genetic testing) and even allow them to select or alter the genetic profile of their offspring (e.g. reproductive genetics). From this point of view, the fact that personalised medicine has in the meantime become intertwined with commercial interests, and even part of a burgeoning industry, is not necessarily a problem. Commercial genetic testing, for instance, could 'democratise DNA', in the words of Linda Avey (one of the founders of 23andMe), and

---

[1] Donna Dickenson, *Me Medicine vs We Medicine: Reclaiming Biotechnology for the Common Good* (New York, NY: Columbia University Press, 2013).

'take genetics out of the protective realm of the scientific community by making it accessible to the lay public'.[2]

However, according to those who are more sceptical of these promises, the emphasis within personalised medicine on the uniqueness, individuality and autonomy of the patient is mostly illusory, in many cases misplaced and in some cases even harmful. First, it could be said that personalised medicine is not truly about the individual, as the term suggests, but instead about genetic types, and thus about membership of genetic groups.[3] Second, critics fear that the concept of the person underlying personalised medicine is too biological. For instance, some point out that pharmacogenetic developments in oncology are better described with the phrase 'biology-driven medicine' than 'personalised medicine'.[4] Moreover, proper medical treatment not only involves knowledge of the patient's genetic profile, but also knowledge of one's personal circumstances, relations and narratives.[5] A third criticism is that the individualistic ideology underlying personalised medicine neglects the importance of more communal approaches in healthcare, as Donna Dickenson argues in her book *Me Medicine vs We Medicine* (2013).

In this chapter I offer a legal-philosophical contribution to the debate on the Me of Me Medicine. If we take personalised medicine's aspirations towards personal autonomy and empowerment seriously, the relevance of a legal perspective becomes visible immediately. As Jenny Reardon describes the ideal typical subject of personalised medicine:

> The preferred subject of human genomic variation research is no longer the 'vulnerable' isolated indigenous population but the 'empowered' person. This person is a rational individual, capable of self-governance and *imbued with rights* – centrally, the right to consume.[6] (emphasis added)

From this perspective, the person in personalised medicine is interconnected with law's understanding of the person as a bearer of legal rights and responsibilities. Indeed, it could be said that one of the reasons why

---

[2] Quoted in Jenny Reardon, 'The "persons" and "genomics" of personal genomics' (2011) 8 (1) *Personalized Medicine* 95–107.

[3] Dickenson, *Me Medicine vs We Medicine*, p. 8; Heather Widdows, *The Connected Self: The Ethics and Governance of the Genetic Individual* (Cambridge: Cambridge University Press, 2013), p. 44.

[4] F. Doz, P. Marvanne and A. Fagot-Largeault, 'The person in personalised medicine' (2013) 49 *European Journal of Cancer* 1159–1160.

[5] Barbara Prainsack, 'Personhood and solidarity: What kind of personalised medicine do we want?' (2014) 11(7) *Personalized Medicine* 651–7.

[6] Reardon, 'The "persons" and "genomics" of personal genomics'.

the rhetoric of personalised medicine has proven to be so powerful, even if many of its promises have failed to come true so far,[7] is that it accords with 'the sacredness of personal choice and individualism'[8] in a society which has adopted the language of individual rights as a dominant way of thinking.

Correspondingly, it can be expected that personalised medicine will give rise to new types of legal claims and responsibilities, such as the oft-invoked right to access genomic information,[9] even if the existence of that right is still legally and ethically controversial.[10] This chapter is premised on the idea that the emergence of these 'genomic rights' also reflects back on the subjects of these rights, and in some cases even calls into existence new types of legal subjects. The reason is that in order to invoke these new types of rights, legal subjects have to take on a certain shape in law.

To explore how certain legal claims in the context of personalised medicine affect law's understanding of the person, I focus on the emergence of new legal rights and new modes of legal subjectivity in a field of law that is already being referred to as 'genomic torts'. One of the most striking illustrations of genomic torts liability is the wrongful life action. Under a wrongful life action, a child who is born with certain genetic disabilities charges that she has been harmed by being brought into existence, as a result of which she now has to live a life full of suffering. This suffering could have been prevented, according to the claimant, if a physician, genetic counsellor or other medical professional had not negligently failed to warn her parents of the genetic impairments with which she would be born.

As I will discuss, the wrongful life action, according to its internal legal logic, enables the child with the genetic disabilities to exercise a radical form of retroactive self-authorship and autonomy. Yet, upon closer inspection, the claim to self-authorship, as implied by wrongful life claims, comes out as deceptive and problematic in several respects. In other words, within the context of wrongful life claims, the discussion on the person in personalised medicine recurs on a legal-philosophical level.

---

[7] Michael J. Joyner and Nigel Paneth, 'Seven questions for personalized medicine' (2015) 314(10) *JAMA* 999–1000.

[8] Dickenson, *Me Medicine vs We Medicine*, p. 24.

[9] E.g. Misha Angrist, 'Personal genomics: Access denied? Consumers have a right to their genomes' (2008) September/October *MIT Technology Review*, www.technologyreview .com/s/410662/personal-genomics-access-denied.

[10] See the chapter by Hogarth, Cockbain and Sterckx in this volume.

This chapter's line of reasoning is as follows. In Section 10.2 I first explore in general terms the interconnections between the Me of Me Medicine on the one hand, and the legal subject on the other hand, through Michel Foucault's and Nikolas Rose's reflections on legal subjectivity in an age of biopower. I use their thoughts to develop the idea that, as the language of personalised medicine and genetic risk becomes a dominant way of thinking in society, it also leaves its marks on the legal system and law's central category: the legal subject. Indeed, personal genomics and the accompanying rhetoric are likely to result in the creation of new 'genomic rights and duties', which are already starting to take shape, especially in the field of tort law (Section 10.3). Through an exploration of the concept of 'genomic negligence' in the context of wrongful life claims (Section 10.4), I demonstrate how the insertion of law into genomic discourse leaves its marks on law's understanding of the person as a bearer of rights and duties (Sections 10.5 and 10.6). I conclude that wrongful life claims are emblematic of a Me Medicine approach to regulating reproductive genetics and genomics in several respects, including its most problematic.

10.2   Legal Subjectivity, Biopower and Personalised Medicine

What are the interconnections between the rhetoric of personalised medicine and the legal language of rights? And how are genetic and genomic understandings of the self affecting the legal concept of the person? To come to an answer to these questions, Michel Foucault's reflections on the relation between biopower and legal subjectivity offer important insights.

As also explained by Huijer and Detweiler in this volume, by 'biopower' Foucault refers to the technologies of power that are centred on life itself, that is, life in its most corporeal and biological aspects. This power over life itself, through the 'administration of bodies and calculated management of life',[11] can be recognised on various levels in society, ranging from education to health, as part of an intricate network of professionals, experts, services and bureaucratic apparatuses.

Originally, biopower emerged in the seventeenth and eighteenth century in the form of 'an anatomo-politics of the human body' and 'a

---

[11] Michel Foucault, *The Will to Knowledge: The History of Sexuality Volume I* (London: Penguin Books, 1998), p. 140.

biopolitics of the population'.[12] However, over the centuries, biopower has manifested itself in various forms and gradations. Indeed, decades after the publication of the first volume of his *History of Sexuality* (1976), Foucault's reflections on biopower seem more relevant than ever, given the multiple biopolitical networks of governance and self-governance which have emerged in response to medical technologies, especially in the field of biomedicine. From genetic counselling to consumer genetics, from medical-ethical committees to medical-professional associations, and from preconception screening programmes to euthanasia laws and protocols, all of these phenomena illustrate to what extent the biological lives of individuals have been inserted into various configurations of control. Indeed, as a consequence of the rise of genetics and other life sciences, contemporary biopolitics even functions at the level of genes and neurochemistry, thereby taking on the form of 'molecular politics'.[13]

The normalising effects of genetic and genomic truth regimes on our self-understanding, and the new modes of subjectivity that they have produced, have in the meantime become the topic of an extensive literature.[14] What has received less attention are the implications of Foucault's thoughts for *legal* subjectivity in an era of biopower. Interestingly, according to Foucault, the rise of biopower in the seventeenth and eighteenth century coincides with the start of a phase of regression of the law and legal models of power.[15] As he argues, in order to come to an understanding of the novelty of the concept of biopower, we have 'to rid ourselves of a juridical and negative representation of power, and cease to conceive of it in terms of law, prohibition, liberty, and sovereignty'.[16] Whereas the traditional, juridico-discursive model of power goes back to the sovereign's 'right to *take* life or let live', biopower refers to a more productive, normalising account of power, 'a power to *foster* life or *disallow* it to the point of death'.[17] Consequently, within biopolitical constellations of power, the legal subject can no longer be at the forefront. As Foucault explains in the following striking sentences:

[12] Ibid., p. 139.
[13] Nikolas Rose, 'The politics of life itself' (2001) 18(6) *Theory, Culture & Society* 1–30, p. 12. Also see the chapter by Huijer and Detweiler in this volume.
[14] E.g. Hub Zwart, 'Genomics and identity: the bioinformatisation of human life' (2009) 12 *Medicine, Health Care and Philosophy* 125–36; Nikolas Rose, *The Politics of Life Itself: Biomedicine, Power, and Subjectivity in the Twenty-First Century* (Princeton, NJ: Princeton University Press, 2007). Also see Zwart's chapter in this volume.
[15] Foucault, *The Will to Knowledge*, p. 144.   [16] Ibid., p. 90.   [17] Ibid., p. 138.

For the first time in history, no doubt, biological existence was reflected in political existence; the fact of living was no longer an inaccessible substrate that only emerged from time to time, amid the randomness of death and its fatality; part of it passed into knowledge's field of control and power's sphere of intervention. Power would no longer be dealing simply with *legal subjects* over whom the ultimate dominion was death, but with *living beings*, and the mastery it would be able to exercise over them would have to be applied at the level of life itself. It was the taking charge of life, more than the threat of death, that gave power its access even to the body.[18] (emphasis added)

What do Foucault's words imply for the functioning of law and legal subjectivity in an age of genetic and genomic regimes of truth? At first sight, his remark that biopower is exercised over *living beings* rather than *legal subjects* seems to suggest that in the context of biopolitics, the notion of legal subjectivity is under pressure. If biopower is exercised over the biological and genetic aspects of life, and if individuals are moulded by the normalising effects of biopolitical institutions, how then can we hold on to the law's implicit ideal of the person as an individual who is capable of making choices and who can be held responsible for his or her actions?[19]

Related concerns can be recognised in current debates on the possibly erosive effects of the life sciences on the foundations of law. If, for example, genetic understandings of the self become more prevalent, and a growing number of individuals' actions and decisions are attributed to genetic and genomic predispositions, what will be left of central legal notions such as 'guilt' and 'intent', or law's foundational belief in *liberté, égalité, fraternité*?[20] From that perspective, it is likely that genomic technologies will lead to a further erosion of responsibility and legal subjectivity, and to new types of determinism and objectification of individuals that are at odds with fundamental rights and principles.

However, upon closer inspection, this account of the relation between genetics and legal subjectivity is not entirely convincing, also from

---

[18] Ibid., p. 143.
[19] In Lon Fuller's famous words: 'To embark on the enterprise of subjecting human conduct to the governance of rules involves of necessity a commitment to the view that man is, or can become, a responsible agent, capable of understanding and following rules, and answerable for his defaults' (Fuller 1964, 162). Also see Giorgio Agamben, 'Identity without the person' in Giorgio Agamben, *Nudities* (Palo Alto, CA: Stanford University Press, 2010), p. 46.
[20] Yuval Noah Harari, *Homo Deus: A Brief History of Tomorrow* (London: Harvill Secker, 2016).

a Foucauldian perspective. As already explained briefly, within Foucault's analysis, power is not understood in primarily negative terms, such as repression, prohibition or objectification; instead, biopower functions in more complex and productive ways, at the level of identity formation, disciplining the individual to behave in certain ways, and producing new forms of self-understanding and subjectivity.

Similarly, it seems that legal subjectivity within the context of personal genomics is not so much eroding, but rather transforming. Indeed, even if risks of genetic determinism have to be taken seriously, what we are witnessing as a result of genomic technologies is in many cases better described as an 'explosion, not an erosion, of responsibility',[21] also on a legal level.

For example, within the context of reproductive genetic testing, doctors are generally said to have an expanded duty of care. According to professional guidelines, they are responsible not only for the well-being of their patients with fertility problems, but also for the well-being of the children who may be born as a result of the fertility treatment.[22] As will be discussed in a later section, wrongful birth and life claims offer a striking illustration of the possible legal consequences of this expanded responsibility: medical professionals can be held liable, both by the parents and by the child itself, if they negligently failed to detect certain genetic risks or genetic abnormalities during pregnancy or fertility treatment. It is clear that under these circumstances, genetic technologies are producing new responsibilities and rights, and therefore new modes of legal subjectivity, rather than merely new types of genetic determinism or objectification of individuals.

Foucault scholar Nikolas Rose arrives at similar conclusions, albeit from a primarily sociological perspective. In his book *The Politics of Life Itself: Biomedicine, Power, and Subjectivity in the Twenty-First Century* (2007), he discusses how, within contemporary practices of genetic testing and genomic knowledge, patients are no longer believed to be passive parties, who are merely subjected to medical treatment and knowledge. Instead, individuals who are 'genetically at risk' are supposed 'to become skilled, prudent and active, an ally of the doctor, a protoprofessional and to take a share of the responsibility for getting themselves better'.[23] In this

---

[21] Michael Sandel, *The Case Against Perfection: Ethics in the Age of Genetic Engineering* (Cambridge, MA: Harvard University Press, 2007), p. 87.

[22] ESHRE, 'The welfare of the child in medically assisted reproduction' (2007) 22(10) *Human Reproduction* 2585–8.

[23] Nikolas Rose, *The Politics of Life Itself: Biomedicine, Power, and Subjectivity in the Twenty-First Century* (Princeton, NJ: Princeton University Press, 2007), p. 110.

process of 'genomic subjectification', individuals are required to take an active role in their own medical trajectory. According to the rhetoric of personalised medicine, patients who find out that they are at genetic risk can take responsibility for their health and use this genomic information to make better-informed choices in life. As they adapt their life plans upon confrontation with their genetic profiles, they are transforming, in Rose's words, into 'somatic individuals', endowed with 'genetic responsibility' towards not only themselves, but also an expanding group of third parties, such as relatives, reproductive partners and future offspring.

Typically, in these novel processes of identity formation, concerns about genetic risk are expressed in terms of rights and duties. In an age of personalised medicine, with its emphasis on patient empowerment and autonomy, somatic individuals, 'even when genetically at risk [...] consider themselves to be creatures of rights, legal subjects whose somatic personhood grants them entitlements as well as obligations'.[24] As a result, new 'genomic' rights and duties are emerging. In Rose's words:

> In this context, where autonomy and choice are paramount, and where genetic information is thought of as containing the potential to transform one's life, the disclosure of genetic risk information gets framed in terms of the language of rights: the right to know of one's kin and children, so that they may have the right to choose versus the right not to know, the right not to be known, the fear of the consequences that that knowledge may bring for one's conduct of one's own life and for one's treatment by others – friends, employers, teachers or insurers.[25]

Given these developments, the legal subject does not seem to be fading into the background at all, as Foucault's words on legal subjectivity and biopower may seem to imply at first. Instead, as also convincingly argued by Rose, legal subjectivity takes on a new form: it becomes part of and interacts with genomic discourse.

This account of the relation between legal subjectivity and biopower also corresponds better with Foucault's own words elsewhere on the functioning of law in an age of biopower. In a crucial paragraph, he writes that by 'juridical regression' he does not mean to imply that the law becomes completely redundant. Instead, his argument is that, ever since the rise of biopower, 'the law operates more and more as a norm, and that the judicial institution is increasingly incorporated into a continuum of

24 Ibid., pp. 124–5.   25 Ibid., p. 128.

apparatuses (medical, administrative, and so on) whose functions are for the most part regulatory'.[26]

In this chapter, I argue that these thoughts also apply to the interaction between the rhetoric of personal genomics and legal discourse. As the language of genetic risk and personalised medicine becomes a more dominant way of thinking in society, the legal system and its basic categories are also incorporated into these new truth regimes. In that process, law's understanding of the person as a bearer of rights and duties is equally changing, as I will illustrate through the concept of genomic negligence and, more specifically, the wrongful life action.

Because Rose's analysis is predominantly sociological, he leaves these legal-philosophical questions undiscussed. To come to a further understanding of these developments, the next section explores the new rights and duties surfacing in the context of what has been called 'genomic torts' or, more precisely, 'genomic negligence'.

10.3   From 'Genetic Responsibility' to 'Genomic Negligence'

It is common knowledge that legal systems are struggling to keep up with technological developments. Genetics and genomics are no exception to that rule. In the absence of direct government regulation of these technological developments, and given the inevitable rise of conflicts in this new field, tort law is starting to fill the regulatory gap. More precisely, tort law can function as a form of indirect regulation of these technologies by confronting health professionals who are assisting individuals in their genetic projects with liability when these professionals engage in negligent behaviour that causes harm to their patients or relevant third parties, such as the patient's family members or offspring.[27]

As early as 1997, Deftos coined the phrase 'genomic torts' to designate the emerging area of tort law that derives, either directly or indirectly, from outcomes and applications of genomics research.[28] The rise of legal claims in this field offers a striking illustration of the ways in which the

[26] Foucault, The Will to Knowledge, p. 144.

[27] Victoria Chico, Genomic Negligence: An Interest in Autonomy as the Basis for Novel Negligence Claims Generated by Genetic Technology (London/New York, NY: Routledge, 2011), p. 16; Radhika Rao, 'How (not) to regulate assisted reproductive technology: Lessons from "Octomom"' (2015) 49(1) Family Law Quarterly, p. 141.

[28] L. J. Deftos, 'Genomic torts: The law of the future – the duty of physicians to disclose the presence of genetic disease to the relatives of their patients with the disease' (1997) 32 University of San Franciso Law Review 105–138.

language of genetic risk and the language of legal rights have indeed started to blend. However, even if roughly 20 years have passed since Deftos' publication, and genomics-based technologies have started to take off in the meantime, many questions remain as to what the exact legal status is of these new legal claims. To what extent and under which circumstances can genomic information give rise to negligence and damage?

In her elaborate study on genomic negligence under English law, legal scholar Victoria Chico offers a legal analysis of four situations that are leading to genomic claims. Each of these four types of genomic claims arises 'due to the culpable carelessness of an individual who has undertaken to assist the aggrieved party in her genetic project'.[29]

The first two situations that Chico identifies relate to genetic risk in the context of reproductive medicine, and were already briefly mentioned in the previous section. If a medical professional fails to detect severe genetic deficiencies in the foetus, or fails to disclose this information to prospective parents, based on which the parents would have decided to abort the child, the parents can claim damages for the birth of their child through a *wrongful birth* action. Second, the child itself can also claim that it has been aggrieved by the medical professional's failure to detect his or her genetic deficiencies (a *wrongful life* action).

The third and fourth situation relate to more general practices of genetic information disclosure. With genetic testing becoming increasingly commonplace, the question arises as to how far the medical professional's duty of care extends under these circumstances. Can or should a physician share information on genetic deficiencies with the patient's genetic relatives, as this information may also indicate certain genetic risks for these parties? Or should medical confidentiality prevail in these circumstances? Additionally, legal claims can be expected from individuals who are confronted with genetic risks or deficiencies about which they would rather have remained ignorant. In these cases, they may invoke what is often called a *right not to know*.

As Chico admits, the legal status of most of these genomic claims is still shrouded in controversy and leaves much room for speculation. Because the case law in this field is still in an embryonic stage of development, much disagreement persists among legal scholars, both in England and worldwide, on the question of whether and to what extent these claims can be recognised under existing systems of negligence law. For example,

---

[29] Chico, *Genomic Negligence*, p. 1.

although much has been written about the right not to know in legal and ethical literature, it is still unclear whether such a right not to know can lead to negligence.[30] According to Chico, the main problem is that genomic negligence causes frictions with the existing legal concept of damage. Her book can, therefore, be understood as an attempt to develop an alternative concept of damage which, unlike traditional concepts of damage, is able to recognise novel grievances in the context of genetic services. Her central argument is that the concept of autonomy is able to fill the current gap in negligence law. According to her line of reasoning, the main harm involved in future genomic negligence claims is interference with the aggrieved party's autonomy. As such, Chico's approach to these novel legal dilemmas is in line with personalised medicine's references to patient empowerment and autonomy.

In this chapter I take a different approach by exploring how genomic negligence claims not only cause frictions with the legal concept of harm, but also with the legal concept of the person. Moreover, by focusing on legal subjectivity, several shortcomings of autonomy-based approaches to these dilemmas can come to light.

As such, this chapter's approach is in line with a more general trend in bioethics and biolaw to rethink the paramount position of the individual in ethics. In this vein, Knoppers and Chadwick argue that developments in human genetic research have caused a shift in ethics: away from the traditional emphasis on values such as autonomy, privacy and informed consent towards more communal values such as reciprocity, mutuality, solidarity, citizenship and universality.[31] Similarly, Widdows proposes to come to a renewed, *interconnected* account of the self to serve as a conceptual aid in the governance of genetic technologies.[32] For example, the aforementioned dilemma, whether medical professionals can be said to be under a duty to disclose a patient's genetic information to the patient's relatives, would not have arisen if patients and their relatives were truly autonomous and independent instead of interconnected and interdependent of each other in the context of genetic testing.

Hereafter, I focus on the first and second type of genomic claims that Chico analyses in her study: wrongful birth and wrongful life claims.

[30] Lee Black, Jacques Simard and Bartha Maria Knoppers, 'Genetic testing, physicians and the law: Will the tortoise ever catch up with the hare?' (2010) 19(1) *Annals of Health Law* 115–120; Chico, *Genomic Negligence*.
[31] Bartha M. Knoppers and Ruth Chadwick, 'Human genetic research: emerging trends in ethics' (2005) 6 *Nature Reviews Genetics* 75–9.
[32] Widdows, *The Connected Self*.

Whereas the concept of genomic negligence is still quite speculative in the third and fourth situation (the failure to disclose genetic information and the disclosure of unwanted genetic information), genomic claims within the context of reproductive genetics have been recognised in several legal systems for quite some time, even if they remain controversial.

10.4   Wrongful Birth and Wrongful Life Actions: Regulating Reproductive Genetics as Me Medicine

Once human reproduction becomes part of a complex of medical-technological interventions, in which multiple parties are involved – ranging from genetic counsellors to gynaecologists and from genetic test developers to embryologists – and several difficult choices have to be made that may have profound consequences for both prospective parents and future children, Sandel's 'explosion of responsibility'[33] does indeed not seem far away. If something goes wrong somewhere along the reproductive chain – for example, because reproductive choices have been negligently frustrated or certain genetic services are performed without due care and attention – both parents and resulting child can turn to tort law for recognition and compensation of their resulting grievances. Probably the most striking examples of tort liability in this area are wrongful birth and wrongful life lawsuits.

Tort law can be regarded as a private law alternative to the more common 'top-down' regulation of reproductive genetics through public law.[34] A typical public law measure within the governance of reproductive genetics is banning the use of these technologies for eugenic or enhancement purposes through criminal law prohibitions. For example, in many European countries PGD for non-therapeutic reasons, such as non-medical sex selection or the creation of 'designer babies', is prohibited by law, and as such constitutes a punishable act.

To some, private law regulation of assisted reproductive technologies (hereafter: ARTs) seems a more appealing option. For example, legal scholar Michele Goodwin proposes to explore the viability of tort law to address the harms resulting from negligent application of

---

[33] Sandel, *The Case against Perfection*.

[34] As is basic knowledge among lawyers, public law concerns those fields of law that, broadly speaking, govern the relationship between the state and its citizens. Examples are criminal law and constitutional law. Private law, on the other hand, regulates the relationships between private parties, through contract law, tort law and property law.

ARTs.[35] According to her, one of the dangers of public law regulation
of these questions is a communitarian approach to reproduction that
'seemingly legitimizes holding reproduction and intimacy hostage to
community values'.[36] Conversely, by delegating the regulation of ARTs
to the judiciary, the government does not have to enter into this legal-
ethical minefield and can remain neutral on several controversial
issues, such as the limits of liberal eugenics. Additionally, Goodwin
argues that private law regulation makes for a fairer distribution of the
financial costs related to accidents that take place in the field of ARTs.
As she argues:

> The issue most important to address is one of fairness with contemporary
> biotechnologies. Who should pay for the mistakes increasingly incurred
> by the use of technology? The disabilities resulting from reckless use of
> ART range from life-threatening conditions to an impaired quality of life.
> The costs incurred in treating and living with severe disabilities is calcul-
> able and, absent recovery from a parent, may be borne entirely by the child
> (into adulthood) or the state [...] Much in the same way that the law
> recognizes personal injury arising from the use of technology, such as
> cars, trains, and planes, so too should the law recognize personal injury
> actions in biotechnology and in ART in particular.[37]

Nevertheless, even if private regulation has certain advantages over
government regulation, it is not without reason that 'tort law [...] is
generally underexplored in the domain of reproductive technologies'.[38]
First, liability for personal injuries arising from transportation technology, to use Goodwin's example, does not raise as many moral questions
as liability for birth injuries arising from reproductive technologies. For
example, under Goodwin's proposal, children would be able to sue their
own parents for irresponsible use of ARTs, which breaks with the legal
tradition of intra-familial immunity, as Goodwin also admits.[39] And in
the case of wrongful birth and life actions, the harm involved is the birth
of a child, which raises concerns on the legal principle of human dignity
(more on this in Sections 5 and 6).

Additionally, also in the case of private law regulation, the state is not
truly and entirely neutral. As legal scholar Radhika Rao points out,
governments are still indirectly involved by allowing tort liability for

---

[35] Michele Goodwin, 'A view from the cradle: Tort law and the private regulation of assisted
reproduction' (2010) 59 *Emory Law Journal* 1039–100, p. 1043.
[36] Michele Goodwin, 'Prosecuting the womb' (2008) 76 *George Washington Law Review*
1657–746, p. 1672.
[37] Goodwin, 'A view from the cradle', p. 1089.   [38] Ibid., p. 1080.   [39] Ibid., p. 1074.

these cases in the first place.[40] Indeed, governments can easily bring an end to wrongful life actions through legislation that rules out the possibility of wrongful life actions. A striking example is the so-called *Loi Anti-Perruche* that was enacted in France after the *Cour de Cassation* had recognised Nicolas Perruche's wrongful life claim.[41] Also, the democratic deficit of private law regulation in comparison to enacted laws needs to be taken into account. Finally, Rao points out that regulation through tort liability delegates decision-making on reproductive matters to judges and juries, thereby increasing the risk of bias and discrimination.[42]

Although I agree with Rao, I choose a different line of argumentation to problematise the use of tort law in this field. Through the lens of negligence, the legal issues involved in reproductive medicine tend to be viewed as disputes between individuals about personal rights and entitlements.[43] Consequently, reproductive genetics is then regarded as a type of *Me Medicine*: Me Medicine for the parents in case of wrongful birth cases, and Me Medicine for the child in wrongful life cases. Moreover, as also will become clear in the next section, central values within Me Medicine, such as personal choice, self-authorship and autonomy, figure prominently within a tort law approach to regulating reproductive genetics. In other words, the choice for private law regulation instead of public law regulation of reproductive genetic testing reflects the choice of a Me Medicine approach. However, like Dickenson, I am concerned that within such a Me Medicine approach we lose sight of the more communal interests that are also at stake.[44] Or, as Reuter writes in an article on the politics of wrongful life:

> in spite of their liberal individualist preoccupation, these cases should not be viewed narrowly as isolated disputes between individuals – that is, not as personal troubles but rather as public issues. In other words, these malpractice suits extend beyond the legal matter of negligence to encompass larger problematics deriving from the normative risk politics that have emerged with contemporary geneticization.[45]

---

[40] Rao, 'How (not) to regulate assisted reproductive technology', p. 141.

[41] *La loi no. 2002–303 du 4 mars 2002 relative aux droits des malades et à la qualité du système de santé* (commonly called '*Loi anti-Perruche*').

[42] Rao, 'How (not) to regulate assisted reproductive technology', p. 142.

[43] Shelley Z. Reuter, 'The politics of "wrongful life" itself: Discursive (mal)practices and Tay-Sachs disease' (2007) 36(2) *Economy and Society* 236–62, p. 245.

[44] Dickenson, *Me Medicine vs We Medicine*, p. 2.

[45] Reuter, 'The politics of "wrongful life" itself', p. 245.

Even if tort law may fill an existing regulatory gap, and even if it can serve as an important incentive against the negligent application of ARTs by fertility doctors, tort liability's internal logic shows several important shortcomings and inconsistencies for the regulation of reproductive genetics when the claimant is the resulting child, as I discuss in the next two sections through an analysis of wrongful life claims.

10.5 Wrongful Life Actions and the Ideal of Self-Authorship

Negligence in the area of reproductive genetics can have far-reaching consequences, not only for the prospective parents, but also for their future child. For example, a doctor mistakenly selects and implants an embryo with a serious genetic disorder as part of preimplantation genetic diagnosis (hereafter: 'PGD'),[46] or she wrongly assumes that there is no reason for prenatal testing, even if there is a family history of a certain genetic diseases. As a consequence of her culpable carelessness, a child is born with severe genetic disorders. Under these circumstances, wrongful birth actions allow the parents to act as aggrieved party, whereas wrongful life actions allow the child to take on this legal role.

Wrongful life claims have been recognised in several legal systems worldwide.[47] However, the number of lawsuits against the medical profession is likely to increase as the number of genetic tests continues to expand. In this chapter, I focus on Dutch and French landmark rulings on wrongful life as representing two distinct directions in the case law on wrongful life.

One of the most puzzling aspects of wrongful life claims is that a child's congenital disabilities, which have not been caused as such by third parties, can legally qualify as a source of damages. The idea is that the child's suffering could have been prevented because, if the prospective parents had been informed about their child's genetic impairments, they would, in all probability, have decided to terminate the pregnancy. The concept of wrongful life claims thus presupposes that under

---

[46] For more on wrongful life claims in these situations, see Kate Wevers, 'Prenatal torts and pre-implantation genetic diagnosis' (2010) 24(1) *Harvard Journal of Law & Technology* 257–80; Rosamund Scott, 'Reconsidering wrongful life in England after 30 years: Legislative mistakes and unjustifiable anomalies' (2013) 72(1) *Cambridge Law Journal* 115–54.

[47] For an overview and comparison, see Ivo Giesen, 'The use and influence of comparative law in "wrongful life" cases' (2012) 8 *Utrecht Law Review* 35–54; Ronen Perry, 'It's a wonderful life' (2007) 93 *Cornell Law Review* 329–400.

circumstances of foreseeable genetic risk, the fact of being given life instead of being aborted can be considered a legal wrong. Under this line of reasoning it becomes possible to perceive reproductive genetic testing as a type of Me Medicine for the child, even if at the moment of genetic testing, the child is not yet born, and therefore not yet even recognised as a legal subject.

Much has been written about wrongful life claims over the years. However, a question that is generally neglected is *what kind of legal concept of the person is presupposed by this legal action*. How is it possible that these children are allowed to use their legal subjectivity to complain about the way in which they were created and became legal subjects in the first place? As will be discussed below, there is something profoundly troubling about wrongful life's depiction of reproductive genetics as a form of Me Medicine for the child. Nevertheless, it cannot be denied that, in line with Me Medicine's allusions to personal choice and individualism, awarding damages for wrongful life can also be defended as promoting the child's autonomy and self-authorship on several levels. I will discuss three levels: economic empowerment; access to the legal system; and retroactive self-authorship.

Firstly and most obviously, the compensation that these children receive for their suffering can help them live their lives in relative economic independence. Awarding damages to the children themselves, and not only to their parents under a wrongful birth action, can be regarded as a welcome supplement, because these children's financial support can then continue when they reach the age of majority or in the unfortunate event of their parents' death. From that perspective, the legal qualification of a child's life as wrongful can be regarded as 'enabling her to live her life in a manner that is as dignified as possible, to the extent that it is possible to realise that through a sum of money', to paraphrase the Dutch Supreme Court's *Baby Kelly* decision.[48] It is clear that within the Dutch court's interpretation, the principle of human dignity is understood as synonymous with the Me Medicine values of empowerment and respect for autonomy.[49]

---

[48] Hoge Raad, 18 March 2005 (*Baby Kelly*), NJ 2006, 606, par. 4.15.

[49] See Beyleveld and Brownsword's well-known distinction between two prevailing interpretations of human dignity: human dignity as empowerment and human dignity as constraint (Deryck Beyleveld and Roger Brownsword, *Human Dignity in Bioethics and Biolaw* [Oxford: Oxford University Press, 2001]). On the Dutch Supreme Court's analysis of human dignity in the *Baby Kelly* case, see Britta van Beers, *Persoon en Lichaam in het Recht: Menselijke Waardigheid en Zelfbeschikking in het Tijdperk van de Medische*

Secondly, also on a more legal level, self-authorship is realised for these children. Because the plaintiffs in these lawsuits are in most cases also mentally disabled, in real life, they would not have been able to voice their complaints. In *legal* reality, however, they are able to function as autonomous subjects. Because they are legally represented by their parents, the judge can, by legal fiction,[50] act as if these children brought suit themselves. For example, both in the *Baby Kelly* and *Perruche* case, the parents initiated the procedure. It could be said that through this legal construction, a voice is given to these disabled children, thereby granting them access to the legal system. From this perspective, wrongful life claims assist in their ascendance as legal subjects despite their mental disabilities, and as such are a legal recognition of these children's dignity.[51]

Finally, but also most controversially, recognition of wrongful life legally assists in what could be called *retroactive* self-authorship. That is, through these lawsuits children can have a say about the process of reproductive decision-making preceding their birth. To a certain extent, this fits with the more general trend in reproductive ethics to take the welfare of future children into account, as already briefly mentioned.[52] During the reproductive treatment, others will necessarily have to speak on behalf of the future children and represent their interests for them. One could say that a wrongful life action allows these children to finally also speak for themselves, albeit retroactively. Do the children in question, now that they are born, actually agree that their interests and welfare were served well by the reproductive decisions that others made on their behalf? Would they have wanted to be born under these circumstances, with such a genome? Under a wrongful life cause of action, the child's answer to these questions is negative.

Interestingly, the argument of self-authorship is also an important argument for those who are critical about the possibilities offered by reproductive genetics. For example, one of German philosopher Jürgen Habermas' main concerns in his book *The Future of Human Nature* is that children who are born as a result of selective or eugenic reproduction

---

Biotechnologie (The Hague: Boom Juridische Uitgevers, 2009), pp. 324–30; and see Giesen, 'The use and influence of comparative law in "wrongful life" cases'.

[50] Elsewhere, I have written more extensively on the legal fictions that are employed in wrongful life actions (Britta van Beers, 'The changing nature of law's natural person: The impact of emerging technologies on the legal concept of the person' (2017) 18(3) *German Law Journal* 559–94).

[51] Muriel Fabre-Magnan, 'Avortement et responsabilité médicale' (2001) *RTD Civil* 285–318, p. 300.

[52] See Section 10.2; and see ESHRE, 'The welfare of the child'.

'may no longer see themselves as the *undivided authors of their own lives* – nor will be called upon as such' (emphasis added).[53] He explains the interference with the child's capacity of self-authorship as a result of reproductive genetics as follows:

> If we see ourselves as moral persons, we intuitively assume that since we are inexchangeable, we act and judge in *propria persona* – that is our own voice speaking and no other. It is for this 'capacity of being oneself' that the 'intention of another person' intruding upon our life history through the genetic program might primarily turn out to be disruptive. The capacity of oneself requires that the person be at home, so to speak, in her own body.[54]

In the light of these words, it seems that, from Habermas' perspective, recognition of children's wrongful life claims should be welcomed as a form of compensation for their parents' intrusion upon their life histories. Wrongful life actions enable these children to take their life and personhood ('propria persona') into their own hands (*self-ownership*) and to write their own life history (*self-authorship*), at least on a legal level. At long last, by being given a legal voice, they are involved in 'the communication process',[55] out of which they were initially excluded through their parents' efforts to create the best possible child.[56]

10.6 'The Best *Me* I Can Possibly Be': From Self-Authorship to Autopoietic Legal Subjects

Upon closer inspection, the notion of self-authorship comes out as deceptive and self-contradictory in the context of wrongful life claims. As already mentioned, in practice, it is often the parents who speak on behalf of the child in a wrongful life claim, thereby reinforcing the intrusion on the child's life history instead of undoing it. Nonetheless, on a more fundamental level, there is something disconcerting about wrongful life's depiction of reproductive genetics as a form of Me Medicine for the child. To explain that, two different interpretations of

---

[53] Jürgen Habermas, *The Future of Human Nature* (Cambridge: Polity Press, 2003), p. 67.
[54] ibid., p. 57.   [55] Ibid., p. 62.
[56] It should be noted at this point that Habermas is critical about parents' wrongful birth claims, which, in his words, seem to suggest that 'the medically unexpected handicap was tantamount to damage to one's property' (ibid., pp. 13–4). Indeed, from the perspective of self-authorship, wrongful birth claims are damaging as they reconfirm on a legal level the parents' intrusion on the child's life history. However, the question remains as to how children's wrongful life claims should be valued from the perspective of self-authorship.

the wrongful life claim should be distinguished, each with its own problematic reading of self-authorship.

10.6.1   Self-Authorship as the Right Not to Be Born

A first possibility is that the court awards damages for the child's entire life. The child not only receives damages for the expenses related to its disabilities, but also for all its living expenses. In the *Baby Kelly* case (2005), the Dutch Supreme Court ('Hoge Raad') chose this direction. A benefit of this approach is that it seems to follow the rules of causality: without the medical failure to detect the genetic impairments, the parents would have known about them and would have had the chance to abort the child. In other words, as a result of the failure, the child is condemned to be born and thus to live its severely disabled life.

Nevertheless, what makes this interpretation controversial is that it presupposes that one can ever have a legal interest in one's own abortion. In other words, under this interpretation of wrongful life, the notion of self-authorship takes on the form of *a right not to be born*.[57] The question is, of course, whether one can one ever have such a right or legal interest. Protection of the child's right would, paradoxically, cause the child not to come into existence in the first place. The philosophical riddles under-lying the supposed right not to be born are well rehearsed in academia as part of what Derek Parfit famously calls the nonidentity problem.[58] One of the more practical aspects of the nonidentity problem, with which judges in wrongful life cases are confronted, is how to assess the damages owed to the child. The traditional logic underlying the law of damages would require judges to compare the child's current situation with the situation in which the harm would not have taken place. However, in this case that would amount to comparing existence with nonexistence, which seems logically impossible.

At the root of this practical problem is the more fundamental question whether one can ever legally argue that nonexistence is preferable to

---

[57] The Dutch Supreme Court explicitly denied that it had recognised a right not to be born (see *Baby Kelly*, paragraph 4.13). In the legal reasoning underlying the ruling, Kelly's claim is interpreted as derived from her parents' right to self-determination. Therefore, within this specific interpretation of wrongful life, children would not be able to sue their parents for wrongful life. However, given the fact that Kelly was awarded damages for her entire life, the conclusion seems inevitable that, if Kelly did not have a right not to be born, she at least had a legal interest in her own abortion, as I have argued elsewhere (Van Beers, *Persoon en Lichaam*, pp. 316–23).

[58] Derek Parfit, *Reasons and Persons* (Oxford: Clarendon Press, 1984).

existence in a liberal democracy committed to protecting each life as having an equal intrinsic worth. Indeed, in many legal systems, recognition of wrongful life claims is deemed to be at odds with the legal principle of human dignity, because it implicitly depicts the child's disabled life as not worth living.[59]

A possible objection against arguments based on human dignity or fears of eugenics, is that wrongful life actions do not rely on other people's value judgement about the child's life or some objective standard of worthwhile life (objective interpretation). Instead, the child's own judgement and experiences can be said to be the starting point of these actions (subjective interpretation). However, even leaving aside the fact that it is often the parents who sue for wrongful life on behalf of their child, this argument does not convince. In order to apply tort law to this situation, the child's suffering has to be legally qualified under the existing system of the law of damages. In Hensel's words, 'a line will have to be drawn somewhere between actionable and non-actionable disabilities'.[60] This makes the question inevitable what kind and which degree of suffering is enough to be able to conclude that the child's life is not worth living and can be legally regarded as a source of damages. In other words, some objective standard is inevitably needed to measure the child's life and to argue that it falls below the threshold of worthwhile life. Additionally, most defenders of wrongful life claims agree that the child's congenital disabilities need to be severe enough in order to justify this legal claim,[61] though it is beyond doubt that discussions on the question what we exactly owe to future children will continue.[62]

These discussions will undoubtedly become even more complex with the prospect of further developments in the field of 'fetal personalised medicine'.[63] For example, fetal whole genome sequencing makes it possible to uncover enormous volumes of genomic data already before birth.

---

[59] E.g. under English law (*McKay* v. *Essex Area Health Authority* [1982] 1 QB 1166); and German law (BVerfGE 88, 203 (296)).

[60] Wendy F. Hensel, 'The disabling impact of wrongful birth and wrongful life actions' (2005) 40 *Harvard Civil Rights – Civil Liberties Law Review* 141–95, p. 182.

[61] Allen Buchanan, Dan Brock, Norman Daniels and Daniel Wikler, *From Chance to Choice: Genetics and Justice* (Cambridge: Cambridge University Press, 2000), pp. 240–1; Scott, 'Reconsidering wrongful life in England after 30 years'.

[62] E.g. Jonathan Glover, *Choosing Children: Genes, Disability, Design* (Oxford: Clarendon Press, 2006); David DeGrazia, *Creation Ethics: Reproduction, Genetics, and Quality of Life* (Oxford: Oxford University Press, 2012).

[63] Diana W. Bianchi, 'From prenatal genomic diagnosis to fetal personalized medicine: progress and challenges' (2012) 18 *Nature Medicine* 1041–51.

If this technology were to become more routinely applied, which degree of risk and what kind of genetic 'abnormality' will then be deemed severe enough to recognise wrongful life claims?

Even from a tort law perspective, it is clear that the Me Medicine values of self-authorship and autonomy will not be able to provide answers to these vexing questions. More generally, it could be said with Hensel that 'once the nondisabled are given authority to judge from a "reasonable person" perspective whether or not the disabled life is worse than no life, the power of individuals with disabilities over their own identity and self-worth is seriously diminished'.[64]

10.6.2   Self-Authorship as the Right to Be Born in a Different Body

According to the second approach to wrongful life, the medical professional in question is liable only for the costs related to the child's disabilities. This interpretation is also at the root of the Cour de Cassation's *Perruche* decision (2000).[65] It presupposes that children such as Nicolas Perruche are wronged, not by the fact of being born, but by their genetic deficiencies. A major advantage of this approach is that no value judgements have to be made about the child's life, only about his genetic disabilities. The child's legal situation no longer needs to be explained in terms of a supposed right not be born or to be aborted. Consequently, objections based on human dignity can be evaded.

Yet this reading of wrongful life claims poses other serious problems. After all, the child's disabilities are inherent to its existence. They were, as such, not caused by third parties, but have a genetic cause. In other words, under the current possibilities of reproductive technologies, it would not have been possible for the child to be born without the genetic deficiencies. Therefore, holding medical professionals liable solely for the genetic impairments implies going against the laws of causality, and even the laws of nature.

As French legal historian Yan Thomas demonstrates in his fascinating analysis of the *Perruche* case, these counterfactual elements go back to a novel legal fiction that is introduced by this interpretation of wrongful life. This legal fiction entails that the child could have been born in a different body and with a different genetic make-up and still be the same person. Of course, the law mobilises legal fictions more generally,

---

[64] Hensel, 'The disabling impact of wrongful birth and wrongful life actions', p. 194.
[65] Cour de Cassation (ass. plén.), 17 November 2000, *JCP* 2000, II, 10438, p. 2293.

also with regard to unborn life.[66] However, what makes the wrongful life claim's legal fiction historically unprecedented is that it calls into existence a completely *fictional legal subject*.[67]

By treating the child's genetic disabilities as a source of damages, even if he could not have been born without them, the child is implicitly allowed to exercise a form of self-authorship that presupposes a *right to be born in a different body*.[68] In order to be able to exercise this novel right, the legal subject becomes dissociated from and even juxtaposed to his flesh-and-blood-counterpart. The result is a Cartesian separation between person and body, and between legal subject and flesh-and-blood human being. As such, the wrongful life claim in its second interpretation offers a striking illustration of the idea that I have a right to be 'the best Me I can possibly be', to use Dickenson's expression,[69] even if this means that 'that better individual [would] actually be someone else – not "Me" any longer'.[70]

Within this reading of wrongful life 'the problem of line drawing'[71] becomes more acute. The limit is no longer set at the minimum of worthwhile living, but becomes even more diffuse. Operating under the legal fiction that the child could have come into existence without genetic deficiencies, wrongful life no longer revolves around the question of worthwhile living, but the question of undesired genetic disabilities. Moreover, as assisted reproductive technologies continue to be develop, the standard will become increasingly difficult to determine.

For example, if, in a near future, human reproduction through 'easy PGD' (a combination of whole genome sequencing and gametogenesis) became the norm for reproduction in society, as Henry Greely predicts in his 2016 book *The End of Sex and the Future of Human Reproduction*, and natural reproduction came to be regarded as too risky for the child,[72] will children start to use wrongful life actions to claim that they have been wronged by being brought into existence the natural way?

---

[66] For example, the *nasciturus*-fiction, which dates back to Roman law, can still be recognised in many contemporary legal systems: An unborn child, if subsequently born alive, is considered as already in existence whenever it is to its own advantage ('nasciturus pro iam nato habetur quotiens de commodo eius agitur' (*Digest* 1.5.7)).

[67] Yan Thomas, *Du Droit de Ne Pas Naître* (Paris: Gallimard, 2002), p. 166.

[68] Thomas, *Du Droit de Ne Pas Naître*, p. 147.

[69] Dickenson, *Me Medicine vs We Medicine*, p. 113.   [70] Ibid., p. 126.

[71] Hensel, 'The disabling impact of wrongful birth and wrongful life actions', p. 181.

[72] Henry Greely, *The End of Sex and the Future of Human Reproduction* (Cambridge, MA: Harvard University Press, 2016).

More importantly, with the currently much discussed technology of human gene editing (CRISPR/Cas9) on the horizon, one of the most important barriers for the recognition of wrongful life claims, namely the impossibility of separating the child from its genetic disabilities, may be lifted in a near future. After all, the right to be born in a different body can no longer be rejected as an outrageous legal fiction as soon as it is technologically possible to genetically engineer children. Indeed, one of the effects of the introduction of human gene editing for reproductive purposes would be that the nonidentity problem can no longer be used as an argument against the recognition of wrongful life claims. In all likelihood, the number of wrongful life claims will then also rise dramatically.

10.6.3 Self-Authorship as Legal Autopoiesis

In both interpretations, the wrongful life claim has far-reaching consequences for the legal concept of the person. In the first interpretation, to make the legal claim for wrongful life, one has to, so to say, distance oneself from one's disabled life in order to be able to make a value judgement about it, as if one were able to occupy an Archimedean point of view. In the second interpretation of wrongful life, the claimant becomes a highly unnatural and disembodied legal being.

Moreover, because both the right not to be born and the right to be born in a different body are given retroactive effect ('retroactive self-authorship'), relating to negligent acts that took place in a period preceding the child's own legal existence, it could be said that wrongful life claims, in both interpretations, ultimately also introduce *self-authorship at the level of legal subjectivity* itself. That is, the child becomes the author of its own legal subjectivity by rejecting the circumstances under which it was given legal subjectivity. The child 'acts in *propria persona*', to use Habermas' words, by being allowed the means to rewrite its own legal subjectivity. In other words, the child uses its legal subjectivity to legally contest the outlines of its own legal subjectivity. Through this act of legal self-constitution,[73] the child's legal *persona* becomes *causa sui*.[74]

The circularity of this act suggests that the idea of self-created legal subjectivity is deeply problematic. Indeed, wrongful life claims, in their

[73] Thomas, *Du Droit de Ne Pas Naître*, p. 165.
[74] Elsewhere, I offer a more elaborate analysis of the legal concept of the person and currently emerging legal claims to rewrite one's own legal persona in various contexts (Van Beers, 'The changing nature of law's natural person').

self-referential conceptualisation of the legal self, can be said to negate the ways in which the legal concept of the person is, at heart, an *intersubjective* or *transsubjective* category. The Roman etymology of the word 'person' can be used to illustrate this.

'Persona' originally stood for the masks worn by actors in Roman theatre. In this vein, the legal concept of the person is generally understood as the role that the law writes for its subjects to play on the stage of law. By accepting this legal role, individuals subject themselves to the legal order. In return, they are protected as free and equal beings.[75] However, in today's legal order, a growing number of individuals demand to be recognised as the authors of their own legal roles. In the words of legal philosopher Dorien Pessers, these individuals

> [...] remove the mask of the intersubjective legal subject, and demand recognition as human beings of flesh and blood who require complete self-determination, as an expression of their individual dignity. They refuse their symbolic transformation into legal subjects, perceiving this transformation as a restriction of their freedom and happiness. In other words, they withdraw from the inter-subjectivity of the law and of what is considered as the supra-individual, general interest. But, does this deprivation not also deprive them – in the same act – from the legal, normative infrastructure upon which their existence depends?[76]

These ambiguities can be equally recognised in the dynamics of wrongful life claims. On an individual level, many of these children will be empowered by the legal recognition of their suffering and the financial compensation. However, on a societal level, wrongful life claims may cause these children more harm than good. By depicting their disabled lives as a source of damages, and by attributing to them a right not to be born or a right to have a different body, the law threatens to stigmatise these children's lives as less worthy of living than 'normal' people's lives.

10.7 Conclusion

How will genomic technologies affect our identities? Will they become a tool to write one's own story, as is suggested by the rhetoric of

---

[75] Alain Supiot, *Homo Juridicus: On the Anthropological Function of the Law* (New York, NY: Verso Books, 2007), pp. 20–1; Dorien Pessers, 'The symbolic meaning of legal subjectivity' in Bart van Klink, Britta van Beers and Lonneke Poort (eds.), *Symbolic Legislation Theory and Developments in Biolaw* (Switzerland: Springer 2016), 201–12; Van Beers, 'The changing nature of law's natural person'.

[76] Pessers, 'The symbolic meaning of legal subjectivity', p. 209.

personalised medicine? Or will they be used as an instrument by other people to decide 'who I am'? As Hub Zwart describes these core questions:

> Who can be regarded as the author of these novel genomics-based iden-
> tities that are envisioned? Will these technologies invite individuals to
> constitute *themselves* as subjects, or will new identities rather *be* produced
> by emerging discursive practices and strategies of classification and
> demarcation?[77]

In this chapter I have explored these questions on a legal-philosophical level, focusing on the effects of genomic technologies for *legal* subjectivity. Emerging legal claims in the recent field of genomic torts suggest that the law is already adopting, to a certain extent, a Me Medicine approach to regulating genomic technologies. As Chico argues, the grievances underlying genomic negligence claims are best explained in terms of an interference with the aggrieved party's autonomy and self-authorship.

Nevertheless, this autonomy-based framework for regulating the dilemmas raised by genomic technologies has important shortcomings. To illustrate and identify several of these problematic aspects, I have discussed the role and meaning of self-authorship within a specific type of genomic negligence claims: wrongful life claims.

In line with Me Medicine's allusions to personal choice and individualism, awarding damages for wrongful life can be defended as promoting the child's autonomy and self-authorship. However, upon closer inspection, the child's claim to self-authorship comes out as deceptive, self-contradictory and even harmful.

The ideal of self-authorship is *deceptive*, because recognition of children's wrongful life claims is practically impossible without a third party's judgement of the value of these children's lives, be it from the judge, the parents or the 'reasonable person'. The notion of self-authorship is also *self-contradictory* because awarding damages for the child's genetic deficiencies is based on the remarkable fiction that the child could have been born in a different body with a different genetic constitution, and still be the same person. Finally, wrongful life's emphasis on self-authorship is *harmful*, because it leads to a disregard of various societal interests and communal values that are also at stake in the regulation of reproductive genetics. Evidently, these interests and values include the parent–child relationship, the place of disabled people in

---

[77] Zwart, 'Genomics and identity', p. 136.

society and the value of human dignity in a legal order that is devoted to the protection of each human life as having an equal intrinsic worth. What has, however, generally received less attention, is that wrongful life's radicalisation of self-authorship also has a major impact on one of law's most important institutions: the legal subject. Whichever reading of the wrongful life claim is chosen, the result is an internally fragmented, surrealistically disembodied and ultimately autopoietic legal subject.

11

I Run, You Run, We Run

A Philosophical Approach to Health and Fitness Apps

MARLI HUIJER AND CHRISTIAN DETWEILER

11.1 Introduction

Since the introduction of the Apple iPhone in 2007 and the App Store that accompanies it, millions of people have downloaded and used health and fitness apps on iPhones, Android phones and other smartphones. In 2016, 102.4 million smartwatches and fitness trackers shipped. Fitbit alone shipped 22.5 million devices in that year.[1] Health and fitness apps, often used in combination with wearable sensing technologies, primarily track physical fitness, sleep, diet, smoking and stress.[2] The predominantly healthy users of these apps aim to acquire knowledge about their behaviour and states in order to maintain or improve their daily functioning and well-being.

How to understand this phenomenon of self-tracking? Are these technologies tools to increase self-knowledge and to empower individuals to better take care of themselves? This position is taken by the global Quantified Self (QS) movement, which understands self-tracking or 'life-logging' practices as a way to acquire 'self-knowledge through numbers'.[3] The Socratic phrase 'Know Thyself' is used to argue that quantified knowledge of the self is the starting point to reach and maintain a healthy and good life.[4] Self-tracking is thus a personalised type of

---

[1] Dan Graziano, 'Fitbit sold more wearables in 2016 than Apple and Samsung combined', *CNET*, 2 March 2017, available at www.cnet.com/news/fitbit-sold-more-wearables-in -2016-than-apple-and-samsung-combined (accessed 2 February 2018).

[2] Eun Kyong Choe, Nicole B. Lee, Bongshin Lee, et al., 'Understanding quantified selfers' practices in collecting and exploring personal data' (2014) *Conference on Human Factors in Computing Systems – Proceedings* 1143–52.

[3] Deborah Lupton, 'M-health and health promotion: the digital cyborg and surveillance society' (2012) 10(3) *Social Theory & Health* 229–44. See also: quantifiedself.com.

[4] Gary Wolf's talk on the Quantified Self at TED@Cannes, www.ted.com/talks/ gary_wolf_the_quantified_self.

'primary prevention', that is, prevention of disease, injury or early death before it ever occurs.

However, self-tracking technologies can also be understood as disciplinary instruments that subject (groups of) individuals to disciplinary regimes in order to reach the highest level of health and well-being for both the individual and the population at large. This critical stance is taken by sociologists, science and technology and human–computer interaction scholars who analyse the health and illness norms inscribed in self-sensing and self-monitoring technologies.[5] Self-tracking is here understood as both a personal and a collective type of primary preventive health. Commercial rather than public goods seem, however, to rule these disciplinary regimes.

In this chapter, we put these two ways of understanding self-tracking technologies into a broader philosophical context. We will first show that understanding the use of these technologies as a form of self-knowledge and self-empowerment is part of a more general discourse of what Donna Dickenson calls Me Medicine, a style of medicine centred on the individual's personal health and well-being. Second, we will show that understanding self-tracking technologies as disciplinary instruments is part of a broader discourse that criticises the so-called 'biopolitical' societal development in which populations and individuals are submitted to health norms that support economic and political goals.[6] Although these disciplinary regimes operate at both the individual (Me) and collective level (We), corporate interests rather than common goods dominate the market of health and fitness apps.

Though it is tempting to be either enthusiastic or to remain critical of self-tracking technologies for health and fitness, we will examine approaches in philosophy that allow us to offer a third alternative. Starting from the assumption that the view of mankind from which

---

[5] Deborah Lupton, 'Self-tracking cultures: towards a sociology of personal informatics' (2014) *Proceedings of the 26th Australian Computer-Human Interaction Conference on Designing Futures: the Future of Design* 77–86; Vera Khovanskaya, Eric P. S. Baumer, Dan Cosley et al., 'Everybody knows what you're doing: a critical design approach to personal informatics' (2013) *Proceedings of the SIGCHI Conference on Human Factors in Computing Systems* 3403–12; Stephen Purpura, Victoria Schwanda, Kaiton Williams, 'Fit4life: the design of a persuasive technology promoting healthy behaviour and ideal weight' (2011) *Proceedings of the SIGCHI Conference on Human Factors in Computing Systems* 423–32.

[6] Michel Foucault, *The Will to Knowledge: The History of Sexuality, Vol. 1* (London: Penguin, 1976); Michel Foucault, *Discipline and Punish: The Birth of the Prison* (London: Penguin, 1977); Nikolas Rose, *The Politics of Life Itself*.

one designs has a bearing on the design itself and on the constellations of humans and technologies that one brings about, we argue for
a design of self-tracking technologies that is predominantly informed
by notions of We Medicine. In this perspective, the users' responsibility for primary prevention is not limited to their own selves, but
encompasses broader common interests and goods related to health
and fitness.

11.2   Me Medicine and Health Apps

In her thought-provoking book *Me Medicine vs We Medicine*, Donna
Dickenson analyses how publicly targeted healthcare has increasingly
been replaced by personalised forms of medicine. Direct-to-consumer
genetic testing, personal tailored drug regimes, personalised pharmacogenetics, private umbilical cord blood banking and enhancement technologies are examples of an ever more individualised healthcare. What
these technologies have in common is an underlying assumption that
'individual' is better than 'social' and that a 'true revolution' is going on in
medicine to make it more individualised.[7] What makes Me Medicine
attractive to patients, physicians, multinational firms, researchers and
even 'presidents of the United States',[8] is that it goes beyond the 'one size
fits all' model for patients. What could be more appealing than physicians
being able to make the most effective medical decisions for individual
patients?

In her philosophical exploration of why people are tempted to buy into
personalised medicine, Dickenson discerns four possible reasons: threat and
promise; narcissism; corporate interests and political neoliberalism; and the
sacredness of personal choice. Dickenson draws on a range of technologies,
such as private umbilical cord banking, direct-to-consumer genetic testing
and enhancement technologies, to illustrate these approaches to understanding Me Medicine. These technologies are not the only ones that
exemplify the shift towards Me Medicine. We argue that activity trackers
and accompanying health and fitness apps also embody the reasons that
people might be tempted to subscribe to personalised medicine.

Threat and promise. The rise of individualised healthcare is inspired
not only by fear of threats such as pollution, toxins, the zika virus and
other contagious diseases, but also by financial or political crises that
make it difficult to find insurance for healthcare. The anxiety that there

[7] Dickenson, *Me Medicine vs We Medicine*, p. 4.   [8] Ibid.

will be no one to help you when you fall ill encourages people to find out all they can about their personal health risks and to minimise the chance of illness. In this perspective, do-it-yourself diagnostic and therapeutic technologies appear to be the best means to prevent diseases and to promote health and fitness.

Health and fitness apps play on the promise to tackle these threats. Optimism and promises about a better personal life seem better strategies to seduce potential users than the pessimistic message of threats.[9] The apps aim to help their users mitigate the risk of a sedentary life by prompting them to be active frequently. For example, one of the latest versions of the Fitbit Charge, the Charge 2, sends users reminders to move, encouraging users to take 250 steps every hour. Fitbit calculates users' 'active minutes' and refers to Centers for Disease Control's recommendations on how much physical activity adults need.[10] Among the recommendations is a minimum amount of activity that adults need. While this does not explicitly indicate a threat, it can leave users feeling uncomfortable if they do not move enough to meet these recommendations.

Narcissism. In a celebrity culture, every person seems to be as newsworthy as celebrities. Each detail of one's life and one's body can be the stuff of drama. Social media provides individuals with the means to express themselves by showing their performances, daily activities, workouts or outputs. Self-expression, self-admiration and self-centred behaviour is stimulated by the likes of digital 'friends'. This sharing on social media platforms could be seen as a type of social bonding, but it is often reached through group closure. People who are 'not like us' are excluded. More in general, the practice of increasing social capital through group closure, which has become ever more common in the USA, might be one of the explanations why there is more 'Me'ness in today's medicine and social policy.[11]

Popular commercial self-tracking technologies invite users to indulge in narcissistic activities. Users are encouraged to track every step, every meal (or snack) they eat and even every hour of sleep. Statistics are often

---

[9] Similarly, the brand for companies selling direct-to-consumer personalised genetic testing is promise rather than threat. See Dickenson, *Me Medicine vs We Medicine*, p. 55.

[10] Fitbit, *What are Active Minutes*, available at: help.fitbit.com/articles/en_US/Help_article/ 1379 (accessed 2 February 2018; Centers for Disease Control and Prevention, *Physical Activity*, available at: www.cdc.gov/physicalactivity/basics/adults/index.htm (accessed 2 February 2018).

[11] Dickenson, *Me Medicine vs We Medicine*, p. 17.

presented back to the user in dashboards, where graph bars and histograms display the past week of steps, active minutes, meals and sleep, for the user to peruse in an attempt to gain 'self-knowledge'. On those activities where a user has exceeded some personal goal, the visualisation of that activity might contain a green element (to indicate goodness) or a star (to indicate achievement). In some cases, a user will earn a badge (e.g. the Trail Shoe badge in Fitbit, which indicates 30,000 steps) to display on her personal profile. Users are encouraged to share these achievements on social media.

Corporate interests and political neoliberalism. Personalised medicine has coincided with the growing dominance of a neoliberal political ideology that aims to limit the state's involvement in healthcare and public wealth and increases the involvement of private corporations. The state is believed to be harmful to free markets, whereas the free market is seen as the 'true creator of wealth'.[12] This dominance of free market economics has affected science and medicine as well: private capital has entered a wide range of medical and scientific activities. Profits can be gained in personalised diagnostic tests, personalised treatments, personalised drug regimens and personalised information.

The immense growth of the personalised health and fitness apps market is a further sign of neoliberalism's influence in Me Medicine. These apps emphasise that, through self-tracking, one can adjust one's behaviour to optimise one's well-being and productivity, echoing the neoliberal focus on self-responsibility.[13] Furthermore, the apps portray health and fitness as things that can be shaped in the first place and should be, supported by consumer products.[14]

Commercial health apps also explicitly play to corporate interests, by offering products for corporations. FitBit, for example, introduced the programme 'Group Health', which allows clients to 'keep employees happy, healthy and engaged by creating an effective wellness program with Fitbit'.[15] This Group Health programme aims to 'improve employee health status' and 'create a culture of well-being'.[16] These are typically among the aims of public health, but here we see these functions shift towards private organisations (facilitated by Fitbit). Essentially, this aligns with policies of 'rolling back the state' and involvement of private

---

[12] Ibid., p. 20.   [13] E.g. Lupton, 'Self-tracking cultures'.
[14] Brad Millington, 'Smartphone apps and the mobile privatization of health and fitness' (2014) 31 *Critical Studies in Media Communication* 479–93.
[15] Fitbit, *Health Solutions*, www.fitbit.com/nl/group-health (accessed 2 February 2018).
[16] Ibid.

organisations in key governmental functions (i.e. public health) – policies Dickenson describes as neoliberalism: 'We the people' has become 'We the market'.[17]

Moreover, the benefits of Fitbit's Group Health programme are framed in terms of the corporate benefits of employee well-being, e.g. '[r]esearch shows that wellness programs can have big benefits for your business'; '[c]ompanies with worksite wellness programs experience an 8% increase in employee productivity';[18] and 'Decrease healthcare costs – CDW Healthcare reports wearable technology could reduce hospital costs by as much as 16% over the course of 5 years.'[19] Inserting these types of interests into the function of health promotion can be seen as a downplaying the notion of the public good.

The sacredness of individual choice. Autonomy, personal choice and self-ownership have become the paramount values both in medical ethics and in society as a whole. Me Medicine relies heavily on the rhetoric of unlimited personal choice. In light of the commodification of medicine, this focus on autonomy and individual choice has transformed into a sacredness of the *consumers'* personal choice, self-engagement and self-care. Communitarian forms of medicine are challenged, because they limit individual choice.

The emphasis on individual choice is clearly prevalent in discourses on digital technology-driven healthcare. As the sociologist Deborah Lupton has observed, patients and lay-persons have become 'participants' who are deliberately and actively involved in self-care. In her view, these discourses also represent the latest version of patient consumerism:

> In contemporary discussions of patient consumerism, the discourse of patient engagement is brought together with that of digital medicine to construct the figure of what I term 'the digitally engaged patient' when lay people are advised that they should use digital technologies as part of patient engagement practices.[20]

Health and fitness apps fit into this focus on individual choice. Wearable activity trackers and accompanying apps, such as FitBit, Jawbone UP and Moov NOW, embrace individual choice and self-engagement even

---

[17] Dickenson, *Me Medicine vs We Medicine*, p. 185. She draws this phrase from Thomas Frank's book *Pity the Billionaire* (2012).

[18] Fitbit, *Health Solutions*, www.fitbit.com/nl/group-health (accessed 2 February 2018).

[19] Fitbit, *Fitbit for Corporate Welness*, www.fitbit.com/content/assets/group-health /FitbitWellness_InfoSheet.pdf (accessed 2 February 2018).

[20] Deborah Lupton, 'The digitally engaged patient: Self-monitoring and self-care in the digital health era' (2013) 11(3) *Social Theory & Health* 256–70, p. 258.

before users purchase an activity tracker: Fitbit sells a whole range of activity trackers (Blaze, Surge, Charge 2, Charge, Alta, Flex 2, One, Zip), some with features beyond counting steps, such as guided breathing sessions, GPS location tracking and heart rate sensing, to suit different users' preferences. Each model is available in its own range of colours and some models include 'special editions' and 'designer collections'. Taglines on the website include 'Only Fitbit gives you the freedom to get fit your way'[21] and 'Fitbit motivates you to reach your health and fitness goals by tracking your activity, exercise, sleep, weight and more',[22] emphasising personal expression alongside fitness and motivation. Individual choice and self-engagement also characterise Google's 'Play Store' and Apple's 'App Store', where users can choose from thousands of apps to help them exercise, maintain a healthful diet or lose weight. Once users install and begin to use such apps, individual choice and engagement remain important. In Fitbit, for example, users are first asked to enter personal information, such as weight and age. The next step is to set personal goals, such as amount of weight to lose, daily amount of exercise. Though the app provides defaults based on recommendations from organisations such as the American Medical Association, the user is still free to set personal goals. This is the user taking 'personal responsibility for detecting and directing [her] own future health'.[23]

Health and fitness apps exemplify Me Medicine in all of the approaches Dickenson identifies: they promise to counter individual health risks, they encourage self-expression, they generate profits for private companies and they focus on individual choice.

11.3   Disciplinary Regimes and Health Apps

Yet, how personalised are health and fitness apps? Certainly, each user views statistics specific to their tracked activity. Users might even get feedback or 'coaching' on their activity in light of their personal goals. However, the overall approach is the same for all users: be active and eat and sleep well to meet goals. It is a 'personal choice' to do as everyone should do. In other words, a 'personal choice' but within a framework (of goal-setting) constructed by the apps' designers.

---

[21] Fitbit, *Why Fitbit*, www.fitbit.com/nl/whyfitbit (accessed 2 February 2018).
[22] Fibit, *Official Site for Activity Trackers & More*, www.fitbit.com/home (accessed 2 February 2018).
[23] Dickenson, *Me Medicine vs We Medicine*, p. 39.

Could it be that these Me Technologies are based on a collective societal and/or economic interest that everyone should act as a responsible citizen? This brings us to the second interpretation of self-tracking technologies: as disciplinary instruments that seduce or force individuals to take responsibility for their own health and fitness.

In *Discipline and Punish*, French philosopher Michel Foucault explains how, from the end of the eighteenth century, individuals became submitted to disciplinary tactics that governed and controlled their movements and behaviours. These disciplinary methods originated in the army, where discipline and dressage had been introduced in the seventeenth century. The success which discipline brought armies engendered a military dream of society: what worked in the army would also work in society.[24] Means of correct training, such as hierarchical observation of individuals, normalising judgements (small penalties, humiliations, corrections, gratifications and ranking) and examinations (combining observation and normalising judgements), were used to transform pupils at school, patients in hospitals, prisoners in prison and labourers in factories into docile bodies.

Activity trackers and health apps match the disciplinary means of correct training, i.e. hierarchical observation, normalising judgement and examination, as described in Foucault's *Discipline and Punish*.

Observation – this is described by Foucault as an 'absolutely indiscreet' surveillance that is 'everywhere and always alert' while simultaneously being absolutely 'discreet', since it functions largely in silence.[25] Tracking activity necessarily involves observation of some kind. Activity trackers can count the wearer's steps (by detecting motion) and, in some cases, measure the wearer's heart rate. The same motion detection can be used to track sleep. Though it is uncertain whether activity trackers actually improve health outcomes,[26] the idea behind the activity they encourage is to get people to be healthier by being more active, which the apps stimulate by giving people 'insights on [their] performance'[27] and reminding them to be active, as discussed above. When reminding users to be active, these apps implicitly inform users that the user's activity is being observed (by the app). When insights on performance

---

[24] Foucault, *Discipline and Punish*, p. 169.   [25] Ibid., p. 177.

[26] E.g. J. M. Jakicic, K. K. Davis, R. J. Rogers, W. C. King, M. D. Marcus, D. Helsel et al., 'Effect of wearable technology combined with a lifestyle intervention on long-term weight loss: the IDEA randomized clinical trial' (2016) 316 *JAMA* 1161.

[27] Fitbit, *Fitbit App*, www.fitbit.com/nl/app (accessed 2 February 2018).

are presented to users, however, it is the user observing themselves. This gives rise to a situation in which data are recorded by an individual about that individual – what Katie Shilton calls 'participatory personal data'.[28] In activity tracking, then, data collection is used both as a means of discipline and self-discipline.

Normative judgement (or normalisation) is described by Foucault as 'a small penal mechanism' that defines and represses behaviours outside the scope of the law, enforces artificial orders, functions as a corrective, prefers rewards above punishment and ranks individuals according to their good or bad behaviour.[29] It refers to the means of achieving discipline through imposing norms. Normalisation is pervasive in activity trackers and their accompanying apps, but is subtle.

A frequently encountered feature of activity tracking apps is a visualisation of activity levels for a certain period (e.g. the last seven days). Such a visualisation often includes a representation of the desired or recommended level of activity. For example, the Fitbit app includes a screen with a histogram of the last seven days of activity, expressed in steps walked. The histogram includes a line at the daily step goal (set by the user or by default). Such a visualisation directly expresses a norm or standard to which the user's activity is compared. Though the user is free to set the daily step goal, there is no option to disable the line that represents it.

Also, the app describes the default goal (10,000 steps) as being based on CDC recommendations, reinforcing the idea that this is a norm or standard to meet. If the user zooms in on a specific day, another histogram is displayed (in two-hour intervals). In this visualisation, bars are coloured according to the level of intensity of the user's activity – red for 'light activity', yellow for 'moderate activity' and green for 'intense activity'. Categorising activity in such a way is also a form of normalising. In this case, the user is not free to set the thresholds of each category. Users are also rewarded for certain achievements, for example, by being awarded a 'badge' for walking 30,000 steps in one day. Such rewards implicitly label certain behaviour as desirable or praiseworthy – in other words, certain behaviour is normalised in these apps.

Health apps also embed normalisation through defaults for various goals. For example, Jawbone's UP app allows users to set goals for hours

---

[28] Katie Shilton, 'Participatory personal data: An emerging research challenge for the information sciences' (2012) 63 Journal of the American Society for Information Science and Technology 1905–15.
[29] Foucault, Discipline and Punish, pp. 177–84.

of sleep, daily steps and weight. The slider with which the user can set hours of sleep also indicates 'average' sleep and 'recommended' sleep, which is the default. Below the slider it says '[t]he National Institutes of Health recommends between 7–8 hours of sleep per night'. The slider to set a daily step goal similarly has indicators for the average and recommended amounts and a text stating '[a]verages based on UP users. Experts recommend 10000 steps a day for an active, healthy lifestyle.' Finally, the weight slider indicates a 'Healthy Range' and the user's current weight. If the user sets a goal below his or her current weight, the text below the slider states

> Lose. Eat 500 calories fewer than you burn in order reach your weight goal. There are also other factors that affect weight loss, like sleep, which you can log in UP. If you stick to that plan, you are likely to reach your [xx] kgs goal in about [x] weeks. Men your height should weigh between [xx] kgs and [xx] kgs according to WHO's BMI formula (Jawbone's UP app).

These defaults, averages and recommendations impose norms on users' goal setting. Even if users choose not to follow apps' recommendations in setting their goals, they still act relative to a norm. As such, their choice of goal is either 'normal' or 'abnormal'. Moreover, once they have set a goal, their activity is judged in relation to that goal and is thus normalised. Even the act of goal-setting is a norm in such apps; activity tracking apps are normalising from the outset.

The final technique of disciplinary control that activity trackers and their apps implement is the *examination*, in which the techniques of hierarchical observation and of normalising judgement are combined. Foucault describes this examination as both a ritual and a 'scientific' way of fixing individual differences, in which each individual is pinned down in his own particularity. The examination is at the centre of the disciplinary power:

> It is the examination which, by combining hierarchical surveillance and normalizing judgment, assures the great disciplinary functions of distribution and classification, maximum extraction of forces and time, continues genetic accumulation, optimum combination of aptitudes and, thereby, the fabrication of seller, organic, genetic and combinatorial individuality.[30]

In health and fitness apps, the examination is embedded through the ways in which the apps process users' self-tracked data (observation) in

---

[30] Ibid., p. 192.

light of the norms the apps include (normalising judgement) to classify the user and their activity. In Fitbit, users' activity is classified as 'intense', 'moderate' or 'light'. Jawbone UP users' sleep is categorised as 'awake', 'light' or 'sound'. Those users' meals get a score and are classified as 'healthy', 'OK' or 'avoid' (if they log food intake). In some cases, apps even actively advise users to change their behaviour. For example, Jawbone UP's 'Smart Coach' feature will tell a user who has slept 3 hours and 58 minutes:

> Last night you only slept for 3 h 58 m. Try for more tonight. Skip that new episode of Dancing with the Stars or The Big Bang Theory. Your body will thank you tomorrow (Jawbone's UP app).

Users are also compared to other users. In the case of Fitbit, the user's activity level is compared to other 'befriended' users and ranked accordingly. Cyclists who use the Strava app can see how they rank in comparison to other users (or 'athletes') on the time it took them to complete a segment of road. Some apps, such as Fitbit, also give users badges for certain achievements, such as new badges for each additional 10,000 steps taken in a day. This comparison to other users, ranking and rewarding achievements exemplifies the examination aspect in health and fitness apps.

What this disciplinary perspective on health and fitness apps discloses is that Me and We Medicine are intertwined: collective norms are taken as default criteria to set personal goals. Disciplinary regimes, especially in the field of health and illness, are always aimed at both the individual and the population at large. In *The Will to Knowledge* (1976), Foucault shows that while health became an ever more important economic value in Western societies, knowledge regimes and disciplinary powers became increasingly oriented toward the optimisation of the health of both the individual and the population. He uses the word 'biopower' to explain the disciplinary forces and policies that incite individuals and society at large to behave as healthily as possible: 'Western man was gradually learning what it meant to be a living species in a living world, to have a body, conditions of existence, probabilities of life, an individual and collective welfare, forces that could be modified and a space in which they could be distributed in an optimal manner'.[31]

Biopower, as a 'political technology of life', evolved over two axes: the one focused on an 'anatomo-politics' of the human body and the other on

[31] Michel Foucault, *The Will to Knowledge*, p. 142.

a 'biopolitics' of the population.[32] In these regimes, the human body became surveyed and disciplined unto the smallest, microphysical level. Today, these disciplinary forces work at an even smaller scale, as the sociologist Nikolas Rose argues in *The Politics of Life Itself*: at the molecular (genetic and neurochemical) level of the human body. The species body, on the other hand, became regulated and controlled in order 'to protect the security of the whole from internal dangers'.[33]

Yet, these disciplinary regimes cannot be understood as either a Me or We type of Medicine. The distinction between strategies governing the individual body and those regulating the species body already became blurred in the nineteenth century, as state authorities and later 'sub-State institutions such as medical institutions, welfare funds, insurance and so on' sought to act upon the population through action upon the human body.[34] The best example to explain this is the political issue of sex, which was at the pivot of the two axes:

> On the one hand it was tied to the disciplines of the body: the harnessing, intensification and distribution of forces, the adjustment and economy of energies. On the other hand, it was applied to the regulation of populations, through all the far-reaching effects of its activity. It fitted in both categories at once, giving rise to infinitesimal surveillances, permanent controls, extremely meticulous orderings of space, indeterminate medical or psychological examinations, to an entire micro-power concerned with the body. But it gave rise as well to comprehensive measures, statistical assessments and interventions aimed at the entire social body or at groups taken as a whole.[35]

Continuing this line of thought, Rose analyses how contemporary citizens have become vehicles of biopolitics themselves. Rather than feeling subjected to this politics of life, individuals consider themselves to be free and autonomous beings who deliberately take responsibility for their individual health and well-being. Rose links Foucault's later work on 'care of the self' to the existing disciplinary health regimes. While Foucault considered 'care of the self' to be a technique to criticise existing knowledge and power regimes and to open up new ways to work on and shape one's self, Rose shows that this strategy also further submits individuals to disciplinary power regimes. Contemporary 'biological citizens' not only enthusiastically engage with their own health, they

---

[32] Ibid., p. 139.   [33] Foucault, 'Society must be defended', p. 249.
[34] Foucault, *The Will to Knowledge*, p. 141. Foucault, 'Society must be defended', p. 250. Rose, *The Politics of Life Itself*, p. 53.
[35] Foucault, *The Will to Knowledge*, pp. 145–6.

even claim to have a right to health and well-being and thus to genetic testing, anti-depressive drugs or enhancing technologies.[36] They are convinced that they have freely chosen to behave as healthily as possible.[37]

Deborah Lupton's sociological critique of self-tracking and 'the quantified self' subscribes to this type of analysis. Lupton argues that 'Foucault's writings on the practices and technologies of the self in neoliberalism are pertinent to understanding the quantified self as a particular mode of governing the self.[38] On this view, citizens voluntarily engage in practices that serve their own interests and conform to those of the state – the responsible citizen self-manages her health through 'self-knowledge' gained through self-tracking ('voluntary self-surveillance').

11.4   We Medicine and Health Apps

Is it possible to develop health and fitness apps that do not conform to Me Medicine? Could health and fitness apps prioritise We Medicine over Me Medicine? What would such apps look like? Dickenson's main goal in *Me Medicine vs We Medicine* is to reclaim medical and bio-technologies for the common good.[39] Rather than focusing on the narcissism, corporate interests and autonomous choice of Me Medicine, she stresses the importance of public health, notions of common interests and common ownership and concepts of mutuality and interrelationships – in short, We Medicine – while dealing with diseases and other conditions that affect our health and fitness.

> Historically, it was not Me Medicine but We Medicine—programs like public vaccination, clean water and screening for tuberculosis—that brought us reduced infant mortality, comparative freedom from contagious disease, and an enhanced lifespan. Yet today, many of these public programs seem to be increasingly distrusted, even detested.[40]

---

[36] Nikolas Rose and Carlos Novas use the term 'biological citizenship' descriptively, 'to encompass all those citizenship projects that have linked their conceptions of citizens to beliefs about the biological existence of human beings, as individuals, as families and lineages, as communities, as population and races and as a species'. See Nikolas Rose and Carlos Novas, 'Biological citizenship' (2002), at p. 3, available at: http://thesp.leeds.ac.uk /files/2014/04/RoseandNovasBiologicalCitizenship2002.pdf (accessed 2 February 2018).

[37] Rose, *The Politics of Life Itself*, pp. 146–7 and 154. See also Nikolas Rose, *Inventing Our Selves: Psychology, Power and Personhood* (Cambridge: Cambridge University Press, 1996).

[38] Lupton, 'The digitally engaged patient', p. 28.

[39] Dickenson, *Me Medicine vs We Medicine*, p. viii.   [40] Ibid., p. 5.

The question, then, is how we, in primary prevention, can make use of health and fitness apps (or similar technologies) to embody We Medicine rather than Me Medicine. Before we can offer proposals for design directions such apps could take, we need to be more specific about what We Medicine means.

Public health programmes such as those mentioned above exemplify what Dickenson calls We Medicine. It encompasses solidarity and altruism ('We factors'[41]) and involves communal action directed towards communal purposes, common possessions or the common good ('working together for what we have in common'). So, in promoting the idea of We Medicine, Dickenson is calling for a return to, or a reclaiming of, the commons – and creating a 'new spirit of togetherness'.[42]

However, Dickenson identifies two threats to the commons that we see in Me Medicine today and that need to be overcome in order to realise We Medicine. First, there is the threat of free riding: that is, individuals endangering the commons (or communal resource) by 'taking more than their fair share'.[43] One example of this is parents who decide to withdraw their children from vaccination programmes. Sufficient individual participation in such programmes creates a communal health resource or commons – population immunity. Individuals who withdraw their children distrust public health and their view is that they alone are responsible for protecting the individual health of their children – a view fed by market populism, according to Dickenson. By not participating in vaccination programmes, these individuals reap the benefits of population immunity (they are protected by it), but they do not contribute to it themselves. Of course, as Dickenson notes, if too many parents were to withdraw their children from vaccination programmes, population immunity would decline and there would be no commons.

The other threat to the commons is the threat of the commons being enclosed to create a wholly or partially private good.[44] Under this threat, commoners who contributed to the commons are now kept from accessing the benefits of that communal resource. Dickenson illustrates this second threat with the example of corporations such as 23andMe owning and deriving (commercial) value from the commons of the human genome. In this case, individuals' access to the benefits of, for example, diagnostic testing based on these commons can be limited by the private owner of those commons.[45]

---

[41] Ibid., p. 207.   [42] Ibid., p. 227.   [43] Ibid., p. 218.   [44] Ibid., p. 218.   [45] Ibid., p. 222.

So, the commons that We Medicine should reclaim, according to Dickenson, can include common goods, such as population immunity, to which individuals contribute through individual actions, such as undergoing vaccination. It can also be information that individuals contribute, such as genome sequencing information, from which all can benefit through, for example, diagnostic testing based on the communal resource.

Above, we discussed how health and fitness apps and activity trackers exemplify many of the reasons for Me Medicine. Do these apps and activity trackers similarly exemplify threats to a commons? If so, what commons do they threaten? The threat of free-riders, exemplified by the vaccine case, does not seem to have an obvious parallel in health and fitness apps – there does not seem to be an equivalent of population immunity (or of free-riding individuals) in health and fitness apps.

A more plausible parallel seems to exist between individual users tracking their activity through a centralised service such as Fitbit and individuals contributing to 23andMe's genotype-phenotype database. The latter was 'created by the labour, cash and bodily materials of thousands of individuals',[46] but belongs to a private firm. Similarly, users of activity trackers spend money on the means to track their activity and labour (exercise) to produce the data on a private firm's servers. Where the genotype–phenotype database captures a communal resource – the genome is something all humans have in common – from which individuals could benefit, the databases in which the daily activity data of millions of individuals are stored captures a communal resource of knowledge about human behaviour. People have activity (or absence thereof), food intake and sleep in common, and while private firms such as Fitbit do not own the activities themselves, they do own the data derived from these activities. So, as in the 23andMe example, private firms are in a position to limit or deny access to a form of communal resource, to sell the data generated by patients to pharmaceutical companies, private firms in health and fitness apps are in a position to decide in what ways they use or exploit these data. In the case of 23andMe, beside marketing their database, they can use their databases to patent gene sequences and to stake patent claims. In 2012, 23andMe was granted a US genetic patent related to Parkinson's disease without making clear to consumers that it was seeking such patents, ultimately undermining

[46] Ibid., p. 222.

consumers' trust in 23andMe.[47] Though it is not immediately clear how Fitbit's databases could be used to seek patents, similar issues could arise if Fitbit attempts to create intellectual property from aggregated data and profit from it.

Dickenson discusses a number of possible responses to these threats, in the form of various collective movements. One of these responses is the charitable trust model. In this model, contributors to a biobank do not gain ownership rights of (samples and related data in) the biobank, but there is a requirement that the trustees act in the interest of the bene-ficiaries – so it would not be possible to profit from the biobank. Another response is for an (indigenous) group to claim the right to determine what is done with its genetic data, often by appealing to traditional communal belief systems.[48]

Promoting the idea of We Medicine in relation to health and fitness apps would mean to start with the question of what health and fitness norms we share and what primary prevention means best fit these norms. In the case of air pollution, for example, rather than digitally alerting citizens and helping them to adapt their behaviour to the amount of pollution (thus intermingling Me and We medicine), designers could start by asking what the best primary prevention measures are to prevent health-endangering forms of air pollution. Citizens could be motivated to work together to improve the quality of the common air. Something similar can be seen in Strava's Metro product.[49] Strava is a service that lets people track their cycling and running activity. Strava Metro anonymises and aggregates this data and licenses it to departments of transportation and related organisations to improve infrastructure for cyclists and pedestrians. Though Strava is using data its users have contributed to create intellectual property, the data is ultimately used to improve peo-ple's safety.

Prioritising We Medicine in the design of health and fitness apps could start from new sorts of communal identification or new kinds of com-munal concerns for prevention of diseases. Initiatives such as Science Commons and FOSTER Open Science, which aim to make research data reusable, better accessible and better integrated, are examples of how

---

[47] Sigrid Sterckx, Julian Cockbain, Heidi Howard et al., '"Trust is not something you can reclaim easily": patenting in the field of direct-to-consumer genetic testing' (2013) 15 *Genetics in Medicine* 382–7.

[48] See also Donna Dickenson, *Property in the Body: Feminist Perspectives* (Cambridge: Cambridge University Press, 2007), chapter 8.

[49] Strava, *Strava Metro*, https://metro.strava.com (accessed 2 February 2018).

communal concerns can be taken as the starting point for digital communitarian associations focused on common goods. Dickenson refers to Richard Titmuss's notion of 'the gift relationship', funding the UK blood donation system, to stress the importance of the sense of identification with a wider collective.[50]

We Medicine in the health and fitness apps area also implies investigating the options for common possessions. On the one hand, non-profit public databases could be built that store and analyse the data of tracking activities. Comparable to the charitable trust model, the interests of the contributors would be represented by the trustees. As far as profits are made, they could be used to further research or other common interests.[51] On the other hand, small group databases could be built, in which members share their activity data and have the right to determine what is done with these.

11.5   Conclusion

Taking Donna Dickenson's contrast between Me and We Medicine as a starting point, the development of health and fitness apps can be seen as both a type of Me Medicine and a disciplinary regime imposing collective norms on the individual.

The most robust explanation for the rise of Me Medicine in this case is, similarly to other fields of medicine, the dominance of corporate interests and a neoliberal public policy. The responsibility for living a healthy and long life is put on the individual and no longer seen as a communal interest.

Yet, it is impossible to draw a strict boundary between Me and We Medicine. Health and fitness apps are also disciplinary technologies in which public, state and sub-state norms or corporate interests are translated into actions on the individual body. However, Me Medicine claims to be superior to We Medicine when primary prevention is at stake. 'Me often markets itself as clinically superior to We', as Dickenson argues – even though the evidence base for this superiority is weak.[52]

Dickenson's plea to resurrect the commons, in this case in digital technologies that support primary prevention goals, invites us to take

---

[50]   Dickenson, *Me Medicine vs We Medicine*, pp. 214–5.

[51]   Dickenson presents the non-profit UK Biobank and PXE International Foundation as examples of a middle way between pure altruism and pure capitalism (*Me Medicine vs We Medicine*, p. 211).

[52]   Ibid., p. 57.

a completely different angle. Developing health and fitness apps from a We Medicine perspective, governed by common rather than corporate interests, would imply that users (contributors) would have an insight into and a say in the norms inscribed in the apps; that they are stimulated to identify with communal values and communal concerns; that they know what data are stored and what algorithms are used to analyse these data; and that they have a right to determine what is done with the collected data.

Designers who are willing to bring in more 'We'-ness in the design of health and fitness apps should be aware that Me Medicine in primary prevention often eclipses We Medicine. So, rather than focusing on promises for a better individual life, on narcissism, corporate interests and self-engagement, designers would have to take communal values and common goods as their starting point for design. Design for We Medicine would involve designing for communities rather than individual users. Active involvement and deliberation of citizens and other users in the design of digital primary preventive medicine technologies could be a way to broaden the normative scope of the good life as aimed for in health and fitness apps. Moreover, designers should be aware that group closures (only sharing data with 'people like us') can further encourage the rise of Me Medicine.

In order to bring more We Medicine into health and fitness apps, designers should also recognise that observation, normalising judgement and examination are part and parcel of data tracking technologies. Each design embodies, often invisibly, norms, values and ideologies.[53] Rather than keeping these invisible or implicit, it would be better to submit the embedded norms, values and ideologies to public scrutiny and discussion.

Finally, designers could respect the 'commons' by building databases in which contributors can share their data and stories without giving up the right to decide about these data, in a form similar to the examples of charitable trust fund models that Dickenson discusses.

---

[53] Bruno Latour, 'Where are the missing masses? The sociology of a few mundane artifacts' (1992) www.bruno-latour.fr/sites/default/files/50-MISSING-MASSES-GB .pdf; Mary Flanagan, Daniel C. Howe and Helen Nissenbaum, 'Embodying values in technology: Theory and practice' in Jeroen van den Hoven and John Weckert (eds.), *Information Technology and Moral Philosophy* (Cambridge: Cambridge University Press, 2008), pp. 322–53; Peter-Paul Verbeek, *Moralizing Technology* (Chicago, IL: University of Chicago Press, 2011).

Although there is still a long way to go to resurrect the commons in medicine and to reclaim the various kinds of medical and bio-technologies for the common good, Dickenson's invitation to look for new ways to create a spirit of togetherness in biomedicine undeniably opens up new perspectives to design, develop and use health and fitness apps with more solidarity and in more altruistic We-oriented ways. Just as user-friendliness became a central aim in the design of digital technology, We-ness could become the focus of health and fitness apps.

12

The Molecularised Me

Psychoanalysing Personalised Medicine and Self-Tracking

HUB ZWART

12.1 Introduction

During the 1990s, new forms of technoscience pervaded postmodern society, exemplified by the Human Genome Project (HGP) in the life sciences and by the Internet in the realm of Information and Communications Technology (ICT). These developments initially focused on the construction of a novel 'We', represented by the transpersonal Human Reference Genome (HRG) in the life sciences and by the World Wide Web (as a decidedly transpersonal enterprise) in ICT. Currently, however, against the backdrop of Next Generation Sequencing (NGS) and the emergence of wearable electronic devices, we witness the advent of yet another revolution, again combining genomics with ICT, which claims to entail a shift of focus from *We* to *Me*. Francis Collins[1] and others herald the advent of a new era of personalised medicine, referred to by Donna Dickenson[2] as *Me Medicine*: a development which allegedly transforms human individuals into bio-citizens, empowering them to become proactive managers of their own wellness and health. These bio-citizens become increasingly involved in new practices of the Self, often referred to as self-monitoring, self-tracking, do-it-yourself (DIY) diagnostics, personal informatics or lifelogging.[3] Such practices assist users in maintaining wellness by closely monitoring personal activities such as exercise, sexuality and diet. Indeed, even the molecular effects

---

[1] F. Collins, *The Language of Life: DNA and the Revolution in Personalised Medicine* (New York: Harper, 2010).

[2] D. Dickenson, *Me Medicine vs We Medicine: Reclaiming Biotechnology for the Common Good* (New York: Columbia University Press, 2013).

[3] D. Lupton, *The Quantified Self: A Sociology of Self-Tracking* (Cambridge: Polity Press, 2016).

of allegedly healthy activities such as laughter on wellness are being studied.[4] Bio-citizens are regarded as valuable repositories of information, and the focus is no longer on various stages of illness or recovery, but rather on wellness as such, and more specifically on the latent subliminal molecular onsets of health challenges during the wellness stage. Or, to phrase it in the terminology of French philosopher of science Gaston Bachelard,[5] the focus of attention has shifted from the *phenomenal* (i.e. physical) aspects of health and disease to the *noumenal* (i.e. the biochemical, biomolecular or microphysical) dimensions.

Although self-monitoring, self-measuring and self-recording have been practiced since ancient times, in the era of wearable devices and sensor-saturated environments a self-tracking culture has gained momentum that is increasingly bent on quantification.[6] Indeed, the combination of digital devices and personalised health information has given rise to the emergence of a numbered or 'quantified' Self,[7] and self-knowledge is increasingly articulated in terms of measurements and numbers, so that bio-citizens are expected to measure and monitor their bodies and their everyday lifeworld in real time, continuously and automatically.

But personal data are never purely personal. Not only because, at least potentially, they may become available to others (developers of devices, data-mining companies, government agencies, cybercriminals and the like[8]), but also because, for these measurements to make sense, they must be compared to transpersonal standards and performance levels, to sociocultural expectations, indeed: to a digital version of the superego, exposing the self-tracking bio-citizen to continuous surveillance and criticism.[9]

In this contribution, the advent of Me Medicine (or personalised medicine) will be assessed from a psychoanalytical perspective. Basically I will argue that Me Medicine entails a molecularisation or

[4] T. Hayashi et al., 'Laughter regulates gene expression in patients with type 2 diabetes' (2006) 75 *Psychotherapy and Psychosomatics*, 62–5.
[5] G. Bachelard, 'Noumène et microphysique' (1932/1970) *Recherches Philosophiques* 55–65: 11–24; G. Bachelard, *L'activité rationaliste de la physique contemporaine* (Paris: Presses Universitaires de France, 1951).
[6] Lupton, *The Quantified Self: A Sociology of Self-Tracking.*   [7] Ibid.   [8] Ibid., p. 4.
[9] H. Zwart, 'The obliteration of life: depersonalisation and disembodiment in the terabyte age' (2016) 35(1) *New Genetics and Society*, 69–89. doi:10.1080/14636778.2016.1143770; H. Zwart, '"Extimate" technologies and techno-cultural discontent: A Lacanian analysis of pervasive gadgets' (2017) 22(1) *Techné: Research in Philosophy and Technology*, 24–54. doi:10.5840/techne20174560.

digitalisation of our conscience as well as of the unconscious: a technification of both the superego and the id. The design of this chapter is as follows. First, I will assess currently emerging self-tracking practices against the backdrop of an extended history of self-directedness, and as the most recent 'epidemic' of the human tendency towards self-obsession. Donna Dickenson already problematises this in psychoanalytic terms, namely as a 'wave of patient narcissism and self-absorption',[10] in combination with capitalism's protean capacity for creating new products. This is not only reflected by personalised genetics as such, moreover, but notably in combination with the latest wave of ICT gadgets (cf. the lower-case *i* in iPods, iPhones, iPads and so on[11]). Subsequently, I will outline how traditional genomics (focused on sequencing the molecularised We) during the first decade of the new millennium gave way to personalised genomics (focused on exploring the molecularised Me). I will explain how new technologies, notably the combination of Next Generation Sequencing (NGS) and wearable devices, give rise to self-tracking practices as part of a global 'citizen health science' movement, exemplified by a paradigmatic laboratory experiment known as the Snyderome. I will indicate how such practices concur with the famous psychoanalytic rule which claims that, in order to achieve self-knowledge, *everything*, however trivial, personal or embarrassing, should be reported. My basic argument will be that, rather than facilitating practices of the self, these self-tracking endeavours expose the individuals involved to a molecularised superego or voice of conscience, continuously imploring them to better their daily habits, so as to exploit and enjoy life to the full.

12.2   Know Thyself 3.0: A Brief Genealogy of Self-Directedness

In *Phaedo*, Socrates tells how his interest in philosophy was aroused by a book entitled *On Nature*, written by Anaxagoras.[12] The reading disappointed him, however. For how was it possible to determine whether the ideas put forward by this author were credible and true? How to determine whether this author was a reliable source of knowledge? Socrates concluded that, in order to understand the

[10] Dickenson, *Me Medicine vs We Medicine*, p. 14.
[11] J. M. Twenge and Keith W. Campbell, *The Narcissism Epidemic. Living in the Age of Entitlement* (New York, NY: Free Press, 2009).
[12] Plato, *Plato I: Euthyphro, Apology, Crito, Phaedo, Phaedrus* [Loeb edition] (Cambridge, MA: Harvard University Press, 1914/1995), pp. 97–9.

external world, we must first of all secure our understanding of ourselves, by critically questioning the reliability of our sense organs and of the human mind. As his maxim he adopted the phrase 'Know Thyself' (γνῶθι σεαυτόν), which was inscribed on the forecourt of the Temple of Apollo at Delphi by the seven sages during the sixth century BC, as recorded by the Greek travelogue writer Pausanias.[13] So, paradoxically, in order to understand nature (external reality, the world, the *object*), we first of all must understand ourselves: we must shift our focus from world to *Self*, from object to *subject*. And dialectics, as a practice of the self, was basically a programme of self-edification via intellectual exercises, meant to transform oneself into a reliable instrument of knowledge.

However, here a second paradox emerged. Within our innermost Self, we discover something else, namely λόγος, the voice of conscience and reason: our inner 'demon', as Socrates called it, or as the Christian author Augustine would later reframe it: God, speaking to us from within ourselves (as *interior intimo meo*, i.e. as something more internal than my innermost Self). So, in our quest for self-knowledge, another shift inevitably takes place: not only from *object* (nature) to *subject* (Self), but also from subject to *Other*: to the inner voice of conscience, or reason, or God, leading the subject upward, as it were. This gave rise to a normative set of questions: how to constitute oneself, not only as a reliable source of knowledge but also as a responsible moral subject? Similar to the dialectical exercises (required for becoming a reliable instrument of knowledge), moral self-edification required a practice of the self as well, consisting of ascetic exercises resulting in self-mastery (ἄσκησις in Greek). Building on Nietzsche and others, this focus on exercise, on practices of the self or auto-plasticity, was taken up by Michel Foucault in the 1980s[14] and more recently by Peter Sloterdijk.[15] The moral and intellectual exercise perspective allows us to see Descartes's *Discourse on Method*, for instance, as a meticulous recording of a self-directed practice, a series of spiritual exercises, grafted on Jesuit models.[16] And indeed, according to Sloterdijk,[17] human history is basically the result of

---

[13] Pausanias, *Guide to Greece Volume I* (London: Penguin, 1971), p. 466.
[14] M. Foucault, *Histoire de la sexualité 2: L'usage des plaisirs* (Paris: Gallimard, 1984); M. Foucault, *Histoire de la sexualité 3: Le souci de soi* (Paris: Gallimard, 1984).
[15] P. Sloterdijk, *Du musst dein Leben ändern: Über Anthropotechnik* (Suhrkamp, 2009).
[16] H. Zwart, *Technocratie en Onbehagen: De Plaats van de Ethiek in het Werk van Michel Foucault* (Nijmegen: Sun, 1995).
[17] Sloterdijk, *Du musst dein Leben ändern*.

THE MOLECULARISED ME   249

millennia of relentless self-experimentation by practicing individuals or
networks of individuals.

In the course of the nineteenth century, self-reflection (i.e. the critical
turn towards the Self) became objectified by a new discipline, namely
psychology (in its various branches and guises), focused on the mental
and behavioural aptitudes of individuals. The Self became the formal
object for scientific psychological assessment and research. Although the
birth of the psychological research subject was already thematised (and
problematised) in Georg Büchner's dramatic classic *Woyzeck*,[18] this
development gained momentum around 1900, when the scientific
reframing of the Self resulted in the emergence of a new type of human
subject: the quantified and objectified Self of test psychology.

This development is convincingly captured by the movie *A Dangerous
Method* (2011), directed by David Cronenberg and casting Michael
Fassbender in the role of Carl Gustav Jung. In his thirties, just before
meeting Freud, Jung conducted association experiments to explore
unconscious psychic 'complexes', employing new experimental devices
such as a galvanometer, but also a *Fünftel-sekundenuhr* (a one-fifth
second time watch) to measure reaction times of patients and/or research
subjects as accurately as possible.[19] Slight, almost imperceptible hesita-
tions in a subject's responses to certain stimuli could provide a window
into these psychic complexes (i.e. particular constellations of ideas, concerns and emotions) which hampered the individuals involved. After the
break with Freud, Jung took up this line of research again, culminating in
his theory of psychological types,[20] which notably differentiates between
'introvert' and 'extrovert' personality types: terms which are still in use,
for instance in the context of the Myers–Briggs personality test. In other
words, test psychology provided new options and new vocabularies for
self-knowledge: a new set of techniques was introduced for opening up
the black box of our inner Self.

Yet here again, a paradox occurs. Terms such as 'introvert' and 'extrovert' only make sense in comparison with certain standards of normalcy.
In other words, in our quest for self-knowledge, we are inevitably

[18] H. Zwart, 'Woyzeck and the birth of the human research subject: genetic disposition and
the nature–nurture debate through the looking-glass of fiction' (2013) 6(3) *Bioethica
Forum*, 97–105.
[19] C. G. Jung, 'Über das Verhalten der Reaktionszeit beim Assoziationsexperimente' in
Gesammelte Werke II. Experimentelle Untersuchungen (Olten und Freiburg im Breisgau:
Walter, 1905/1979), pp. 239–289.
[20] C. G. Jung, *Psychologische Typen* (Leipzig and Stuttgart: Rascher, 1921/1925).

confronted with a standardised, normalised *Other*, with a societal standard or optimum which we may aspire to reach: defined by those who *designed* the test.

In the early twentieth century, such psychological and psychoanalytical techniques were still regarded as *dangerous methods*, as the title of the movie indicates, but nowadays psychological vocabularies and techniques have become more firmly embedded in everyday language and social practices. They have become *domesticated*, so to speak, becoming household terms. Perhaps the same will happen to the molecular-digital repertoire of genome-speak during the coming years.

In this chapter I argue that personalised medicine, or Me Medicine, may indeed be regarded as yet another turn towards self-knowledge, albeit employing bio-molecular and digital terms and techniques. Self-tracking devices purport to provide access to our molecularised unconscious. The research platform MyFinder, for instance, established by Takashido Kido in Tokyo, explicitly aims to make intelligent agents more aware of their 'subconscious' processes, signals and behaviours, via daily self-monitoring.[21] In other words: self-tracking purports to offer a more direct window into unconscious mechanisms, bypassing more traditional language-based techniques such as psychotherapy, dream analysis or free associations on a Freudian couch.[22] Again, words are increasingly replaced by quantification, by measurements, by *numbers*.

But once again we are faced with a paradox, I argue. At the heart of this quest for a personalised (i.e. molecularised, quantified and sequenced) Self of the terabyte age, we encounter a (big) Other: a molecularised voice of conscience, confronting us with demands and expectations, in accordance with the pervasive neoliberal rationality and its entrepreneurial logic, which entails a neoliberal imperative of wellness and sexuality as well. For, as Žižek[23] convincingly argues, building on Lacan, neo-liberal bio-citizens are faced with a rather demanding imperative: they are expected to *enjoy* life relentlessly and to the full.

---

[21] http://takashikido.info

[22] H. Zwart, 'The genome as the biological unconscious – and the unconscious as the psychic "genome": A psychoanalytical rereading of molecular genetics' (2013) 9(2) *Cosmos and History: the Journal of Natural and Social Philosophy*, 198–222.

[23] S. Žižek, *Organs without Bodies: On Deleuze and Consequences* (London/New York, NY: Routledge, 2004/2012), p. 299.

12.3   The Personal (= $1,000 dollar) Genome and Its Pioneers (Venter, Collins, Crichton)

One of the first individuals who had his personal genome sequenced was genomics pioneer Craig Venter. Some years after launching a privately funded human genome sequencing endeavour of his own (in competition with the publicly funded programme led by Francis Collins), he published an autobiographical account of the genomics revolution entitled *A Life Decoded: My Genome: My Life*.[24] For anyone interested in contemporary life sciences research and personalised medicine, this ego-document is simply inescapable: a must-read. In the author's own language, it is 'a tale of seemingly impossible quests and grand objectives', but also of 'great rivalries and bitter disputes', of 'battles of ideologies, morals and ethics', of 'clashes of egos'.[25] The story relates (in an engaging manner) how the human genome epic swept the author 'from peaks of incredible exhilaration as I marshalled a relatively small but dedicated army of scientists, computers and robots to achieve what seemed almost impossible, and then plunged me into black pits of depression as I faced opposition from Nobel laureates and senior government officials, my colleagues, and even my wife'.[26] Interestingly, moreover, the book contains a systematic reflection on the relationship between personal genes and biographical vicissitudes. In separate boxes, dedicated to specific genes which Venter discovered on his own genome, the author notably singles out genes that are allegedly associated with behavioural characteristics, such as thrill-seeking behaviour, attention deficit hyperactivity disorder (ADHD) and stress-coping. Thus, Venter is a genomics pioneer in more than one sense. He is one of the first individuals who explicitly began to think about himself in terms of genes and genomics techniques. In Venter's case, autobiography and the genome are connected in more than one way.

At the same time, there is an obvious incongruence between Venter's genetic boxes and the story of his life. For if a lesson can be derived from the latter at all, it would be that the vicissitudes of scientists and their projects are the outcome of a horrendously complex constellation of interacting factors so that, narratively speaking, the explanatory (let alone predictive) power of certain (behavioural or personality) genes can be regarded as negligible. What seems absent in Venter's

---

[24] J. C. Venter, *A Life Decoded: My Genome: My Life* (New York, NY: Viking/Penguin, 2007).
[25] Ibid., p. 2.   [26] Ibid., p. 2.

reconstruction, for instance, while figuring prominently in the psychology of types developed by Carl Gustav Jung[27] mentioned above, is that,
even if certain predispositions of individuals (say, an inclination towards
risk-seeking, or rather the lack thereof) can be associated with the presence or absence of certain genes, there will at the same time be
a tendency in the human beings involved to 'compensate' for their
deviances, so that extrovert persons, for instance, will invest time and
effort in becoming more focused, while introverts will learn to develop
interest in others, and so on. Indeed, even if some level of explanatory
power can be granted to specific genes, the 'nurture' dimension (education, societal interaction, relationships and the like) is likely to compensate for geneticised 'nature'.

But the issue of rethinking health and biographies from a personalised
genomics perspective was also taken up by Venter's competitor Francis
Collins, former director of the publicly funded Human Genome Project
(HGP) and now Director of the National Institutes of Health (NIH), in
his book *The Language of Life: DNA and the Revolution in Personalised
Medicine*.[28] Although Collins still sees the HGP as 'one of the boldest
scientific efforts that humankind has ever mounted',[29] at the same time
he observes that genomics enthusiasm has more or less evaporated.
The revolution is still raging, he maintains, but will not be realised by
the discovery of the human sequence as such. Rather, the impact of
genomics will become visible via the subsequent stage of Next
Generation Sequencing (NGS) and personalised medicine:

> Healthy individuals are increasingly able to discover some of their body's
> inner secrets and take appropriate action. The potential for individual
> prediction is beginning to spill out to the general public, offering the
> opportunity to take more control of your fate ... None of this is happen-
> ing overnight, [but] without question, man's knowledge of man is under-
> going the greatest revolution since Leonardo.[30]

But as soon as Collins comes up with concrete examples, the revolutionary fervour rapidly evaporates.[31] One of the examples given by Collins is
the impact of the personalised genomics revolution on assessing personality traits. Through the focus on personality and behaviour, the genomics revolution moves beyond clinical settings and enters into the daily

---

[27] C. G. Jung, *Psychologische Typen*.   [28] F. Collins, *The Language of Life*.
[29] Ibid., p. 299.   [30] Ibid., p. 5.
[31] H. Zwart, 'Francis Collins: The Language of Life' (Book Review) (2011) 6(3) *Genomics,
Society & Policy*, 67–76.

lifeworld of healthy individuals, he argues. Will information derived from NGS and personalised genome sequencing in the near future replace (or at least complement) existing techniques such as the Myers–Briggs personality test? Will pre-employment genetic screening (PEGS), for example, become accepted practice, testing candidates (for their own benefit) for genes associated with stress tolerance, for instance? In recent years, a number of genes associated with personality traits have indeed entered the stage, Collins remarks, notably genes allegedly associated with novelty seeking, harm avoidance, reward dependence and persistence. As Collins points out, however, although some of these genes may have some effects, the contribution of each of them will be so infinitesimally small that predictability claims of personality traits based on DNA testing 'should be taken with considerable scepticism'.[32] The same holds for the genetic basis for male 'infidelity' as a personality trait: 'Do not be misled ... the actual influence on the behaviour on an individual male [of such a gene] is quite modest, and should certainly not be used in mate selection or as an excuse for cheating [on] one's partner'.[33] Thus, compared to the soaring claims made in the introduction to his book, the actual evidence provided for the 'next' genomics revolution is remarkably slight.

In the novel *Next* (a reference perhaps to NGS), science novel author Michael Crichton[34] takes the argument one step further by using his novel as an ethical laboratory for exploring the emerging future. Series of lifeworld experiments are conducted in the form of multiple storylines: what will happen if personalised genomics information proliferates into society and increasingly affects the ways in which individuals think and speak about themselves? *Next* explores in an imaginative manner the impact of personalised bio-information on self-understanding and identity-formation by showing a number of individuals actively engaged in redefining themselves on the basis of their genetic profile. Their narratives revolve around a number of 'genes for' – i.e. recently identified genes that supposedly co-determine behavioural characteristics such as the 'maturity' gene, the 'novelty-seeking' (or thrill-seeking) gene, the 'sociability' gene and the 'infidelity' gene. The absence of the maturity gene, for instance, serves to explain an individual's propensity for drug addiction. Various practices of the Self, ranging from paternity testing and partner selection up to taking a stand in court, are articulated in terms of

---

[32] Ibid., p. 200.   [33] Ibid., p. 204.
[34] M. Crichton, *Next* (New York, NY: Harper Collins, 2006).

genomics-speak. Thus, the moral of the story is that, in the near future, bio-citizens may indeed use the absence or presence of certain genes in their genomes to identify themselves, as easily perhaps as we currently speak about ourselves as introverts or extroverts. In the end, however, although there are various traceable connections between storylines and ongoing research programmes,[35] Crichton's novel seems to ridicule rather than to endorse the genomics revolution by taking the logic of behavioural and personality genomics to the point of absurdity.

Things continue to evolve rapidly, though, and in the current situation, because of the *combination* of personalised genome information with self-tracking practices, involving wearable devices, the revolution finally appears to gain momentum (in high-income parts of the world, that is).

12.4   The Snyderome

In 2012, Michael Snyder and his team at the Department of Genetics at Stanford University published the 'integrative Personal Omics Profile' (iPOP) of a single individual, a 54-year-old male volunteer whom they had closely monitored over the course of 14 months.[36] This longitudinal case study resulted in a comprehensive omics portrait ('high resolution'), combining 'deep sequencing' (of the subject's genotype) with more than 3 billion measurements of molecules (i.e. the subject's phenotype). Although the research subject was a 'healthy individual', the project evolved into a case history (*Krankengeschichte*) as two minor viral infections, together with (unexpected) evidence of the subject's propensity for diabetes, constituted the dramatic highlights of the story.

Soon, it turned out that the 'male volunteer' of this $N = 1$ experiment (surrounded by qualified personnel and costly equipment) was none other than Michael Snyder himself, the department chair, now acting as his own research subject of choice, turning his body into an omics laboratory. The experiment resulted in what has been referred to as the Snyderome, or even the 'narcissome'.[37] Snyder himself made it known that he plans to remain a study subject for life, adding new sources of

[35] H. Zwart, 'Next' (Book review) (2007) 3(1) *Genomics, Society & Policy*, 48–51.

[36] R. Chen, G. I. Mias, J. Li-Pook-Than et al., 'Personal omics profiling reveals dynamic molecular and medical phenotypes' (2012) 148 *Cell* 1293–1307. doi:10.1016/j.cell.2012.02.009.

[37] C. Dennis, 'The rise of the narciss-ome: Profiles of a researcher's genes, proteins and more show personalized genomic medicine in action' (2012) *Nature News*. doi:10.1038/nature.2012.10240.

information as the process unfolds, including data procured from body samples such as breath, urine, faeces ('stool microbiome') and saliva. Psychoanalytically speaking, the focus of molecularised self-tracking consistently seems to be on bodily waste materials, released via various erogenous zones.

But another, perhaps more striking parallel with psychoanalysis can be pointed out as well. Insofar as the Snyderome can indeed be regarded as a prototypical version of an emerging practice of the self, a window into the future, an intriguing scenario evolves. Individuals will be requested to monitor and report, with evenly poised attention, *everything* about themselves, however trivial, embarrassing or indiscreet it may seem, so that they may learn and communicate things about their moods and bodies which even they do not know themselves. Such practices of self-tracking adhere to the psychoanalytic rule that, in order to probe one's symptoms, *everything*, however trivial or personal, is relevant. Or, as Freud himself phrased it: 'We instruct the patient to ... report to us whatever internal observations he is able to make [taking care not to] exclude any of them, whether on the ground that it is too *disagreeable* or too *indiscreet* to say, or that it is too *unimportant* or *irrelevant*'.[38] Seemingly trivial details (the bagatelle) often prove highly significant. The Freudian credo that full coverage (full transparency) is essential, and that nothing is too trivial or too embarrassing to report, applies to microbiome research as well. But again, articulation and verbalisation give way to measurements and quantification. Rather than on verbal symptoms (slips of the tongue, word finding problems and the like) the focus will be on peaks and dips in self-tracking diagrams.

As a case study of Me Medicine, the Snyderome involves a self-tracking pioneer, committed to measuring *everything*, even those dimensions of bodily functioning that may seem too trivial, too personal or too unpleasant to record, resulting in an *integrative Personal Omics Profile* (iPOP), a comprehensive omics portrait (extremely high resolution) of a single individual. This portrait is highly personal and highly impersonal at the same time, however, as the living individual is both captured and lost in data.[39] It is not a portrait in the sense of a recognisable image, but

---

[38] Freud, S., 'Vorlesungen zur Einführung in die Psychoanalyse' in *Gesammelte Werke XI* (London: Imago, 1917/1940), p. 297.

[39] The Snyderome project is also a testbed for the latest omics technologies. Besides chairing a prominent genetics department, Snyder is also involved in high-tech omics companies such as Personalis, GenapSys and Illumina; Zwart, 'The obliteration of life: depersonalisation and disembodiment in the terabyte age'.

a decidedly technical and symbolic form of self-portrayal, so that the individual involved runs the risk of becoming obliterated in meaningless data litter.

Snyder's idea is that, via high-resolution self-monitoring, future biocitizens will become the proactive managers of their own health condition (rather than hypochondriacs). Longitudinal multi-omics analysis will allow them to take medicine into their own hands, with doctors acting as mere advisors (with whom we will communicate via websites and portals) rather than as 'dictators'. For those who want a look into the future of health: visit the Stanford lab. Or, as science author Jon Cohen phrases it: Michael Snyder takes axioms such as 'know thyself' and 'heal thyself' to the next technological level by taking an extraordinarily detailed look at one's body, employing a slew of recent technological advances.[40] The Snyder experiment purports to provide a window into the future where individuals will not only monitor huge amounts of body molecules in a detailed manner, but will also heavily wire themselves, so as to register pulse, heartbeat, stress (transpiration) and numerous other indicators continuously. Thus, the focus of attention is displaced from the familiar (domesticated) weight scale to a plethora of high-tech wearable gadgets. Measurements of thousands of factors can be integrated through devices such as iPhones and compared with big data references, available 24/7 at open-source repositories (vast science clouds), so that self-diagnostics can be translated into every-day options (such as diet and exercise). The Snyderome project suggests that especially the aetiology of mystery symptoms (such as unexplained fatigue) can from now on be elucidated, while expert science will become democratised into citizen science.

12.5　Citizen Health Science: An Enticing Future?

The Snyderome heralds the advent of a new form of self-directedness. It exemplifies the idea of self-monitoring, self-tracking and data sharing with the help of wearable devices, currently evolving into a new practice of the Self known as 'citizen health science', a term which refers to non-professionals providing professional scientists with observations and measurements, notably by collecting health records on personal health and wellness information.[41] Fitness trackers, smart watches and other

---

[40] Jon Cohen, 'Examining his own body, Stanford geneticist stops diabetes in its tracks', *Science* (16 March 2012), www.sciencemag.org/news/2012/03/examining-his-own-body-stanford-geneticist-stops-diabetes-its-tracks.

[41] A. Bowser and L. Shanley, 'New visions in citizen science' (2013) *Commons Lab: Woodrow Wilson International Center for Scholars*; E. Vayena and J. Tasioulas, 'We the

health applications (or apps) claim to convert smartphones into electronic stethoscopes, ultrasound machines, diagnostic hearing devices, skin cancer detectors, blood test platforms and other medical devices (cf. Huijer and Detweiler in this volume). This development is facilitated by increased global connectivity and technological innovations such as online crowd-sourcing, big data strategies and computational analytics in combination with societal developments, such as the growing do-it-yourself culture relying on smartphones and similar mobile technologies. Thus, citizen health science is symptomatic of a high degree of global internet penetration in combination with the conviction that citizens should be empowered to actively participate in self-management and scientific research.[42]

The challenge now is to provide a preliminary assessment or diagnostics of this development. In terms of neo-liberal Me Medicine, the wave of high-resolution self-monitoring will be presented as empowerment, no doubt, although due attention will also be given to issues such as privacy, informed consent, data management and other mainstream bioethics items. What can a psychoanalytic (or depth ethics) perspective add to such an analysis? In this final section, three aspects of self-monitoring will be highlighted, as building blocks for a psychoanalytical assessment, namely: (a) its focus on radical transparency (as a molecular version of the Freudian maxim to give away *everything*); (b) the specific attention that is given to sexuality and excrements (i.e. the tendency of self-tracking practices to survey everyday existence through genital and excremental grids); and finally (c) the paradoxical (or rather: dialectical) relationship between self-tracking egos and their molecularised conscience or superego, their personalised panopticon.

First of all, as pointed out above, self-tracking techniques request individuals to monitor and report (with evenly poised attention) *everything* about themselves, however trivial or personal, embarrassing or indiscreet it may seem. Thus, the Freudian maxim is transferred to the physical wellness domain. And while Freudian psychotherapy has been regarded as 'automatic talking', in reference to automatic writing (*écriture automatique*, an artistic practice of the Self adopted by

scientists: a human right to citizen science' (2015) 28 *Philosophy and Technology* 479–485. doi:10.1007/s13347-015-0204-0; M. Rothstein, J. Wilbanks and K. Brothers, 'Citizen science on your smartphone: An ELSI research agenda' (2015) 43(4) *The Journal of Law Medicine & Ethics* 897–903.
[42] Vayena and Tasioulas, 'We the scientists: a human right to citizen science'.

surrealists and modernist authors[43]), the self-reporting practices of the present are becoming fully atomised, with the help of gadgets. Somewhere in this stream of data something may show up that raises our suspicion as a remarkable or even revelatory symptom, pointing to something which the individuals themselves may be completely unaware of (such as a subliminal viral infection or a propensity to diabetes).

Moreover, from a psychoanalytical perspective it is striking that, besides physical exercise and food intake, sexual activity likewise has become a key target for self-tracking. While Mozart's Don Giovanni relied on the services of his assistant Leporello to keep a quantified account of his conquests and exploits (640 in Italy, 231 in Germany, 100 in France, 91 in Turkey and 1,003 in Spain), this role is now taken up by digital automation, in the form of mobile apps employed to track (specific features of) sexual behaviour, such as calories burned. This association suggests that, in the neoliberal present, sexual activity is seen as a kind of self-centred physical exercise, rather than as an aristo-cratic game, and comparable to running or swimming.[44]

No less interesting, psychoanalytically speaking, are self-monitoring practices concerning the gut microbiome, i.e. the millions of microor-ganisms (E-coli and others) inhabiting our intestines, responsible for our metabolism, functioning as benign intruders, but regarding us merely as their ecosystem. A symptomatic exemplification of the emergence of citizen health science is provided by the ubiome.com website, which encourages individuals worldwide to explore their microbiome (the gut dimension of their personal Snyderome), sharing the information and becoming 'part of the process' (i.e. of massive health data collecting and sharing). The website provides a sample kit containing 'everything you need to swab and submit your microbiome. Whether for your mouth, ears, nose, gut or genitals, your kit will allow you to learn more about your microbiome. You swipe the sample swab across the corresponding site and send the kit back to us'.[45] Not coincidentally, I would argue, these 'corresponding sites' happen to coincide with what psychoanalytic ter-minology labels as 'erogenous zones'. Indeed, visitors are persuaded to join the initiative with nudging slogans such as 'Compare yourself with others who have a microbiome like yours', 'How does your microbiome

---

[43] H. F. Ellenberger, *The Discovery of the Unconscious* (London: Lane/Penguin, 1970); Zwart, 'The genome as the biological unconscious'.

[44] D. Lupton, 'Quantifying the body: Monitoring and measuring health in the age of mhealth technologies' (2013) 23(4) *Critical Public Health* 393–403.

[45] http://ubiome.com

compare to cutting-edge scientific research?' and 'Explore Your Microbiome, get sequenced'.[46] For instance, users are enabled to follow the effects of a vegetarian diet or exercise on their faeces.

Seen from a psychoanalytical perspective, it is especially remarkable how, in recent years, human excrements have become a focal point of attention in biomedical research, no less than in psychoanalytic case studies of the past.[47] Life scientists worldwide have taken to studying the gut microbiome, and human stool is now increasingly used as a diagnostic tool (for detecting colon cancer). The microbiome emerges as something which is both 'me' and 'not me': both familiar and repellent, both detestable and valuable, both an item of waste and a gift (a source of highly valuable data), an assessment which concurs with psychoanalytic Freudian views.

Thus, self-monitoring may be seen as a high-tech molecularised practice of the Self, allowing individuals to take daily existence more emphatically into their own hands by becoming more aware of things which so far had been hidden. Once again, however, the paradox emerges. Rather than allowing individuals to refashion their own lives, they are requested to compare their daily performances with quantified expectations. Health apps provide reference data (i.e. standards for normality) and can easily become a ubiquitous electronic panopticon:[48] a molecularised version of the super-ego, the voice of conscience of the terabyte age. On a daily basis, computer monitors will be telling individuals that they must change their lives,[49] representing the vertical dimension of human existence (oriented towards systematically improving themselves). They must work on themselves and keep a close watch on themselves to optimise somatic functioning and to live up to health and normalcy standards, and/or to postpone the impacts of unhealthy lifestyles and ageing.

Me Medicine aims to provide data-rich characterisations of individuals, at various stages of health and disease via a comprehensive, high-density portrayal of a person's health status, combining static data (e.g. gene sequence) with dynamic information (concerning lifestyle, responses and environmental challenges for instance). Whereas traditional medicine focuses on processes from the onset of illness towards recovery or death, this new type of Me Medicine reverses the focus of attention, closely monitoring the human body from wellness to early onset stages of disease. In the near future, patients may even pay for their

---

[46] Ibid.   [47] Zwart, '"Extimate" technologies and techno-cultural discontent'.
[48] M. Foucault, Surveiller et punir: naissance de la prison (Paris: Gallimard, 1975).
[49] Sloterdijk, Du musst dein Leben ändern.

healthcare (offered to them at no cost) with their data: the new currency of the upcoming petabyte age.[50]

But again, rather than to practices of the Self, this development gives rise to a digitalised and personalised panopticon: a molecularised version of the voice of conscience; as computers from now on inform us (on a daily basis) that we must change our life: the superego of the terabyte age. And eventually perhaps, rather than achieving self-determination (by translating continuous measurements into lifestyle *options*), individuals will rather be drowned in data, so that lifestyle options will submerge in indigestible data litter.

In conclusion, self-monitoring may indeed be regarded as a new chapter in the long history of practices of self-directedness and self-observation. Moreover, in preliminary assessments of this emerging development (discussed above), three positions can be distinguished. Some voices (such as Francis Collins and Michael Snyder) emphasise the *knowledge* dimension, i.e. the extent to which these techno-scientific contrivances produce extremely high-resolution portraits of our selves: much more detailed and reliable than previous sources of information (such as introspection, spiritual exercises or personality tests). Others (critics) will be inclined to emphasise the *power* dimension, however. From this perspective, lifestyle gadgets easily become a personalised panopticon, urging individuals to adapt themselves to societal expectations in their daily private lives. Finally, advocates or adepts of the Me Medicine wave are likely to applaud this development in terms of self-determination and empowerment. As Foucault[51] convincingly argued, however, phenomena such as self-monitoring can only be adequately assessed if all three axes of analysis are included; if all three dimensions are taken into consideration. Self-monitoring emerges at the intersection of three types of practices: practices of knowledge, of power and of the Self. Rather than concluding that we ought to be *in favour of* or *against* self-monitoring devices, a differential assessment is called for, mapping the interacting pros and cons in three directions. And precisely because self-monitoring is part of a broader socio-cultural and techno-scientific transition, such an assessment will become part of and contribute to a comprehensive diagnostics of the present.

[50] C. Elliott, *White Coat, Black Hat: Adventures on the Dark Side of Medicine* (Boston: Beacon Press, 2011).
[51] Foucault, *Histoire de la sexualité 2*.

BIBLIOGRAPHY

Abouna, George M., 'Negative impact of trading in human organs on the development of transplantation in the Middle East' (1993) 25(3) *Transplant Proceedings* 2310–2313

Agamben, Giorgio, 'Identity without the person' in Giorgio Agamben, *Nudities* (Palo Alto, CA: Stanford University Press, 2010) 46–54

Agarwal, M. B., 'Umbilical cord blood transplantation: newer trends' (2006) 54 *Journal of the Association of Physicians of India* 143–147

Alzheimer's Association, 'Alzheimer's and dementia testing for earlier diagnosis' www.alz.org/research/science/earlier_alzheimers_diagnosis.asp

Alzheimer's Association, 'For healthcare professionals: frequently asked questions about beta-amyloid imaging' (2013) www.alz.org/documents_custom/hps_auc_faq.pdf

Ambagtsheer, Frederike and Weimar, Willem, 'A criminological perspective: why prohibition of organ trade is not effective and how the Declaration of Istanbul can move forward' (2012) 12(3) *American Journal of Transplantation* 571–575

American Academy of Pediatrics (AAP), 'Policy statement: cord blood banking for potential future transplantation' (2007) 119(1) *Pediatrics* 165–170

American College of Obstetricians and Gynecologists (ACOG), *Committee Opinion 648* (December 2015)

American Society of Human Genetics, 'ASHG opposes H.R.1313, the preserving employee wellness programs act: bill would undermine genetic privacy protections' (8 March 2017), www.ashg.org/press/201703-HR1313.html

Anderson, Elizabeth, 'The ethical limitations of the market' (1990) 6(2) *Economics and Philosophy* 179–205

Anderson, Elizabeth, *Value in Ethics and Economics* (Cambridge, MA: Harvard University Press, 1995)

Andorno, Roberto, 'The right not to know: an autonomy-based approach' (2004) 30(5) *Journal of Medical Ethics* 435–9

Andorno, Roberto, 'Human dignity and human rights as a common ground for a global bioethics' (2009) 34(3) *Journal of Medicine and Philosophy* 223–40

Andrews, Lori and Nelkin, Dorothy, 'Whose body is it anyway? Disputes over body tissue in a biotechnology age' (1998) 351(9095) *The Lancet* 53–7

Angrist, Misha, 'Personal genomics: access denied? Consumers have a right to their genomes' (September/October 2008) MIT Technology Review, www.techno logyreview.com/s/410662/personal-genomics-access-denied/.

Anker, Ashley E. and Feeley, Thomas H., 'Estimating the risks of acquiring a kidney abroad: a meta-analysis of complications following participation in transplant tourism' (2012) 26(3) *Clinical Transplantation* E232–41

Annas, George J., 'The prostitute, the playboy, and the poet: rationing schemes for organ transplantation' (1985) 75(2) *American Journal of Public Health* 187–9

Arnold, Robert, Bartlett, Steven, Bernat, James et al., 'Financial incentives for cadaver organ donation: an ethical reappraisal' (2002) 73(8) *Transplantation* 1361–7

Aronowitz, Alexis A., *Human Trafficking, Human Misery: The Global Trade in Human Beings* (Greenwood Publishing Group, 2009)

Arora, K. S. and Blake, V., 'Uterus transplantation: the ethics of moving the womb' (2015) 125(4) *Obstetrics and Gynecology* 971–4

Ashby-Mitchell, K., Burns R., Shaw J. and Anstey K., 'Proportion of dementia in Australia explained by common modifiable risk factors' (2017) 9(1) *Alzheimers Research and Therapy* 11

Bachelard, G., 'Noumène et microphysique' (1932/1970) *Recherches Philosophiques* 55–65: 11–24

Bachelard G., 'L'activité rationaliste de la physique contemporaine' (Paris: Presses Universitaires de France, 1951)

Bakdash, Tarif and Scheper-Hughes, Nancy, 'Is it ethical for patients with renal disease to purchase kidneys from the world's poor?' (2006) 3(10) *PloS Medicine* e349

Ballen, Karen, 'Challenges in umbilical cord blood stem cell banking for stem cell reviews and reports' (2010) 6(8) *Stem Cell Review and Reports* 8–14

Ballen, Karen, 'Update on cord blood transplantation' (2017) 6 *F1000Research* 1556. doi:10.12688/f1000research.11952.1

Balzer, David, *Curationism: How Curating Took Over the World and Everything Else* (London: Pluto Press, 2015)

Barritt, Jacob A., Brenner, Carol A., Malter, Henry E. and Cohen, Jacques, 'Mitochondria in human offspring derived from ooplasmic transplantation' (2001) 16(3) *Human Reproduction* 513–6

Baylis, Françoise, 'Human nuclear genome transfer (so-called mitochondrial replacement): clearing the underbrush' (2017) 31(1) *Bioethics* 7–19. doi:10.1111/bioe.12309

'The ethics of creating children with three genetic parents' (2013) 26 *Reproductive Biomedicine Online* 531–4

Baylis, Francoise and Cattapan, Alana, 'Personalized medicine and the politics of human nuclear genome transfer' in Britta van Beers, Sigrid Sterckx and Donna Dickenson (eds.), *Personalised Medicine, Individual Choice and the Common Good* (Cambridge: Cambridge University Press, 2018)

Beard, T. Randolph and Leitzel, Jim, 'Designing a compensated-kidney donation system' (2014) 77(3) *Law and Contemporary Problems* 253–87

Beck, Ulrich, *Risk Society: Towards a New Modernity* (New Delhi: Sage, 1992)

Beck, Ulrich, *World Risk Society* (Cambridge: Polity Press, 1999)

Becker, Gary S. and Elias, Julio J., 'Cash for kidneys: the case for a market for organs' (18 January 2014) *The Wall Street Journal*

Becker, Gary S. and Elias, Julio J., 'Introducing incentives in the market for live and cadaveric organ donations' (2007) 21(3) *Journal of Economic Perspectives* 3–24

Benagiano, G., Landeweerd, L. and Brosens, I., 'Medical and ethical considerations in uterus transplantation' (2013) 123(2) *International Journal of Gynecology and Obstetrics* 173–7

Benjamin, Caroline, 'Findings from the National Consent Evaluation' (2016) www.genomicsengland.co.uk/consent-evaluation-findings, accessed 6 November 2017

Bennett, Becki, 'What does consent mean for Generation Genome?' (18 September 2017) *BioNews*, www.bionews.org.uk/page_886840.asp, accessed 6 November 2017

Bentham, Jeremy, *Theory of Legislation*, ed. Etienne Dumont and Richard Hildreth (Holmes Beach, FL: Gaunt, [1802] 2011)

Bentham, Jeremy, *A Fragment on Government and an Introduction to the Principles of Morals and Legislation*, ed. Wilfried Harrison (Oxford: Basil Blackwell, [1789] 1967)

Beyleveld, Derek and Brownsword, Roger, *Human Dignity in Bioethics and Biolaw* (Oxford: Oxford University Press, 2001)

Bharadwaj, Aditya, *Local Cells, Global Science: The Proliferation of Stem Cell Technologies in India* (London: Routledge, 2009)

Bianchi, Diana W., 'From prenatal genomic diagnosis to fetal personalized medicine: progress and challenges' (2012) 18 *Nature Medicine* 1041–51

Biller-Andorno, Nikola and Capron, Alexander M., '"Gratuities" for donated organs: ethically indefensible' (2011) 377(9775) *The Lancet* 1390–1

Binswanger, Harry, 'FDA says, "No gene test for you: you can't handle the truth"' (26 November 2013) *Forbes*, www.forbes.com/sites/harrybinswanger/2013/11/26/fda-says-no-gene-test-for-you-you-cant-handle-the-truth/#780b3d4e4156, accessed 28 January 2018

Björkmann, Barbro, 'Why we are not allowed to sell that which we are encouraged to donate' (2006) 15(1) *Cambridge Quarterly of Healthcare Ethics* 60–70

Black, Lee, Simard, Jacques and Knoppers, Bartha Maria, 'Genetic testing, physicians and the law: will the tortoise ever catch up with the hare?' (2010) 19(1) *Annals of Health Law* 115–20

Blake, L., Jadva, V. and Golombok, S., 'Parent psychological adjustment, donor conception and disclosure: a follow-up over 10 years' (2014) 29(11) *Human Reproduction* 2487–96

Blennow, K., de Leon, M. J. and Zetterberg, H., 'Alzheimer's disease' (2006) 368 *The Lancet* 387–403

Blennow, K. and Zetterberg, H., 'Cerebrospinal fluid biomarkers for Alzheimer's disease' (2009) 18(2) *Journal of Alzheimer's Disease* 413–7

Bode, M. and Kristensen, D. B., 'The digital doppelgänger within: a study on self-tracking and the quantified self movement' in D. Bajde and R. Canniford (eds.), *Assembling Consumption* (Oxford/New York: Routledge, 2015)

Bodkin, Henry, 'Three-parent baby born to infertile couple in world first' (18 January 2017), *The Telegraph*, www.telegraph.co.uk/science/2017/01/18/three-parent-baby-born-infertile-couple-world-first

Bonython, Wendy Elizabeth and Arnold, Bruce Baer, 'Direct to consumer genetic testing and the libertarian right to test' (2017) *Journal of Medical Ethics*. doi: 10.1136/medethics-2016-103778

Borry, Pascal, van Hellemondt, R.E., Sprumont, D. et al., 'Legislation in direct-to-consumer genetic testing in seven European countries' (2012) 20(7) *European Journal of Human Genetics* 715–21

Boyer, J. Randall, 'Gifts of the heart … and other tissues: legalizing the sale of human organs and tissues' (2012) 1 *Brigham Young University Law Review* 313–40

Brady, Diane, 'Do genetic tests need doctors? FDA defends its challenge to 23andMe' (2013) 27 November *Bloomberg Businessweek*

Bramstedt, Katrina A. and Xu, Jun, 'Checklist: passport, plane ticket, organ transplant' (2007) 7(7) *American Journal of Transplantation* 1698–1701

Brännström, M., Johannesson, L., Dahm-Kähler, P. et al., 'First clinical uterus transplantation trial: a six-month report' (2014) 101(5) *Fertility and Sterility* 1228–36

Brännström, M., Bokström, H., Dahm-Kähler, P. et al., 'One uterus bridging three generations: first live birth after mother-to-daughter uterus transplantation' (2016) 106(2) *Fertility and Sterility* 261–6.

Brännström, M., Johannesson, L., Bokström, H. et al., 'Livebirth after uterus transplantation' (2015) 385(9968) *The Lancet* 607–16

Bray, Michelle B., 'Personalizing personality: toward a property right in human bodies' (1990) 69(1) *Texas Law Review* 209–44

Brecher, Bob, 'The kidney trade: or, the customer is always wrong' (1990) 16(3) *Journal of Medical Ethics* 120–3

Bromfield, N. and Smith Robati, K., 'Global surrogacy, exploitation, human rights and international private law: a pragmatic stance and policy recommendations' (2014) 1 *Global Social Welfare* 123–35

Brown, Nik, Kraft, Andrew and Martin, Paul, 'The promissory pasts of blood cells' (2006) 1 *Biosocieties* 329–48

Brown, Nik and Kraft, Andrew, 'Blood ties – banking the stem cell promise' (2006) 3/4 *Technology Analysis and Strategic Management* 313–27

Brown, Nik, Machin, Laura and McLeod, Danae, 'The immunitary bioeconomy: the economisation of life in the international cord blood market' (2011) 30 *Social Science and Medicine* 1–8

Brownsword, Roger, 'An interest in human dignity as the basis for genomic torts' (2003) 42(3) *Washburn Law Journal* 413–87

'What the world needs now: techno-regulation, human rights and human dignity' in Roger Brownsword (ed.), *Human Rights* (Oxford: Hart, 2004), pp. 203–34

'Human dignity, biolaw, and the basis of moral community' (2010) 21(4) *Journal International de Bioéthique* 21–40

Buchanan, Allen, Brock, Dan, Daniels, Norman and Wikler, Daniel, *From Chance to Choice: Genetics and Justice* (Cambridge: Cambridge University Press, 2000).

Budiani-Saberi, Debra A., 'Organ trafficking and transplant tourism' in Vardit Ravitsky, Autumn Fiester and Arthur L. Caplan (eds.), *The Penn Center Guide to Bioethics* (New York, NY: Springer, 2009), pp. 699–708

Budiani-Saberi, Debra A. and Columb, Seán, 'A human rights approach to human trafficking for organ removal' (2013) 16(4) *Medicine, Health Care, and Philosophy* 897–914

Budiani-Saberi, Debra A. and Delmonico, Francis L., 'Organ trafficking and transplant tourism: a commentary on the global realities' (2008) 8(5) *American Journal of Transplantation* 925–9

Budiani-Saberi, Debra A. and Karim, Kabir, 'The social determinants of organ trafficking: a reflection of social inequity' (2009) 4(1) *Social Medicine* 48–51

Budiani-Saberi, Debra A. and Mostafa, Amir, 'Care for commercial living donors: the experience of an NGO's outreach in Egypt' (2011) 24(4) *Transplant International* 317–23

Bundeskartellamt, 'Bundeskartellamt initiates proceeding against Facebook on suspicion of having abused its market power by infringing data protection rules' (2016)

Burke, W. et al., 'Extending the range of public health genomics: what should be the agenda for public health in an era of genome-based and "personalized" medicine?' (2010) 12 *Genetics in Medicine* 785–91

Butler, Merlin G. and Menitove, Jay E., 'Umbilical cord blood banking: an update' (2011) 28 *Journal of Assisted Reproduction and Genetics* 669–76. doi: 10.1007/s10815-011-9577-x

Cahill, Damien and Konings, Martijn, *Neoliberalism* (Cambridge: Polity Press, 2017)

Caldicott, Fiona, 'Review of Data Security, Consent and Opt-Outs' (2016) www.gov.uk/government/uploads/system/uploads/attachment_data/file/535024/data-security-review.PDF, accessed 6 November 2017

Callaway, Ewen, 'UK sets sights on gene therapy in eggs' (2012) 481(7382) *Nature News* 419. doi:10.1038/481419a

Caplan, Arthur L., 'Organ transplantation: the challenge of scarcity' in Vardit Ravitsky, Autumn Fiester and Arthur L. Caplan (eds.), *The Penn Center Guide to Bioethics* (New York, NY: Springer, 2009), pp. 679–87

Caplan, Arthur L., Perry, Constance M., Plante, Lauren A. et al. 'Moving the womb' (2007) 37 *Hastings Center Report* 18–20

Capron, Alexander M., Danovitch, Gabriel M. and Delmonico, Francis L., 'Organ markets: problems beyond harm to vendors' (2014) 14(10) *American Journal of Bioethics* 23–5

Caulfield, Tim and Kaye, Jane, 'Broad consent in biobanking: reflections on seemingly insurmountable dilemmas' (2009) 10 *Medical Law International* 85–100

Centers for Disease Control and Prevention (CDC), *How Much Physical Activity Do Adults Need? | Physical Activity | CDC* (no date) Available at: www.cdc.gov/physicalactivity/basics/adults/index.htm (accessed 2 February 2018).

Centers for Medicaid and Medicare, 'Decision Memo for Beta Amyloid Positron Emission Tomography in Dementia and Neurodegenerative Disease' (CAG-00431 N). (2013) www.cms.gov/medicare-coverage-database/details/nca-decision-memo.aspx?NCAId=265.

Chadwick, Ruth F., 'The market for bodily parts: Kant and duties to oneself' (1989) 6(2) *Journal of Applied Philosophy* 129–39

Chaudhary, Vivek, 'Argentina uncovers patients killed for organs' (1992) 304 (5834) *British Medical Journal* 1073–4

Chelsea and Westminster Hospital, 'West London Genomic Medicine Centre', www.chelwest.nhs.uk/about-us/research-development/west-london-genomic-medicine-centre, accessed 6 November 2017

Chen, R., Mias, G. I., Li-Pook-Than., J. et al., 'Personal omics profiling reveals dynamic molecular and medical phenotypes' (2012) 148 *Cell* 1293–307. doi:10.1016/j.cell.2012.02.009

Chen, Jonathan H. and Asch, Steven M., 'Machine learning and prediction in medicine – Beyond the peak of inflated expectations' (2017) 376(26) *New England Journal of Medicine* 2507–9

Cherry, Mark J., 'Is a market for human organs necessarily exploitative?' (2000) 14 (4) *Public Affairs Quarterly* 337–60

Cherry, Mark J., *Kidney for Sale by Owner: Human Organs, Transplantation, and the Market* (Washington, DC: Georgetown University Press, 2005)

Chico, Victoria, *Genomic Negligence: An Interest in Autonomy as the Basis for Novel Negligence Claims Generated by Genetic Technology* (London/New York, NY: Routledge, 2011)

Childress, James F., 'The body as property: some philosophical reflections' (1992) 24(5) *Transplant Proceedings* 2143–8

Chinnery, Patrick F., 'Mitochondrial disorders overview' in Roberta A. Pagon, Margaret P. Adam, Holly H. Ardinger et al. (eds.), *GeneReviews* (Seattle, WA: University of Washington, 1993), www.ncbi.nlm.nih.gov/books/NBK1224/

Choe, E. K. et al., 'Understanding quantified-selfers' practices in collecting and exploring personal data' in *Proceedings of the SIGCHI Conference on Human Factors in Computing Systems* (New York, NY: ACM (CHI '14)) pp. 1143–52. doi: 10.1145/2556288.2557372

Chugh, Kirpal S. and Jha, Vivekanand, 'Commerce in transplantation in third world countries' (1996) 49(5) *Kidney International* 1181–6

Claiborne, Anne, English, Rebecca and Kahn, Jeffrey, *Mitochondrial Replacement Techniques: Ethical, Social, and Policy Considerations*. Edited by National Academies of Sciences, Engineering, and Medicine, Institute of Medicine, Board on Health Sciences Policy, and Committee on the Ethical and Social Policy Considerations of Novel Techniques for Prevention of Maternal Transmission of Mitochondrial DNA Diseases (Washington, DC: National Academies Press, 2016)

Clamon, Joseph B., 'Tax policy as a lifeline: encouraging blood and organ donation through tax credits' (2008) 17(1) *Annals of Health Law* 67–99

Cohen, Cynthia, 'Selling bits and pieces of humans to make babies: "The Gift of the Magi" Revisited' (1999) 24(3) *Journal of Medicine and Philosophy* 288–306

Cohen, I.G. 'Sperm and egg donor anonymity' in Leslie Francis (ed.), *The Oxford Handbook of Reproductive Ethics* (Oxford: Oxford University Press, 2016)

Cohen, Jacques, Scott, Richard, Schimmel, Tim et al., 'Birth of infant after transfer of anucleate donor oocyte cytoplasm into recipient eggs' (1997) 350(9072) *The Lancet* 350 186–7. doi:10.1016/S0140-6736(05)62353-7

Cohen, Lawrence, 'Where it hurts: Indian material for an ethics of organ transplantation' (1999) 128(4) *Daedalus* 135–65

Cohen, Lloyd R., 'Increasing the supply of transplant organs: the virtues of a futures market' (1989) 58(1) *George Washington Law Review* 1–51

Collins, Francis, *The Language of Life: DNA and the Revolution in Personalized Medicine* (New York: Harper Collins, 2010)

Cool, A. 'Detaching data from the state: biobanking and building Big Data in Sweden' (2015) *BioSocieties* 1–19

Cookson, Clive, 'UK researchers secure licence for "three-parent" baby procedure' (16 March 2017) *Financial Times*, www.ft.com/content/a4c7e0ba-0a41-11e7-ac5a-903b21361b43

Coscia, L. A., Constantinescu, S., Davison, J. M. et al., 'Immunosuppressive drugs and fetal outcome: best practice and research' (2014) 28(8) *Clinical Obstetrics and Gynecology* 1174–87

Couzin-Frankel, Jennifer, 'Science gold mine, ethical minefield' (2009) 324(5924) *Science* 166–8

'Unanswered questions surround baby born to three parents' (27 September 2016) *Science*, www.sciencemag.org/news/2016/09/unanswered-questions-surround-baby-born-three-parents

Cozzi, Emanuele, Biancone, Luigi, López-Fraga, Marta et al., 'Long-term outcome of living kidney donation' (2016) 100(2) *Transplantation* 270–1

Craven, Lyndsey, Elson, Joanna L, Irving, Laura et al., 'Mitochondrial DNA disease: new options for prevention' (2011) 20(R2) *Human Molecular Genetics* R168–174. doi:10.1093/hmg/ddr373

Craven, Lyndsey, Herbert, Mary, Murdoch, Alison et al., 'Research into policy: a brief history of mitochondrial donation' (2016) 34(2) *Stem Cells* 265–7. doi:10.1002/stem.2221

Craven, Lyndsey, Tuppen, Helen A., Greggains, Gareth D. et al., 'Pronuclear transfer in human embryos to prevent transmission of mitochondrial DNA disease' (2010) 465(7294) *Nature* 82–85. doi:10.1038/nature08958

Crichton, Michael, *Next* (New York, NY: Harper Collins, 2006)

Critchley, Christine R., Nichol, Dianne, Otlowski, Margaret F. A. et al., 'Predicting intention to biobank: a national survey' (2012) 22 *European Journal of Public Health* 139–44

Cronin, David C., II and Elias, Julio J., 'Operational organization of a system for compensated living organ providers' in Sally Satel (ed.), *When Altruism Isn't Enough: The Case for Compensating Kidney Donors* (Washington, DC, AEI Press, 2008), pp. 34–49

Curnutte, Margaret, 'Regulatory controls for direct-to-consumer genetics tests: a case study on how the FDA exercised its authority' (2017) 36(3) *New Genetics and Society* 209–26

Cutas, Daniela-Ecaterina, 'Looking for the meaning of dignity in the Bioethics Convention and the Cloning Protocol' (2005) 13(4) *Health Care Analysis* 303–13

Daniluk, J. C., '"If we had it to do over again. . .": couples' reflections on their experiences of infertility treatments' (2001) 9(2) *The Family Journal* 122–33

Danovitch, Gabriel M. and Leichtman, Alan B., 'Kidney vending: the "Trojan horse" of organ transplantation' (2006) 1(6) *Clinical Journal of the American Society of Nephrology* 1133–5

Danovitch, Gabriel M., 'Who cares? Impact of commercialized kidney transplantation on the doctor-patient relationship' in Willem Weimar, Michael Bos and Jan van Busschbach (eds.), *Organ Transplantation: Ethical, Legal and Psychosocial Aspects. Towards a Common European Policy* (Lengerich: Pabst, 2008), pp. 49–54

Danske Regioner, *Handleplan for Bedre Brug af Sundhedsdata i Regionerne* (Copenhagen: Danske Regioner, 2015) pp. 1–19

Handlingsplan for Personlig Medicin (Copenhagen: Danske Regioner, 2015)

Sundhedsdata i Spil (Copenhagen: Danske Regioner, 2015)

Datta, A. K., Selman, T. J., Kwok, T. et al., 'Quality of information accompanying on-line marketing of home diagnostic tests' (2008) 101(1) *Journal of the Royal Society of Medicine* 34–8

Davies, Sally, *Generation Genome: Annual Report of the Chief Medical Officer* (London: Department of Health, 2016) www.gov.uk/government/uploads/system/uploads/attachment_data/file/631043/CMO_annual_report_generati on_genome.pdf, accessed 6 November 2017

Day, Sara, Coombes, R. Charles and McGrath-Lone, Louise, 'Stratified, precision or personalised medicine? Cancer services in the "real world" of a London hospital' (2017) 39 *Sociology of Health and Illness* 143–58

Dedding, C., van Doorn, R., Winkler, L. et al, 'How will e-health affect patient participation in the clinic? A review of e-health studies and the current evidence for changes in the relationship between medical professionals and patients' (2011) 72(1) *Social Science & Medicine* 49–53

Deftos, L. J., 'Genomic torts: the law of the future – the duty of physicians to disclose the presence of genetic disease to the relatives of their patients with the disease' (1997) 32 *University of San Francisco Law Review* 105–38

DeGrazia, David, *Creation Ethics: Reproduction, Genetics, and Quality of Life* (Oxford: Oxford University Press, 2012)

Delmonico, Francis L., Arnold, Robert, Scheper-Hughes, Nancy et al., 'Ethical incentives – not payment – for organ donation' (2002) 346(25) *New England Journal of Medicine* 2002–5

Delmonico, Francis L., Danovitch, Gabriel M., Capron, Alexander M. et al., '"Proposed standards for incentives for organs donation" are neither international nor acceptable' (2012) 12(7) *American Journal of Transplantation* 1954–5

Delmonico, Francis L. and Scheper-Hughes, Nancy, 'Why we should not pay for human organs' (2003) 38(3) *Zygon* 689–98

Demme, Richard A., 'Ethical concerns about an organ market' (2010) 102(1) *Journal of the National Medical Association* 46–50

Demsetz, Harold, 'Toward a theory of property rights' (1967) 57(2) *The American Economic Review* 347–59

Dennis, C., 'The rise of the narciss-ome: profiles of a researcher's genes, proteins and more show personalized genomic medicine in action' (2012) *Nature News*. doi:10.1038/nature.2012.10240

Department of Business, Innovation and Skills (DBIS), *Industrial Strategy: Government and Industry in Partnership: Strategy for UK Life Sciences: One*

Year On (2013) www.gov.uk/government/collections/industrial-strategy-gov
ernment-and-industry-in-partnership, accessed 6 November 2017

Department of Health (DoH), 'Jeremy Hunt confirms commitment to balance patient safety and privacy' (2013) www.gov.uk/government/news/
jeremy-hunt-confirms-commitment-to-balance-patient-safety-and-priv
acy-2, accessed 6 November 2017

Department of Health (DoH), 'Your data – Better security, better choice, better
care. Government response to the National Data Guardian for Health Care's
Review of data security. Consent and opt-outs and the Care Quality
Commission's Review "Safe data, safe care"' (2017) www.gov.uk/govern
ment/uploads/system/uploads/attachment_data/file/627493/Your_data_bett
er_security_better_choice_better_care_government_response.pdf, accessed 6
November 2017

De Vries, Raymond G., Tomlinson, Tom, Kim, H. Myra et al., 'The moral concerns
of biobank donors: the effect of non-welfare interests on willingness to
donate' (2016) 12 *Life Sciences, Society and Policy* 3

Dickenson, Donna L., 'Commodification of human tissue: implications for feminist and development ethics' (2002) 2(1) *Developing World Bioethics* 55–63

'The lady vanishes: what's missing from the stem cell debate' (2006) 3(1–2)
Journal of Bioethical Inquiry 43–54. doi:10.1007/s11673-006-9003-8

Property in the Body: Feminist Perspectives (Cambridge: Cambridge University
Press, 2007, 2nd ed. 2017)

Body Shopping: The Economy Fuelled by Flesh and Blood (Oxford: Oneworld
Publications, 2008)

Me Medicine vs. We Medicine: Reclaiming Biotechnology for the Common Good
(New York, NY: Columbia University Press, 2013)

'The commercialization of human eggs in mitochondrial replacement research'
(2013) 19(1) *The New Bioethics: A Multidisciplinary Journal of Biotechnology
and the Body* 18–29

'The common good' in Roger Brownsword, E. Scotford and K. Yeung (eds.), *The
Oxford Handbook of Law, Regulation and Technology* (Oxford: Oxford
University Press, 2017), pp. 135–52

Dillard, C. J, 'Rethinking the procreative right' (2007) 10 *Yale Human Rights and
Development* 1

DiMauro, Salvatore and Davidzon, Guido, 'Mitochondrial DNA and disease'
(2005) 37(3)*Annals of Medicine* 222–32. doi:10.1080/07853890510007368

'Does mobile health matter?' (2017) 390(2216) *The Lancet.* doi:10.1016/S0140-
6736(17)32899-429165258

Domar, A. D., Zuttermeister, P. C. and Friedman, R. 'The psychological impact of
infertility: a comparison with patients with other medical conditions' (1993)
14 *Journal of Psychosomatic Obstetrics and Gynaecology* 45

Domínguez-Gil, Beatriz, Delmonico, Francis L., Shaheen, Faissal A. M. et al., 'The critical pathway for deceased donation: reportable uniformity in the approach to deceased donation' (2011) 24(4) *Transplant International* 373–8

Douzinas, Costas, 'The paradoxes of human rights' (2013) 20(1) *Constellations* 51–67

Dove, E. S., Tassé, A.-M. and Knoppers, B. M, 'What are some of the ELSI challenges of international collaborations involving biobanks, global sample collection, and genomic data sharing and how should they be addressed?' (2014) 12(6) *Biopreservation and Biobanking* 363–4

Doz, F., Marvanne, P. and Fagot-Largeault, A., 'The person in personalised medicine' (2013) 49 *European Journal of Cancer* 1159–60

Duggal, Rishi, Brindle, Ingrid and Bagenal, Jessamy, 'Editorial: Digital healthcare: regulating the revolution' (2018) *British Medical Journal* 360:k6. doi: 10.1136/bmj.k6

Duncan, D. E., *Experimental Man: What One Man's Body Reveals about His Future, Your Health and Our Toxic World* (Hoboken, NJ: Wiley, 2009)

Duster, T., *Backdoor to Eugenics* (New York, NY: Routledge, 2003)

Duxbury, Neil, 'Do markets degrade?' (1996) 59(3) *Modern Law Review* 331–48

Dworkin, Gerald, 'Markets and morals: the case for organ sales' in Gerald Dworkin (ed.), *Morality, Harm and the Law* (Boulder, CO, Westview Press, 1994), pp. 155–61

Ellenberger, H. F., *The Discovery of the Unconscious* (London: Lane/Penguin, 1970)

Elliott, C., *White Coat, Black Hat: Adventures on the Dark Side of Medicine* (Boston, MA: Beacon Press, 2011)

Engel, Margaret, 'Va. doctor plans company to arrange sale of human kidneys' (19 September 1983) *The Washington Post*

Erin, Charles A. and Harris, John, 'An ethical market in human organs' (2003) 29 (3) *Journal of Medical Ethics* 137–8

Ernster, Lars, Ikkos, Denis and Luft, Rolf, 'Enzymatic activities of human skeletal muscle mitochondria: a tool in clinical metabolic research' (1959) 184 *Nature* 1851–4

Ethics Committee of The Transplantation Society, 'The consensus statement of the Amsterdam Forum on the Care of the Live Kidney Donor' (2004) 78(4) *Transplantation* 491–2

'The ethics statement of the Vancouver Forum on the Live Lung, Liver, Pancreas, and Intestine Donor' (2006) 81(10) *Transplantation* 1386–7

Etzioni, Amitai, 'Organ donation: a communitarian approach' (2003) 13(1) *Kennedy Institute of Ethics Journal* 1–18

European Society of Human Reproduction and Embryology (ESHRE), 'The welfare of the child in medically assisted reproduction' (2007) 22(10) *Human Reproduction* 2585–8

Evans, Barbara J., 'The First Amendment right to speak about the human genome' (2014) 16(3) *University of Pennsylvania Journal of Constitutional Law* 549–63

Evans, John H., 'Commodifying life? A pilot study of opinions regarding financial incentives for organ donation' (2003) 28(6) *Journal of Health Politics, Policy and Law* 1003–32

Expert Group on Dealing with Ethical and Regulatory Challenges of International Biobank Research, *Biobanks for Europe: A Challenge for Governance* (2012)

Eyal, Nir, Frenk, Julio, Goodwin, Michele B. et al., 'An open letter to President Barack Obama, Secretary of Health and Human Services Sylvia Mathews Burwell, Attorney General Eric Holder and Leaders of Congress' (11 September 2014), www.ustransplantopenletter.org/openletter.html

Fabre, Cécile, *Whose Body is it Anyway? Justice and the Integrity of the Person* (Oxford: Oxford University Press, 2006)

Fabre-Magnan, Muriel, 'Avortement et responsabilité médicale' (2001) *RTD Civil* 285–318

Falk, Marni J., Decherney, Alan and Kahn, Jeffrey P., 'Mitochondrial replacement techniques – implications for the clinical community' (2016) 374(12) *New England Journal of Medicine* 1103–6. doi:10.1056/NEJMp1600893

Federal Trade Commission, 'FTC notifies Facebook, WhatsApp of privacy obligations in light of proposed acquisition' (2014)

Fernandez, Conrad V., Gordon, Kevin, Van den Hof, Michiel et al., 'Knowledge and attitudes of pregnant women with regard to collection, testing and banking of cord blood stem cells' (2003) 168(6) *Canadian Medical Association Journal* 695–8.

Fisk, Nicholas M. and Atun, Rifat, 'Public-private partnership in cord blood banking' (2008) 336 *British Medical Journal* 642–4

Fitbit (n. d.) *Fitbit App & Dashboard*. Available at: www.fitbit.com/nl/app. (Accessed 2 February 2018)

Fitbit for Corporate Wellness. Available at: www.fitbit.com/content/assets/group-health/FitbitWellness_InfoSheet.pdf (Accessed 2 February 2018)

Fitbit Health Solutions. Available at: www.fitbit.com/nl/group-health (Accessed 2 February 2018)

Fitbit Official Site for Activity Trackers & More. Available at: www.fitbit.com/home (Accessed 2 February 2018)

Help article: What are active minutes? Available at: http://help.fitbit.com/articles/en_US/Help_article/1379 (Accessed 2 February 2018).

Why Fitbit. Available at: www.fitbit.com/nl/whyfitbit (Accessed 2 February 2018)

Flanagan, M., Howe, D. C. and Nissenbaum, H. (2008), 'Embodying values in technology: theory and practice' in Jeroen van den Hoven and John Weckert (eds.), *Information Technology and Moral Philosophy* (Cambridge: Cambridge University Press, 2008), pp. 322–53

Forster, Katie, 'First "three-parent babies" to be born this year as licence approved for new fertility technique' (16 March 2017) *The Independent*, www.indepen dent.co.uk/life-style/health-and-families/health-news/three-3-parent-babies-latest-licence-approved-ivf-fertility-technique-hfea-dna-mitochondrial-a7632916.html

Foster, Charles, *Human Dignity in Bioethics and Law* (Oxford: Hart, 2011)

'Dignity and the use of body parts' (2014) 40(1) *Journal of Medicine and Ethics* 44–7

Foucault, Michel, *Surveiller et Punir: Naissance de la Prison* (Paris: Gallimard, 1975)

'Governmentality' in Graham Burchell, Colin Gordon and Peter Miller (eds.), *Histoire de la Sexualité: L'usage des Plaisirs* (Paris: Gallimard, 1984), vol. 2

Histoire de la Sexualité Le souci de Soi (Paris: Gallimard, 1984), vol. 3

The Foucault Effect: Studies in Governmentality (London: Harvester Wheatsheaf, 1991) pp. 87–104

The Will to Knowledge: The History of Sexuality (London: Penguin Books, 1998), vol. 1

'Society Must Be Defended': Lectures at the Collège de France, 1975–1976 (London: Macmillan, 2003)

Fox, N. S., Stevens, C., Cuibotariu, R. et al., 'Umbilical cord blood collection: do patients really understand?' (2007) 35 *Journal of Perinatal Medicine* 314–21

Frank, L., 'When an entire country is a cohort' (2000) 287(5462) *Science* 2398–9

'The epidemiologist's dream: Denmark' (2003) 301(5630) *Science* 163

Freeman, George, 'Written statement to Parliament: Review of health and care data security and consent' (2016) www.gov.uk/government/speeches/review-of-health-and-care-data-security-and-consent, accessed 6 November 2017

Freud, S., 'Vorlesungen zur Einführung in die Psychoanalyse' in *Gesammelte Werke* XI (London: Imago, 1917/1940)

Friedlaender, Michael M., 'The right to sell or buy a kidney: are we failing our patients?' (2002) 359(9310) *The Lancet* 971–3

Fuller, Lon L., *The Morality of Law* (New Haven, CT: Yale University Press, 1962)

Garrison, Nanibaa' A., Sathe, Nila, A., Matheny Antommaria et al., 'A systematic literature review of individuals' perspectives on broad consent and data sharing in the United States' (2016) 18(7) *Genetics in Medicine* 663–71

Geijsen, N., Horoschak, M., Kim, K. et al., 'Derivation of embryonic germ cells and male gametes from embryonic stem cells' (2004) 427(6970) *Nature* 148–54

Genetics and Public Policy Center, *Survey of Direct-to-Consumer Testing Statutes and Regulations* (Washington, DC: Genetics and Public Policy Center, 2007) https://repository.library.georgetown.edu/bitstream/handle/10822/511162/DTCStateLawChart.pdf, accessed 29 January 2018

Genomics England, 'FAQs about how we are working with industry' (2014) www
.genomicsengland.co.uk/working-with-industry/working-with-industry-
faqs/, accessed 6 November 2017

'100,000 Genomes Project gains ethical approval to offer NHS patients further
information about their genomic results' (2015) www.genomicsengland.co
.uk/100k-genomes-projectp-gains-ethical-approval-to-offer-nhs-patients-
further-information-about-their-genomic-results/, accessed 6 November
2017

George, Thomas, 'The case against kidney sales' (2001) XI(1) *Issues in Medical
Ethics* 49–50

Gerrand, Nicole, 'The misuse of Kant in the debate about a market in human body
parts' (1999) 16(1) *Journal of Applied Philosophy* 59–67

Ghahramani, Nasrollah, Rizvi, S., Hasan, Adibul et al., 'Paid donation: a global
view: outcomes of paid donation in Iran, Pakistan and Philippines' (2012) 19
(4) *Advances in Chronic Kidney Disease* 262–8

Giddens, Anthony, *The Consequences of Modernity* (Cambridge: Polity Press,
1991)

'Risk and responsibility' (1999) (1) *Modern Law Review* 1–10

Giesen, Ivo, 'The use and influence of comparative law in "wrongful life" cases'
(2012) 8 *Utrecht Law Review* 35–54

Gill, Michael B. and Sade, Robert M., 'Paying for kidneys: the case for repealing
prohibition' (2002) 12(1) *Kennedy Institute of Ethics Journal* 17–46

Glendon, Mary A., *Rights Talk: The Impoverishment of Political Discourse* (New
York, NY: Free Press, 1991)

Glover, Jonathan, *Choosing Children: Genes, Disability, Design* (Oxford: Clarendon
Press, 2006)

Gneezy, Uri, *The W Effect of Incentives* (Chicago, IL: University of Chicago
Business School, 2003)

Gneezy, Uri and Rustichini, Aldo, 'A fine is a price' (2000) 29(1) *Journal of Legal
Studies* 1–17

Goldacre, Ben, 'Care.data is in chaos. It breaks my heart' (28 February 2014) *The
Guardian*

Golombok, S., Readings, J., Blake, L. et al., 'Families created through surrogacy:
mother–child relationships and children's psychological adjustment at age 7'
(2011) 47(6) *Developmental Psychology* 1579

Goodwin, Michele, 'Prosecuting the womb' (2008) 76 *George Washington Law
Review* 1657–746

'A view from the cradle: tort law and the private regulation of assisted reproduction' (2010) 59 *Emory Law Journal* 1039–100

(ed.), *Baby Markets: Money and the New Politics of Creating Families* (New York,
NY: Cambridge University Press, 2010)

Gorman, Gráinne S., Grady, John P., Yi Ng et al., 'Mitochondrial donation – how many women could benefit?' (2015) 372(9) *New England Journal of Medicine* 885–7. doi:10.1056/NEJMc1500960

Gottweis, Herbert, 'Governing genomics in the 21st century: between risk and uncertainty' (2005) 24(2) *New Genetics and Society* 175–94

Government Accountability Office, *Direct-to-Consumer Genetics Tests: Misleading Test Results Are Further Complicated by Deceptive Marketing and Other Questionable Practices* (Washington, DC: Government Accountability Office, 2010), pp. 8–9

Goyal, R., Dragoni, N. and Spognardi, A., 'Mind the tracker you wear: a security analysis of wearable health trackers' (2016) 31st ACM Symposium on Applied Computing (SAC'16)

Goyal, Madhav, Mehta, Ravindra L., Schneiderman, Lawrence et al., 'Economic and health consequences of selling a kidney in India' (2002) 288(13) *Journal of the American Medical Association* 1589–93

Grace, Jamie and Taylor, Mark J., 'Disclosure of confidential patient information and the duty to consult: the role of the Health and Social Care Information Centre' (2013) 21(3) *Medical Law Review* 415–47

Grande, D., Mitra, N., Shah, A. et al., 'The importance of purpose: moving beyond consent in the societal use of personal health information' (2014) 161(2) *Annals of Internal Medicine* 855–62

Graziano, D. (2017) 'Fitbit sold more wearables in 2016 than Apple and Samsung combined' *CNET*. Available at: www.cnet.com/news/fitbit-sold-more-wearables-in-2016-than-apple-and-samsung-combined/ (Accessed 2 February 2018)

Greasley, Kate, 'A legal market in organs: the problem of exploitation' (2012) 40(1) *Journal of Medical Ethics* 51–6

'Property rights in the human body: commodification and objectification' in Imogen Goold, Kate Greasley, Jonathan Herring et al. (eds.), *Persons, Parts and Property: How Should We Regulate Human Tissue in the 21st Century?* (Oxford: Hart, 2014), pp. 67–87

Greely, Henry, *The End of Sex and the Future of Human Reproduction* (Cambridge, MA: Harvard University Press, 2016)

Green, Robert C. and Farahany, Nita A., 'Regulation: the FDA is overcautious on consumer genomics' (2014) 505 *Nature* 286–7

Griffin, Anne, 'Kidneys on demand' (2007) 334(7592) *British Medical Journal* 502–5

Gross, Jed A., 'E Pluribus UNOS: The National Organ Transplant Act and its postoperative complications' (2008) 8(1) *Yale Journal of Health Policy, Law, and Ethics* 145–252

Gruben, Vanessa, 'Women as patients, not spare parts: examining the relationship between the physician and women egg providers' (2013) 25(2) *Canadian Journal of Women and the Law* 249–83

Gupta, Jyotsna A., 'Exploring Indian women's reproductive decision-making regarding prenatal testing' (2010) 12(2) *Culture, Health and Sexuality* 191–204

Gymrek, Melissa, McGuire, Amy L., Golan, David et al., 'Identifying personal genomes by surname inference' (2013) 6117 *Science* 321–4

Habermas, Jürgen, *The Future of Human Nature* (Cambridge: Polity Press, 2003).

Haimes, Erica and Taylor, Ken, 'Rendered invisible? The absent presence of egg providers in U.K. debates on the acceptability of research and therapy for mitochondrial disease' (2015) 33(4) *Monash Bioethics Review* 360–78. doi:10.1007/s40592-015-0046-7

'Sharpening the cutting edge: additional considerations for the UK debates on embryonic interventions for mitochondrial diseases' (2017) 13(1) *Life Sciences, Society and Policy.* doi:10.1186/s40504-016-0046-2

Haken, Jeremy, *Transnational Crime in the Developing World* (Washington, DC: Center for International Policy, 2011)

Hamburg Commissioner for Data Protection and Freedom of Information, *Administrative Order Against the Mass Synchronization of Data Between FaceBook and WhatsApp* (2016)

Hamzelou, Jessica, 'World's first baby born with new "3 parent" technique' (2016) *New Scientist*, www.newscientist.com/article/2107219-exclusive-worlds-first-baby-born-with-new-3-parent-technique/

Hansen, A., 'Danish sperm donor passed neurofibromatosis on to five children' (2012) 345 *British Medical Journal* (Online) e6570

Hansen, T., 'Parenthood and happiness: a review of folk theories versus empirical evidence' (2012) 108(1) *Social Indicators Research* 29–64

Harari, Yuval Noah, *Homo Deus: A Brief History of Tomorrow* (London: Harvill Secker, 2016)

Hardy, J. and Selkoe, D. J., 'The amyloid hypothesis of Alzheimer's disease: progress and problems on the road to therapeutics' (2002) 297(5580) *Science* 353–6

Harris, Curtis E. and Alcorn, Stephen P., 'To solve a deadly shortage: economic incentives for human organ donation' (2001) 16(3) *Issues in Law and Medicine* 213–33

Haskett, Dorothy R., 'Mitochondrial diseases in humans' (2014) *The Embryo Project Encyclopedia.* https://embryo.asu.edu/pages/mitochondrial-diseases-humans

Hauskeller, Christine and Beltrame, Lorenzo, 'Hybrid practices in cord blood banking: Rethinking the commodification of human tissues in the bioeconomy' (2016) 35(3) *New Genetics and Society* 228–45

Haw, Jennie, 'The trouble with biological insurance' (4 November 2013) *Impact Ethics*

Hayashi, K., Ogushi, S., Kurimoto, K. et al., 'Offspring from oocytes derived from in vitro primordial germ cell–like cells in mice' (2012) 338(6109) *Science* 971–5

Hayashi, T. et al., 'Laughter regulates gene expression in patients with type 2 diabetes' (2006) 75 *Psychotherapy and Psychosomatics* 62–5

Hays, Rebecca and Daker-White, Gavin, 'The care.data consensus? A qualitative analysis of opinions expressed on Twitter' (2015) 15 *BMC Public Health* 838

Hedgecoe, Adam, *The Politics of Personalised Medicine: Pharmacogenetics in the Clinic* (Cambridge: Cambridge University Press, 2004)

Hegel, Georg W.F., *Elements of the Philosophy of Right*, ed. Allen W. Wood (Cambridge: Cambridge University Press, [1821] 2012)

Helén, I., 'Risk management and ethics in high-tech antenatal care' in R. Bunton and A. Petersen (eds.), *Genetic Governance: Health, Risk and Ethics in the Biotech Era* (London: Routledge, 2005), pp. 47–63

Henaghan, M., 'International surrogacy trends: how family law is coping' (2013) 7(3) *Australian Journal of Adoption*. Available at: www.nla.gov.au/openpub lish/index.php/aja/article/view/3188)

Hensel, Wendy F., 'The disabling impact of wrongful birth and wrongful life actions' (2005) 40 *Harvard Civil Rights – Civil Liberties Law Review* 141–95

Herbrand, Cathy, 'Mitochondrial replacement techniques: who are the potential users and will they benefit?' 31(1) *Bioethics* 46–54. doi:10.1111/bioe.12311

Herholz, K. and Ebmeier, K., 'Clinical amyloid imaging in Alzheimer's disease' (2011) 10 *Lancet Neurology* 667–70

Herring, Jonathan and Chau, Pak-Lee, 'Interconnected, inhabited and insecure: why bodies should not be property' (2014) 40(3) *Journal of Medical Ethics* 39–43

Hester, Micah, 'Why we must leave our organs to others' (2006) 6(4) *American Journal of Bioethics* W23–8

Hetherington, K., 'Secondhandedness: consumption, disposal, and absent presence' (2004) 22 *Environment and Planning D: Society and Spaces* 157–73

Hill, Thomas E. Jr., *Respect, Pluralism, and Justice: Kantian Perspectives* (Oxford, Oxford University Press, 2000)

Hippen, Benjamin E., 'In defense of a regulated market in kidneys from living vendors' (2005) 30(6) *Journal of Medicine and Philosophy* 593–626

'Organ sales and moral travails: lessons from the living kidney vendor program in Iran' (2008) *Cato Institute Policy Analysis* No. 614

Hodges, Sarah, 'Umbilical cord blood banking and its interruptions: notes from Chennai, India' (2013) 42(4) *Economy and Society* 651–70

Hodson, Richard and Cookson, Clive, 'NHS launches genetic sequencing centres to develop treatments' (22 December 2014) *Financial Times*

Hoeyer, Klaus,'Denmark at a crossroad? Intensified data sourcing in a research radical country' (2016) 29 *The Ethics of Biomedical Big Data* 73–93

Hoeyer, K. and Lynöe, N., 'Is informed consent a solution to contractual problems? A comment on the article "Icelandic Inc.? On the ethics of commercial population genomics" by Jon F. Merz, Glenn E. McGee and Pamala Sankar' (2004) 58(6) Social Science and Medicine 1211

Hof, Robert, '"We are going for change": a conversation with 23andMe CEO Anne Wojcicki' (15 August 2014) Forbes

Hogle, Linda F., 'Data-intensive resourcing in healthcare' (2016) BioSocieties 1(22)

Hogle, Linda F., 'The ethics and politics of infrastructures: Creating the conditions of possibility for Big Data in medicine' in B. D. Mittelstadt and L. Floridi (eds.), The Ethics of Biomedical Big Data (Springer, 2016), pp. 397–427

Holmberg, C., Bischof, C. and Bauer, S., 'Making predictions: computing populations' (2013) 38(3) Science, Technology, & Human Values 398–420

Holt, I. J., Harding, A. E. and Morgan-Hughes, J. A., 'Deletions of muscle mitochondrial myopathies' (1988) 331 Nature 717–9

Holland, Suzanne, 'Contested commodities at both ends of life: buying and selling gametes, embryos, and body tissues' (2001) 11 Kennedy Institute of Ethics Journal 263–84

Honoré, A. M., Making Law Bind: Essays Legal and Philosophical (Oxford: Clarendon Press, 1987)

Hood, L. and Flores, M., 'A personal view on systems medicine and the emergence of proactive P4 medicine: predictive, preventive, personalized and participatory' (2012) 29(6) New Biotechnology 613–24

Hottois, Gilbert, 'Dignity of the human body – a philosophical and critical approach' in Peter Kemp, Jacob Rendtorff and Niels Mattsson Johansen (eds.), Bioethics and Biolaw. Vol. II: Four Ethical Principles (Copenhagen: Rhodos, 2000), pp. 87–102

Hübner, K., Fuhrmann, G., Christenson, L. K. et al., 'Derivation of oocytes from mouse embryonic stem cells' (2003) 300(5623) Science 1251–6

Hughes, Paul M., 'Constraint, consent, and well-being in human kidney sales' (2009) 34(6) Journal of Medicine and Philosophy 606–31

HUGO (Human Genome Organization), Summary of Principles Agreed at the International Strategy Meeting on Human Genome Sequencing ('Bermuda Statement') (London: Wellcome Trust, 1996).

Human Genetics Commission, Genes Direct (London: Department of Health, 2003)

Hurley, Jennifer L., 'Cashing in on the transplant list: An argument against offering valuable compensation for the donation of organs' (2004) 4(1) Journal of High Technology Law 117–37

Hutchon, David, 'Commercial cord blood banking – immediate clamping is not safe' (2006) 333 British Medical Journal 919

Hyslop, Louise A., Blakeley, Paul, Craven, Lyndsey et al., 'Towards clinical application of pronuclear transfer to prevent mitochondrial DNA disease' (2016) 534 (7607) Nature 383–6. doi:10.1038/nature18303

Ibarreta, Dolores and Hogarth, Stuart, 'Quality issues in clinical genetic services: regulatory issues and international conventions' in U. Kristofferson, J. Schmidtke and J. Cassiman (eds.), *Quality Issues in Clinical Genetic Services* (Dordrecht: Springer, 2010), pp. 243-9

Indian Council for Medical Research and Department of Biotechnology, *National Guidelines for Stem Cell Research* (New Delhi: Indian Council for Medical Research and Department of Biotechnology, October 2017)

Inhorn, M. C., 'Making Muslim babies: IVF and gamete donation in Sunni versus Shi'a Islam' (2006) 30(4) *Culture, Medicine and Psychiatry* 427-50

Inston, N., Gill, D., Al-Hakim, A. et al., 'Living paid organ transplantation results in unacceptably high recipient morbidity and mortality' (2005) 37(2) *Transplant Proceedings* 560-2

Ioannidis, John, 'Informed consent, Big Data, and the oxymoron of research that is not research' (2013) 13(4) *American Journal of Bioethics* 40-2

'Evidence-based medicine has been hijacked: a report to David Sackett' (2016) 73 *Journal of Clinical Epidemiology* 82-6

IQVIA, 'The growing value of digital health in the United Kingdom: evidence and impact on human health and the healthcare system' (7 November 2017). www.iqvia.com/institute/reports/the-growing-value-of-digital-health (accessed 11 February 2018)

Jakicic, J. M., Davis, K. K., Rogers, R. J. et al., 'Effect of wearable technology combined with a lifestyle intervention on long-term weight loss: The IDEA randomized clinical trial' (2016) 316(11) *Journal of the American Medical Association* 1161-71. doi:10.1001/jama.2016.12858

Janssens, A. C. J. W., Gwinn, M., Bradley, L. A. et al., 'A critical appraisal of the scientific basis of commercial genomic profiles used to assess health risks and personalize health interventions' (2008) 82 *American Journal of Human Genetics* 593-9

Jayaprakasan, Kanna, Herbert, Mary, Moody, Ellis et al., 'Estimating the risks of ovarian hyperstimulation syndrome (OHSS): implications for egg donation for research' (2007) 10(3) *Human Fertility* 183-7. doi:10.1080/14647270601021743

Jha, Vivekanand and Chugh, Kirpal S., 'The case against a regulated system of living kidney sales' (2006) 2(9) *Nature Clinical Practice Nephrology* 466-7

Johannesson, L., Kvarnström, N., Mölne, J. et al. (2015). 'Uterus transplantation trial: 1-year outcome' (2015) 103(1) *Fertility and Sterility* 199-204

Johnson, Karen L., 'The sale of human organs: implicating a privacy right' (1987) 21(3) *Valparaiso University Law Review* 741-62

Jones, Owen, *The Establishment: And How They Get Away With It* (London: Allan Lane, 2014)

Joint Society of Obstetricians and Gynaecologists of Canada, and Canadian Fertility Andrology Society Clinical Practice Guidelines Committee, 'The diagnosis and management of ovarian hyperstimulation syndrome' (2011) 33 (11) *Journal of Obstetrics and Gynaecology Canada* 1156–62

Joyner, Michael J. and Paneth, Nigel, 'Seven questions for personalized medicine' (2015) 314(10) *Journal of the American Medical Association* 999–1000

Juengst, Eric, McGowan, Michelle L., Fishman, Jennifer R. et al., 'From "personalized" to "precision" medicine: the ethical and social implications of rhetorical reform in genomic medicine' (2016) 46 *Hastings Center Report* 21–33

Jung, C. G., 'Über das Verhalten der Reaktionszeit beim Assoziationsexperimente' in *Gesammelte Werke II. Experimentelle Untersuchungen* (Olten und Freiburg im Breisgau: Walter, 1905/1979), pp. 239–89

Kahn, Jeffrey P., 'Three views of organ procurement policy: moving ahead or giving up?' (2003) 13(1) *Kennedy Institute of Ethics Journal* 45–50

Kahn, Jeffrey P. and Delmonico, Francis L., 'The consequences of public policy to buy and sell organs for transplantation' (2004) 4(2) *American Journal of Transplantation* 178–80

Kaimal, A. J., Smith, C. C., Laros, R. K. Jr et al., 'Cost-effectiveness of private umbilical cord blood banking: Comment' (2010) 11(5) *Obstetrics and Gynecology* 1090

Kant, Immanuel, *Lectures on Ethics*, ed. Peter Heath (Cambridge: Cambridge University Press, 2008)

Kant, Immanuel, *Groundwork of the Metaphysics of Morals*, ed. Mary J. Gregor and Jens Timmerman (Cambridge: Cambridge University Press, [1785] 2012)

Kant, Immanuel, *The Metaphysics of Morals*, ed. Mary J. Gregor (Cambridge, Cambridge University Press, [1797] 2012)

Kass, Leon R., *Toward a More Natural Science: Biology and Human Affairs* (New York, Free Press, 1985)

Kass, Leon R., 'Organs for sale? Propriety, property, and the price of progress' (1992) 107 *Public Interest* 65–86

Kass, Leon R., *Life, Liberty and the Defense of Dignity: The Challenge for Bioethics* (San Francisco: Encounter Books, 2004)

Kaushik, A., Jayant R. D., Tiwari S. et al., 'Nano-biosensors to detect beta-amyloid for Alzheimer's disease management' (2016) 80 *Biosens Bioelectron* 273–87

Kelly, Emily R., 'International organ trafficking crisis: solutions addressing the heart of the matter' (2013) 54(3) *Boston College Law Review* 1317–49

Kerstein, Samuel J., 'Autonomy, moral constraints, and markets in kidneys' (2009) 34(6) *Journal of Medicine and Philosophy* 573–85

Kerstein, Samuel J., 'Kantian condemnation of commerce in organs' (2009) 19(2) *Kennedy Institute of Ethics Journal* 147–69

Kesselheim, A., Treasure, C. L. and Joffe, S., 'Biomarker-defined subsets of common diseases: policy and economic implications of Orphan Drug Act coverage' (2016) 14(1) *PLoS Med.* e1002190

Kettis-Lindblad, Åsa, Ring, Lena, Viberth, Eva et al., 'Genetic research and donation of tissue samples to biobanks: what do potential sample donors in the
Swedish general public think?' (2006) 16(4) *European Journal of Public Health*
433–40

Khovanskaya, V., Baumer, E. P. S., Cosley, D. et al., '"Everybody knows what you're
doing": a critical design approach to personal informatics' in *Proceedings of
the SIGCHI Conference on Human Factors in Computing Systems* (New York,
NY: ACM CHI '13, 2013) pp. 3403–12. doi:10.1145/2470654.2466467

Klunk, W., Engler, H., Nordberg, A. et al., 'Imaging brain amyloid in Alzheimer's
disease with Pittsburgh Compound-B' (2004) 55(3) *Annals of Neurology*
306–19

Knapton, Sarah, 'Newcastle University gets green light to create three-parent
babies' (16 March 2017) *The Telegraph*, www.telegraph.co.uk/science/2017/
03/16/newcastle-university-gets-green-light-create-three-parent-babies

Knoppers, Bartha M. and Chadwick, Ruth, 'Human genetic research: emerging
trends in ethics' (2005) 6 *Nature Reviews Genetics* 75–9

Knoppers, Bartha M. and Özdemir, Vural, 'The concept of humanity and bioge-
netics' in Britta van Beers, Luigi Corrias and Wouter Werner (eds.),
Humanity across International Law and Biolaw (Cambridge: Cambridge
University Press, 2014)

Kolata, Gina, 'Birth of baby with three parents' DNA marks success for banned
technique' (27 September 2016) *The New York Times*

Koplin, Julian, 'Assessing the likely harms to kidney vendors in regulated organ
markets' (2014) 14(10) *American Journal of Bioethics* 7–18

Krumholz, H. M., 'Big Data and new knowledge in medicine: the thinking, training, and tools needed for a learning health system' (2014) 33(7) *Health Affairs*
1163–70

Latour, B., 'Where are the missing masses?' (1992) Available at: www.bruno-latour.fr/
sites/default/files/50-MISSING-MASSES-GB.pdf (Accessed 2 February 2018)

Laurie, Graeme, *Genetic Privacy: A Challenge to Medico-Legal Norms* (Cambridge:
Cambridge University Press, 2002)

Laurie, Graeme, Mallia, Pierre, Frenkel, David A. et al., 'Interests in genetic
research? Managing access to biobanks: how can we reconcile individual
privacy and public interests in genetic research?' (2010) 10(4) *Medical Law
International* 315–37

Lavee, J., Ashkenazi, T., Stoler, A. et al., 'Preliminary marked increase in the
national organ donation rate in Israel following implementation of a new
organ transplantation law' (2013) 13(3) *American Journal of Transplantation*
780–5

Lavee, Jacob and Brock, Dan W., 'Prioritizing registered donors in organ allocation: an ethical appraisal of the Israeli Organ Transplant Law' (2012) 18(6)
Current Opinion in Critical Care 707–11

Lavee, Jacob and Stoler, Avraham, 'Reciprocal altruism: the Impact of resurrecting
an old moral imperative on the national organ donation rate in Israel' (2014)
17(3) *Law and Contemporary Problems* 323–36

Laxton, A. and Lozano A., 'Deep brain stimulation for the treatment of Alzheimer
disease and dementias' (2013) 80(S28) *World Neurosurgery* e21–S28

Lee, Hyo-Sang, Hong Ma, Cervera Juanes, Rita, Tachibana, Masahito et al., 'Rapid
mitochondrial DNA segregation in primate preimplantation embryos precedes somatic and germline bottleneck' (2012) 1(5) *Cell Reports* 506–15.
doi:10.1016/j.celrep.2012.03.011

Li, I., Dey, A. and Forlizzi, J., 'A stage-based model of personal informatics systems'
in *Proceedings of the SIGCHI Conference on Human Factors in Computing
Systems* (New York, NY: ACM (CHI '10) (2010)), pp. 557–66. doi:10.1145/
1753326.1753409

Linford, Jake, 'The Kidney Donor Scholarship Act: how college scholarships can
provide financial incentives for kidney donation while preserving altruistic
meaning' (2009) 2(2) *Saint Louis University Journal of Health Law and Policy*
265–326

Link, Daniel C., Schettpelz, L.G., Shen, D. et al., 'Identification of a novel PT3
cancer susceptibility mutation through whole-genome sequencing of a
patient with therapy-related AMI' (2011) 305 *Journal of the American
Medical Association* 1568–76

Lipworth, Wendy, Mason, Paul, Kerridge, Ian et al., 'Ethics and epistemology in big
data research' (2017) 14(4) *Journal of Bioethical Inquiry* 489–500

Lista, S., Dubois, B. and Hampel, H., 'Paths to Alzheimer's disease prevention:
from modifiable risk factors to biomarker enrichment strategies' (2015) 19(2)
Journal of Nutrition Health & Aging 154–63

Littlejohns, T., Henley W. E., Lang, I. A. et al., 'Vitamin D and the risk of dementia
and Alzheimer disease' (2014) 83(10) *Neurology* 920–28

Lock, M., *The Alzheimer Conundrum: Entanglements of Dementia and Aging*
(Princeton, NJ: Princeton University Press, 2015)

Locke, John, *Two Treatises of Government*, ed. Peter Laslett (Cambridge:
Cambridge University Press, [1690] 1967)

Loi, Michele, 'Nobody's data but mine' (2017) *Journal of Medical Ethics*.
doi:10.1136/medethics-2017–104188

López-Fraga, Marta, Van Assche, Kristof, Domínguez-Gil, Beatriz et al., 'Human
trafficking for the purpose of organ removal' in Ryszard Piotrowicz, Conny
Rijken and Baerbel H. Uhl (eds.), *Routledge Handbook of Human Trafficking*
(London: Routledge, 2017), pp. 120–34

Lothian, Judith and DeVries, Charlotte, *The Official Lamaze Guide: Giving Birth
with Confidence* (New York, NY: Meadowbrook Press, 2010, 2nd ed.)

Love, Andrew J., 'Replacing our current system of organ procurement with a futures
market: Will organ supply be maximized?' (1997) 37(2) *Jurimetrics* 167–86

Luft, Rolf, Ikkos, Denis, Palmieri, Genaro et al., 'A case of severe hypermetabolism of nonthyroid origin with a defect in the maintenance of mitochondrial respiratory control: a correlated clinical, biochemical, and morphological study' (1962) 41(9) *Journal of Clinical Investigation* 1776–804

Lupton, Deborah, *Risk* (London: Routledge, 1999)

'M-health and health promotion: The digital cyborg and surveillance society' (2012) 10(3) *Social Theory and Health* 229–44. doi:10.1057/sth.2012.6

'Quantifying the body: monitoring and measuring health in the age of Mhealth technologies' (2013) 23(4) *Critical Public Health* 393–403

'The digitally engaged patient: self-monitoring and self-care in the digital health era' (2013) 11(3) *Social Theory & Health* 256–70. doi:10.1057/sth.2013.10

'Self-tracking cultures: towards a sociology of personal informatics' in *Proceedings of the 26th Australian Computer-Human Interaction Conference on Designing Futures: The Future of Design* (New York, NY: ACM (OzCHI '14) 2014), pp. 77–86. doi:10.1145/2686612.2686623

The Quantified Self: A Sociology of Self-Tracking (Cambridge: Polity Press, 2016)

Mahoney, Julia D., 'Should we adopt a market strategy to increase the supply of transplantable organs?' in Wayne N. Shelton and John Balint (eds.), *The Ethics of Organ Transplantation* (New York, NY: Elsevier, 2001), pp. 65–88

Major, Rupert W. L., 'Paying kidney donors: time to follow Iran?' (2008) 11(1) *McGill Journal of Medicine* 67–9

Malarkey, Mary A., 'Letter to Dr. John Zhang from the Director Office of Compliance and Biologics Quality Center for Biologics Evaluation and Research of the United States Food and Drug Administration (FDA)' (4 August 2017) www.fda.gov/downloads/BiologicsBloodVaccines/GuidanceCompliance RegulatoryInformation/ComplianceActivities/Enforcement/UntitledLetters/UCM570225.pdf

Maliszewska-Cyna, E., Lynch, M, Oore, J. J. et al., 'The benefits of exercise and metabolic interventions for the prevention and early treatment of Alzheimer's Disease' (2017) 14(1) *Current Alzheimer Research* 47–60

Malmqvist, Erik, 'A further lesson from existing kidney markets' (2014) 14(10) *American Journal of Bioethics* 27–9

'Are bans on kidney sales unjustifiably paternalistic?' (2014) 28(3) *Bioethics* 110–18

Maron, B. J., Lesser, J. R., Schiller, N. B. et al., 'Implications of hypertrophic cardiomyopathy transmitted by sperm donation' (2009) 302 *Journal of the American Medical Association* 1681–4

Martin, Dominique, *Beyond the Market: A New Approach to the Ethical Procurement of Human Biological Materials*, PhD dissertation (The University of Melbourne, 2011)

Martin, Paul, Brown, Nik and Turner, Andrew, 'Capitalizing hope: the commercial development of umbilical cord blood stem cell banking' (2008) 27(2) New Genetics and Society 127–43

Matas, Arthur J., 'Design of a regulated system of compensation for living kidney donors' (2008) 22(3) Clinical Transplantation 378–84

Matas, A., Ambagtsheer, J. A. E., Gaston, R. et al., 'A realistic proposal – incentives may increase donation –we need trials now!' (2012) 12(7) American Journal of Transplantation 1957–8

Matas, Arthur J., Hippen, Benjamin and Satel, Sally, 'In defense of a regulated system of compensation for living donation' (2008) 13(4) Current Opinion in Organ Transplantation 379–85

Matesanz, Rafael, Domínguez-Gil, Beatriz, Coll, Elisabeth et al., 'Spanish experience as a leading country: what kind of measures were taken?' (2011) 24(4) Transplant International 333–43

Maxmen, Amy, 'Pharmacogenetics: playing the odds' (2011) 474 Nature S9–S10

Mayer-Schönberger, V. and Cukier, K., Big Data: A Revolution That Will Transform How We Live, Work and Think (London: John Murray, 2013)

Mayrhofer, M.T., 'About the new significance and the contingent meaning of biological material and data in biobanks' (2013) 35(3) History and Philosophy of the Life Sciences 449–67

McKenna, David and Sheth, Jayesh, 'Umbilical cord blood: current status and promise for the future, review article' (2011) 134(3) Indian Journal of Medical Research 261–9

McLeod, Carolyn and Baylis, Françoise, 'Feminists on the inalienability of human embryos' (2006) 21(1) Hypatia 1–14

Mehrabian, S., Alexopoulos, P., Ortner, M. et al., 'Cerebrospinal fluid biomarkers for Alzheimer's disease: the role of apolipoprotein E genotype, age, and sex' (2015) 11 Neuropsychiatric Disease and Treatment 3105–10

Melo-Martin, Immaculada de, 'The art of medicine – vulnerability and ethics: considering our Cartesian hangover' (2009) 373 Lancet 1244–45

Menendez-Gonzalez, M. 'Routine lumbar puncture for the early diagnosis of Alzheimer's disease. Is it safe?' (2014) 6(65) Frontiers in Aging Neuroscience 1–2

Mertes, H., 'Gamete derivation from stem cells: revisiting the concept of genetic parenthood' (2014) 40 Journal of Medical Ethics 744–7

Merz, J. F., McGee, G. E. and Sankar, P., '"Iceland Inc."? On the ethics of commercial population genomics' (2004) 58(6) Social Science and Medicine 1201–09

Microsoft, The Fourth Paradigm (Microsoft Research, 2009)

Millington, B., 'Smartphone apps and the mobile privatization of health and fitness' (2014) 31(5) Critical Studies in Media Communication 479–93. doi:10.1080/15295036.2014.973429

Ministeriet for Sundhed og Forebyggelse (Denmark) *National Strategi for Adgang til Sundhedsdata* (Copenhagen: Ministeriet for Sundhed og Forebyggelse, 2014), pp. 1–2

Mitalipov, Shoukhrat and Wolf, Don P., 'Clinical and ethical implications of mitochondrial gene transfer' (2014) 25(1) *Trends in Endocrinology and Metabolism* 5–7. doi:10.1016/j.tem.2013.09.001

Mittelstadt, B. D. and Floridi, L., 'The ethics of Big Data: current and foreseeable issues in biomedical contexts' (2016) 22(2) *Science and Engineering Ethics* 303–41

Mjøen, Geir, Hallan, Stein, Hartmann, Anders et al., 'Long-term risks for kidney donors' (2014) 86(1) *Kidney International* 162–7

Moggio, Maurizio, Colombo, Irene, Peverelli, Lorenzo et al., 'Mitochondrial disease heterogeneity: a prognostic challenge' (2014) 33(2) *Acta Myologica* 86–93

Moore, Jennifer, 'Kant's ethical community' (1992) 26(1) *The Journal of Value Inquiry* 51–71

More, S., Beach, J. and Vince, R., 'Early detection of amyloidopathy in Alzheimer's mice by hyperspectral endoscopy' (2016) 57 *Investigative Ophthalmology and Visual Science* 3231–8

Morelli, Mario, 'Commerce in organs: a Kantian critique' (1999) 30(2) *Journal of Social Philosophy* 315–24

Morris, Peter J., 'Transplantation – a medical miracle of the 20th century' (2004) 351(26) *New England Journal of Medicine* 2678–80

Moss, R., 'Comment on article by Lay, Kat, "NHS to share opt-out patients' data"' (19 September 2017) *The Times*

Motluk, Alison, 'Is egg donation dangerous?' (2012) 46 *Maisonneuve* 26–33

Mourad, Selma, Brown, Julie and Farquhar, Cindy, 'Interventions for the prevention of OHSS in ART cycles: an overview of Cochrane reviews' in *Cochrane Database of Systematic Reviews* (Hoboken, NJ: John Wiley and Sons, 2017). doi:10.1002/14651858.CD012103.pub2

Mullin, Emily, 'The fertility doctor trying to commercialize three-parent babies' (13 June 2017), *MIT Technology Review*, www.technologyreview.com/s/608033/the-fertility-doctor-trying-to-commercialize-three-parent-babies/

Munzer, Stephen R., 'Kant and property rights in body parts' (1993) 6(2) *Canadian Journal of Law and Jurisprudence* 319–41
   'An uneasy case against property rights in body parts' (1994) 11(2) *Social Philosophy and Policy* 259–86

Murray, Thomas H., 'On the human body as property: the meaning of embodiment, markets, and the meaning of strangers' (1987) 20(4) *University of Michigan Journal of Law Reform* 1055–88

Muzaale, Abimereki D., Massie, Allan B., Wang, Mei C. et al., 'Risk of end-stage renal disease following live kidney donation' (2014) 311(6) *Journal of the American Medical Association* 579–86

Naqvi, S. A., Rizvi, S. A., Zafar, M. N. et al., 'Health status and renal function evaluation of kidney vendors: a report from Pakistan' (2008) 8(7) *American Journal of Transplantation* 1444–50

NASDAQ, 'Alzheimer's takes another hit as Pfizer ends research in this area' (8 January 2018), www.nasdaq.com/article/alzheimers-takes-another-hit-as-pfizer-ends-research-in-this-area-cm901602

Nasir, Muhammad, Nasir, Tehmina, Khan, Hira Ashraf et al., 'Organ trafficking. do you want a society where the destitute become a store for the wealthy?' (2013) 20(2) *The Professional Medical Journal* 177–81

National Bioethics Advisory Commission (US), *Research Involving Human Biological Materials: Ethical Issues and Policy Guidance (Executive Summary)* (1999) https://bioethicsarchive.georgetown.edu/nbac/hbm_exec.pdf, accessed 6 November 2017

National Commission for the Protection of Human Subjects of Biomedical and Behavioral Research (US), *The Belmont Report – Ethical Principles and Guidelines for the Protection of Human Subjects of Research* (1979) www.hhs.gov/ohrp/regulations-and-policy/belmont-report/index.html, accessed 6 November 2017

National Health Service (NHS) England, 'Genomics' (2012) www.england.nhs.uk/ourwork/qual-clin-lead/personalisedmedicine/genomics/, accessed 6 November 2017

'Privacy impact assessment: care.data' (2014) www.england.nhs.uk/wp-content/uploads/2014/04/cd-pia.pdf, accessed 6 November 2017

'Letter dated 10 December 2015, responding to a Freedom of Information Request by Dr Neil Bhatia' (10 December 2015) www.whatdotheyknow.com/request/single_national_gp_dataset_2, accessed 6 November 2017

'Enabling evidence-based continuous improvement. The Target Architecture. Connecting care settings and improving patient experience' (2017) https://medconfidential.org/wp-content/uploads/2017/09/2017-07-13-Target-Architecture.pdf, accessed 6 November 2017

National Public Radio, 'Pfizer halts research into Alzheimer's and Parkinson's treatments' (2018) www.npr.org/sections/thetwo-way/2018/01/08/576443442/pfizer-halts-research-efforts-into-alzheimers-and-parkinsons-treatments

Nayernia, K., Nolte, J., Michelmann, H. W. et al., 'In vitro-differentiated embryonic stem cells give rise to male gametes that can generate offspring mice' 11 *Developmental Cell* 125–32

Negroponte, N., *Being Digital* (New York, NY: Vintage Books, 1995)

Newson, Ainsley J., Wilkinson, Stephen and Wrigley, Anthony, 'Ethical and legal issues in mitochondrial transfer' (2016) 8(6) *EMBO Molecular Medicine* 589–91. doi:10.15252/emmm.201606281

Ng, P., Murray, S. S., Levy, S. et al., 'An agenda for personalized medicine' (2009) 461 *Nature* 724–6

Nicol, Dianne and Critchley, Christine R., 'Benefit sharing and biobanking in Australia' (2012) 21(5) *Public Understanding of Science* 534–55

Nik-Khah, Edward, 'Neoliberal pharmaceutical science and the Chicago School of Economics' (2014) 44(4) *Social Studies of Science* 489–517

Nilstun, Tore and Herméren, Göran, 'Human tissue samples and ethics–attitudes of the general public in Sweden to biobank research' (2006) 9(1) *Medicine, Health Care and Philosophy* 81–6

Nisker, Jeff, 'The latest thorn by any other name: germ-line nuclear transfer in the name of "mitochondrial replacement"' (2015) 37(9) *Journal of Obstetrics and Gynaecology Canada* 829–31. doi:10.1016/S1701-2163(15)30156-0

Nordfalk, F., *Forskerbeskyttelsen i Danmark 1995–2014.* (Copenhagen: Københavns Universitet, 2015), pp. 1–79

Nordfalk, K. and Hoeyer, K., 'The rise and fall of an opt out system' (2018) *Scandinavian Journal of Public Health*, Published online.

Nuffield Council on Bioethics, *Human Bodies: Donation for Medicine and Research* (London: Nuffield Council on Bioethics, 2011)
  Novel Techniques for the Prevention of Mitochondrial DNA Disorders: An Ethical Review (London: Nuffield Council on Bioethics, 2012)

O'Hara, Kieron, *Transparent Government, Not Transparent Citizens: A Report on Privacy and Transparency for the Cabinet Office* (Southampton: University of Southampton, 2011)

Olsen, L., Aisner, D. and McGinnis, J. M., *The Learning Healthcare System: Workshop Summary* (Washington, DC: The National Academies Press, 2007)

Organisation for Economic Co-operation and Development (OECD), Best Practice Guidelines for Quality Assurance in Molecular Genetic Testing (2007) www.oecd.org/dataoecd/43/6/38839788.pdf

Organization for Security and Co-Operation in Europe, *Trafficking in Human Beings for the Purpose of Organ Removal in the OSCE Region: Analysis and Findings, Occasional Paper Series 6* (Vienna: Office of the Special Representative and Co-ordinator for Combating Trafficking in Human Beings, 2013)

Oye, K. A., Jain, G., Amador, M., Arnaout, R. et al., 'The next frontier: Fostering innovation by improving health data access and utilization' (2015) 98(5) *Clinical Pharmacology & Therapeutics* 514–21

Ozkan, O., Akar, M. E., Ozkan, O. et al., 'Preliminary results of the first human uterus transplantation from a multiorgan donor' (2013) 99(2) *Fertility and Sterility* 470–6

Parfit, Derek (1984) *Reasons and Persons* (Oxford: Oxford University Press, 1984)

Pariser, E., *The Filter Bubble* (London: Penguin, 2011)

Pascalev, Assya, de Jong, Jessica, Ambagtsheer, Frederike et al., 'Trafficking in human beings for the purpose of organ removal: a comprehensive literature review' in Frederike Ambagtsheer and Willem Weimar (eds.), *Trafficking in Human Beings for the Purpose of Organ Removal: Results and Recommendations* (Lengerich: Pabst, 2016), pp. 15–68

Patra, Prasanna and Sleeboom-Faulkner, Margaret, 'Following the banking cycle of UCB in India: the disparity between pre-banking persuasion and post-banking utilization' (2016) 35(3) *New Genetics and Society* 267–88

Pattinson, Shaun D., *Medical Law and Ethics* (London: Sweet and Maxwell, 2014)

Pausanias, *Guide to Greece* (London: Penguin, 1971), vol. 1

Pennings, G., 'Measuring the welfare of the child: in search of the appropriate evaluation principle' (1999) 14 *Human Reproduction* 1146–50

Pearson, Elaine, *Coercion in the Kidney Trade? A Background Study on Trafficking in Human Organs Worldwide* (Deutsche Gesellschaft für Technische Zusammenarbeit, 2004)

Percer, Beth, 'Umbilical cord blood banking: Helping parents make informed choices' (2009) 13(3) *Nursing for Women's Health* 216–23

Perry, Ronen, 'It's a wonderful life' (2007) 93 *Cornell Law Review* 329–400

Pessers, Dorien, 'The symbolic meaning of legal subjectivity' in Bart van Klink, Britta van Beers and Lonneke Poort (eds.), *Symbolic Legislation Theory and Developments in Biolaw* (Switzerland: Springer 2016), 201–12

Philips, A., '"Only a click away" – DTC genetics for ancestry, health, love . . . and more: a view of the business and regulatory landscape' (2016) 8 *Applied and Translational Genomics* 16–22

Pierce, Robin, 'Complex calculations: ethical issues in involving at-risk healthy individuals in dementia research' (2010) 36(9) *Journal of Medical Ethics* 553–7

Piketty, Thomas, *Capital in the Twenty-First Century* (Cambridge, MA: Harvard University Press, 2014)

Plato, *Plato I: Euthyphro, Apology, Crito, Phaedo, Phaedrus* [Loeb edition] (Cambridge, MA: Harvard University Press, 1914/1995)

Pollock, Allyson M., Macfarlane, Alison and Godden, Sylvia, 'Dismantling the signposts to public health? NHS data under the Health and Social Care Act' (2012) 344 *British Medical Journal* e2364

Porter, M., Kerridge, I. H. and Jordens, C. F. C. '"Good Mothering" or "Good Citizenship"? Conflicting values in choosing whether to donate or store umbilical cord blood' (2012) 9 *Bioethical Inquiry* 41–7

Posner, Richard, *Economic Analysis of Law* (Boston, MA: Little, Brown and Company, 1972)

'Practice Committee of the American Society for Reproductive Medicine, "Ovarian hyperstimulation syndrome"' (2008) 90(S1) *Fertility and Sterility* 88–93

Prainsack, Barbara, '"Negotiating life": The regulation of human cloning and embryonic stem cell research in Israel' (2006) 36(2) *Social Studies of Science* 173–205
'The "We" in the "Me": solidarity and health care in the era of personalized
medicine' (2018) 43(1) *Science, Technology and Human Values* 21–44
'Personhood and solidarity: what kind of personalised medicine do we want?'
(2014) 11(7) *Personalized Medicine* 651–7
Prainsack, B., Reardon, J., Hindmarch, H. et al., 'Personal genomes: misdirected
precaution' 456 *Nature* 34–5
Prasad, R., 'Public cord-blood banking becomes a reality in Chennai' (1 January
2009) *The Hindu*
Precision Medicine Initiative (PMI) Working Group Report to the Advisory
Committee to the Director, NIH, *The Precision Medicine Initiative Cohort
Program – Building a Research Foundation for 21st Century Medicine* (17
September 2015)
ProtEProbe, 'Nanosensors for the diagnosis of Alzheimer's disease', http://cordis
.europa.eu/result/rcn/188315_en.html
'Public genomes: the future of the NHS?' (2017) 390 *The Lancet* 203
Purpura, S., Schwanda, V., Williams, K., 'Fit4Life: the design of a persuasive
technology promoting healthy behavior and ideal weight' in *Proceedings of
the SIGCHI Conference on Human Factors in Computing Systems* (New York,
NY: ACM (CHI '11), 2011), pp. 423–32. doi:10.1145/1978942.1979003
Quantified Self, *Quantified Self – Self Knowledge Through Numbers, Quantified Self.*
(2018) http://quantifiedself.com/ (Accessed 2 February 2018)
Rabinow, Paul, *Artificiality and Enlightenment: From Sociobiology to Biosociality.
Essays on the Anthropology of Reason* (Princeton, NJ: Princeton University
Press, 1996)
Radcliffe Richards, Janet, 'Nephrarious goings on: kidney sales and moral argu-
ments' (1996) 21(4) *Journal of Medicine and Philosophy* 375–416
Radin, Margaret J., 'Market-inalienability' (1987) 100(8) *Harvard Law Review*
1849–937
Reinterpreting Property (Chicago, IL: University of Chicago Press, 1993)
*Contested Commodities: The Trouble with Trade in Sex, Children, Body Parts,
and Other Things* (Cambridge, MA: Harvard University Press, 1996)
Ram, Natalie, 'Assigning rights and protecting interests: constructing ethical and
efficient legal rights in human tissue research' (2009) 23(1) *Harvard Journal of
Law and Technology* 119–77
Rao, Radhika, 'Property, privacy, and the human body' (2000) 80(2) *Boston
University Law Review* 359–460
'Genes and spleens: property, contract, or privacy rights in the human body?'
(2007) 35(3) *Journal of Law, Medicine and Ethics* 371–82
'How (not) to regulate assisted reproductive technology: lessons from
"Octomom"' (2015) 49(1) *Family Law Quarterly* 137–47

Rasmussen, L. I., 'Danmark er et diagnosesamfund' (27 March 2016) *Politiken*, pp. 4–6

Reardon, J., 'The "persons" and "genomics" of personal genomics' (2011) 8(1) *Personalized Medicine* 95–107

Reardon, Sara, 'Genetic details of controversial "three-parent baby" revealed' (2017) 544(7648) *Nature News* 17. doi:10.1038/nature.2017.21761

Regeringen, *Jo Før – Jo Bedre: Tidlig Diagnose, Bedre Behandling og Flere Gode Leveår for Alle* (Copenhagen: The Danish Government, 2014)

Reuter, Shelley Z., 'The politics of "wrongful life" itself: discursive (mal)practices and Tay-Sachs disease' (2007) 36(2) *Economy and Society* 236–62

Richards, M., Anderson, R., Hinde, S. et al., *The Collection, Linking and Use of Data in Biomedical Research and Health Care: Ethical Issues*. London: Nuffield Council on Bioethics, 2015

Rippon, Simon, 'Imposing options on people in poverty: the harm of a live donor organ market' (2012) 40(3) *Journal of Medical Ethics* 145–50

'Organ markets and harms: a reply to Dworkin, Radcliffe Richards and Walsh' (2014) 40(3) *Journal of Medical Ethics* 155–6

Roberts, Michelle, 'IVF: first three-parent baby born to infertile couple' (18 January 2017) *BBC News*, www.bbc.com/news/health-38648981

Robertson, J. A., 'Embryos, families, and procreative liberty: the legal structure of the new reproduction' (1985) 59 *Southern California Law Review* 939–1041

'Impact of uterus transplant on fetuses and resulting children: a response to Daar and Klipstein' (2016) 3 *Journal of Law and the Biosciences* 710

Roche, Patricia, A., 'The property/privacy conundrum over human tissue' (2010) 22(3) *HEC Forum* 197–209

Rose, Nikolas (1998) *Inventing Our Selves: Psychology, Power and Personhood* (Cambridge: Cambridge University Press, 1998)

'The politics of life itself' (2001) 18(6) *Theory, Culture and Society* 1–30

The Politics of Life Itself: Biomedicine, Power, and Subjectivity in the Twenty-First Century (Princeton, NJ: Princeton University Press, 2007)

Rose, Nikolas and Novas, C., 'Biological citizenship' in A. Ong and S. J. Collier (eds.), *Global Assemblages: Technology, Politics, and Ethics as Anthropological Problems* (Malden: Blackwell, 2005), 439–64

Roski, J., Bo-Linn, G. W. and Andrews,T. A., 'Creating value in health care through big data: opportunities and policy implications' (2014) 33(7) *Health Affairs* 1115–22

Ross, Lainie Friedman, 'Saving lives is more important than abstract moral concerns: Financial incentives should be used to increase organ donation – con' (2009) 88(4) *Annals of Thoracic Surgery* 1056–9

Rothman, Sheila M. and Rothman, David J., 'The hidden cost of organ sale' (2006) 6(7) *American Journal of Transplantation* 1524–8

Rothstein, M., Wilbanks, J. and Brothers, K., 'Citizen science on your smartphone: an ELSI research agenda' (2015) 43(4) *Journal of Law, Medicine and Ethics* 897–903

Rouchi, Alireza H., Ghaemi, Fatemeh and Aghighi, Mohammad, 'Outlook of organ transplantation in Iran: a time for quality assessment' (2014) 8(3) *Iranian Journal of Kidney Diseases* 185–8

Rubinstein, Pablo, 'Why cord blood?' (2006) 67 *Human Immunology* 398–404

Rubio, J. H. 'Family ties: a Catholic response to donor-conceived families' 21(2) *Christian Bioethics* 181–98

Rulli, Tina, 'What is the value of three-parent IVF?' (2016) 46(4) *Hastings Center Report* 38–47. doi:10.1002/hast.594

Sabatello, Maya and Appelbaum, Paul S., 'The precision medicine nation' (2017) 47 (4) *Hastings Center Report* 19–29

Sajjad, Imran, Baines, Lyndsay S., Patel, Prem et al., 'Commercialization of kidney transplants: a systematic review of outcomes in recipients and donors' (2008) 28(5) *American Journal of Nephrology* 744–54

Sample, Ian, 'First UK licence to create three-person baby granted by fertility regulator' (16 March 2017), *The Guardian*, www.theguardian.com/science/ 2017/mar/16/first-licence-to-create-three-person-baby-granted-by-uk-ferti lity-regulator

Samuel, Gabrielle Natalie and Farsides, Bobbie, 'The UK's 100,000 Genomes Project: manifesting policymakers' expectations' (2017) 36(4) *New Genetics and Society* 336–53

Sandel, Michael J., *The Case Against Perfection: Ethics in the Age of Engineering* (Cambridge, MA: Harvard University Press, 2007)

  What Money Can't Buy: The Moral Limits of Markets (London: Allen Lane, 2012)

Sanderson, Saskia C., Diefenbach, Michael A., Zinberg, Randi et al., 'Willingness to participate in genomics research and desire for personal results among under-represented minority patients: a structured interview study' (2013) 4(4) *Journal of Community Genetics* 469–82

Sankar, T., Chakravarty, M., Bescos, A. et al., 'Deep brain stimulation influences brain structure in Alzheimer's disease' (2015) *Brain Stimulation* 645–54

Santoro, Pablo, 'From (public?) waste to (private?) value: the regulation of private cord blood banking in Spain' (2009) 22(1) *Science Studies* 3–23, www.science technologystudies.org/system/files/Santoro.pdf. (accessed 10 December 2012)

Satel, Sally (ed.), *When Altruism Isn't Enough: The Case for Compensating Kidney Donors* (Washington, DC: AEI Press, 2008)

  'You've heard of Trump steaks, now Trump kidneys' (15 November 2016) *Forbes*

Satel, Sally and Cronin, David C., II, 'Time to test incentives to increase organ donation' (2015) 175(8) *Journal of the American Medical Association Internal Medicine* 1329–33

Satz, Debra, 'The moral limits of markets: the case of human kidneys' (2008) 108(3) *Proceedings of the Aristotelian Society* 269–88

Why Some Things Should Not Be for Sale: The Limits of Markets (Oxford: Oxford University Press, 2010)

Saunders, M. K., 'In Denmark, Big Data goes to work' (2014) 33(7) *Health Affairs* 1245

Savulescu, Julian, 'For and Against: No consent should be needed for using leftover body material for scientific purposes. Against' (2000) 325 *British Medical Journal* 648

'Is the sale of body parts wrong?' (2003) 29(3) *Journal of Medical Ethics* 138–9

Savulescu, J. and Kahane, G., 'The moral obligation to create children with the best chance of the best life' (2009) 23(5) *Bioethics* 274–90

Say, Rebecca E., Whittaker, Roger G., Turnbull, Helen E. et al., 'Mitochondrial disease in pregnancy: a systematic review' (2011) 4(3) *Obstetric Medicine* 90–94

Scheper-Hughes, Nancy, 'The global traffic in human organs' (2000) 41(2) *Current Anthropology* 191–224

'Commodity fetishism in organs trafficking' in Nancy Scheper-Hughes and Loïc Wacquant (eds.), *Commodifying Bodies* (London: Sage, 2002), pp. 31–62

'Keeping an eye on the global traffic in human organs' (2003) 361(9369) *The Lancet* 1645–8

'Black market organs: inside the trans-Atlantic transplant tourism trade' (3 June 2005) *LIP Magazine*

Schlitt, Hans J., 'Paid non-related living organ donation: horn of plenty or Pandora's box?' (2002) 359(9310) *The Lancet* 906–7

Scott, Rosamund, 'Reconsidering wrongful life in England after 30 years: legislative mistakes and unjustifiable anomalies' (2013) 72(1) *Cambridge Law Journal* 115–54

Semrau, Luke, 'Misplaced paternalism and other mistakes in the debate over kidney sales' (2017) 31(3) *Bioethics* 190–8

Lopeti Senituli and Margaret Boyes, 'Whose DNA? Tonga and Iceland, Biotech, Ownership, and Consent' in James V. Lavery, Christine Grady, Elizabeth R. Wahl and Ezekiel J. Emanuel (eds.), *Ethical Issues in International Biomedical Research: A Casebook* (Oxford: Oxford University Press, 2007), pp. 53–63.

Sevigny, J., Chiao, P., Bussière, T. et al., 'The antibody aducanumab reduces Aβ plaques in Alzheimer's disease' (2016) 537 *Nature* 50–56

Shanner, L., 'The right to procreate: when rights claims have gone wrong' (1995) 40 *McGill Law Journal* 823–74

Shell, Susan M., 'Kant's concept of human dignity as a resource for bioethics' in The President's Council on Bioethics (ed.), *Human Dignity and Bioethics: Essays Commissioned by the President's Council on Bioethics* (Washington, DC: 2008), pp. 333–49

Shilton, K., 'Participatory personal data: an emerging research challenge for the information sciences' (2012) 63(10) *Journal of the American Society for Information Science and Technology*, 1905–15. doi:10.1002/asi.22655

Shrivastav, Snehlata, 'Cord blood banking takes off in Nagpur' (16 May 2012) *Times News Network (TNN)*

Sifferlin, A., 'Exclusive: First US baby born after a uterus transplant' (1 December 2017), *Time*, http://time.com/5044565/exclusive-first-u-s-baby-born-after-a-uterus-transplant/

Silverman, E. and Skinner, J., 'Medicare upcoding and hospital ownership' (2004) 23 *Journal of Health Economics* 369–89

Simmel, G., 'The stranger' in K. Wolff (ed.), *The Sociology of Georg Simmel* (New York, NY: Free Press, 1950), pp. 402–8

Singer, Peter, 'Altruism and commerce: a defense of Titmuss against Arrow' (1973) 2(3) *Philosophy and Public Affairs* 312–20

Singh, Nancy, 'C(h)ords of Life' (2010) www.chillibreeze.com/articles_various/Umbilical-cord-banking-in-India-310.asp. (accessed 20 December 2012)

Skolbekken, John Arne, Ursin, Lars Ø., Solberg, Berge et al., 'Not worth the paper it's written on? Informed consent and biobank research in a Norwegian context' (2005) 15 *Critical Public Health* 335–47

Sloterdijk, P., *Du Musst Dein Leben Ändern: Über Anthropotechnik* (Suhrkamp, 2009)

Smajdor, A. and Cutas, D., 'Will artificial gametes end infertility?' (2015) 23 *Health Care Analysis* 134–47

Smerdon, U. R., 'Crossing bodies, crossing borders: international surrogacy between the United States and India' (2008) 39 *Cumberland Law Review* 15–85

Smith, Adam, *The Wealth of Nations* (Oxford: Oxford University Press, 2008)

Smith, P. C., 'Reflecting on "Analytical perspectives on performance-based management: an outline of theoretical assumptions in the existing literature"' (2015) 10(4) *Health Economics, Policy and Law* 1–5

Snyder, Jeremy, 'Easy rescues and organ transplantation' (2009) 21(1) *HEC Forum* 27–53

Society for Assisted Reproductive Technology, *National Summary Report* (2014) www.sartcorsonline.com/rptCSR_PublicMultYear.aspx?reportingYear=2014

Sperling, R., Aisen P. S., Beckett, L. A. et al., 'Toward defining the preclinical stages of Alzheimer's disease: recommendations from the National Institute on Aging-Alzheimer's Association workgroups on diagnostic guidelines for Alzheimer's disease' (2011) 7(3) *Alzheimers and Dementia* 280–92

Springate, David, 'Health database could help avoid another pharma scandal' (2014) *The Conversation*, https://theconversation.com/health-database-could-help-avoid-another-pharma-scandal-23730, accessed 6 November 2017

Stauch, Marc and Wheat, Kay, *Text, Cases and Materials on Medical Law and Ethics* (London: Routledge, 2015)

Steering Committee of the Istanbul Summit, 'Organ trafficking, transplant tourism and commercialism: The Declaration of Istanbul' (2008) 372(9632) *The Lancet* 5–6

Sterckx, Sigrid and Cockbain, Julian, *Exclusions from Patentability: How Far Has the European Patent Office Eroded Boundaries?* (Cambridge: Cambridge University Press, 2012)

   'The ethics of patenting in genetics – a second enclosure of the commons?' in Gabriele Werner-Felmayer, Barbara Prainsack and Silke Schicktanz (eds.), *Genetics as Social Practice – Transdisciplinary Views on Science and Culture* (Farnham: Ashgate, 2014), pp. 129–44

Sterckx, Sigrid, Cockbain, Julian, Howard, H. et al., '"Trust is not something you can reclaim easily": patenting in the field of direct-to-consumer genetic testing' (2013) 15(5) *Genetics in Medicine* 382–7

Sterckx, Sigrid, Rakic, Vojin and Cockbain, Julian, '"You hoped we would sleep-walk into accepting the collection of our data": controversies surrounding the UK care.data scheme and their wider relevance for biomedical research' (2015) 19 *Medicine, Health Care and Philosophy* 177–90

Stone, M. A., Redsell, S. A., Ling, J. T. et al., 'Sharing patient data: competing demands of privacy, trust and research in primary care' (2005) 55(519) *British Journal of General Practice* 783–9

Strava (n. d.) *Strava Metro*. Available at: http://metro.strava.com (accessed 2 February 2018)

Strategisk Alliance for Register – og Sundhedsdata, *Eksempelsamling. Brug af Sundhedsdata i Forskning Til Gavn for Patient og Borger* (Copenhagen: www.sum.dk, 2016)

Sullivan, M. J., 'Banking on cord blood stem cells' (2008) 8 *Nature Reviews Cancer* 554–63

Sunstein, Cass R., 'Incommensurability and valuation in law' (1994) *Michigan Law Review* 779–861

Supiot, Alain, *Homo Juridicus: On the Anthropological Function of the Law* (New York, NY: Verso Books, 2007).

Suryanarayan, Deepa, 'Young Mumbai women go for cord blood banking' (9 May 2010) *Mumbai Agency: Daily News and Analysis (DNA)*

Suter, E. A., Seurer, L. M., Webb, S. et al., 'Motherhood as contested ideological terrain: essentialist and queer discourses of motherhood at play in female–female co-mothers' talk' (2015) 82(4) *Communication Monographs* 458–83

Sutton, Agneta M., 'Commodification of body parts' (2002) 235 *British Medical Journal* 114

Swanson, Kara W., *Banking on the Body: The Market in Blood, Milk and Sperm in Modern America* (Cambridge, MA: Harvard University Press, 2014)

Tabarrok, Alexander, 'The organ shortage. a tragedy of the commons?' in Alexander Tabarrok (ed.), *Entrepreneurial Economics: Bright Ideas from the Dismal Science* (Oxford: Oxford University Press, 2002), pp. 107–11

Tachibana, Masahito, Amato, Paula, Sparman, Michelle et al., 'Towards germline gene therapy of inherited mitochondrial diseases' (2013) 493(7434) *Nature* 627–31. doi:10.1038/nature11647

Tachibana, Masahito, Sparman, Michelle, Sritanaudomchai, Hathaitip, 'Mitochondrial gene replacement in primate offspring and embryonic stem cells' (2009) 461(7262) *Nature* 367–72. doi:10.1038/nature08368

Taylor, James S., *Stakes and Kidneys: Why Markets in Human Body Parts are Morally Imperative* (Burlington, VT: Ashgate, 2005)

Teeman, Tim, 'Married to Mr Google' (4 February 2012) *The Times*, www.thetimes.co.uk/articlemarried-to-mr-google-nc6qc5znkwt

Teo, Bernard, 'Is the adoption of more efficient strategies of organ procurement the answer to persistent organ shortage in transplantation?' (1992) 6(2) *Bioethics* 113–29

Testa, G., Anthony, T., McKenna, G. J. et al., 'Deceased donor uterus retrieval: a novel technique and workflow' (2018) 18 *American Journal of Transplantation* 679–83. doi:10.1111/ajt.14476

Thomas, Yan, *Du Droit de Ne Pas Naître* (Paris: Gallimard, 2002)

Thygesen, L. C. and Ersbøll, A. K., 'Danish population-based registers for public health and health-related welfare research: introduction to the supplement' (2011) 39 (Suppl7) *Scandinavian Journal of Public Health* 8–10

'When the entire population is the sample: strengths and limitations in register-based epidemiology' (2014) 29(8) *European Journal of Epidemiology* 551–8

Tingley, Kim, 'The brave new world of three-parent IVF' (27 June 2014) *The New York Times*, www.nytimes.com/2014/06/29/magazine/the-brave-new-world-of-three-parent-ivf.html

Titmuss, Richard, *The Gift Relationship: From Human Blood to Social Policy* (London: Allen and Unwin, 1970)

Tiwari, Shashank S., *The Ethics and Governance of Stem Cell Clinical Research* (2013) PhD Thesis, University of Nottingham, Institute for Science and Society, www.eprints.nottingham.ac.uk/14585/1/602957. Accessed 20 September 2016.

Toft, O.N.M., *Blixt Kræver Samråds-svar i Data-sag* (Altinget, 2016)

Tong, Allison, Chapman, Jeremy R., Wong, Germaine et al., 'The experiences of commercial kidney donors: thematic synthesis of qualitative research' (2012) 25(11) *Transplant International* 1138–49

Toyooka, Y., Tsunekawa, N., Akasu, R. et al., 'Embryonic stem cells can form germ cells in vitro' (2003) 100(20) *Proceedings of the National Academy of Sciences* 11457–62

Tsai, Meng-Kun, Yang, Ching-Yao, Lee, Chich-Yuan et al., 'De novo malignancy is associated with renal transplant tourism' (2011) 79(8) *Kidney International* 908–14

Tullock, John and Lupton, Deborah, *Risk and Everyday Life* (London: Sage, 2003)

Tuppen, Helen A. L., Blakely, Emma L., Turnbull, Douglass M. et al., 'Mitochondrial DNA mutations and human disease' (2010) 1797(2) *Biochimica et Biophysica Acta* 113–28. doi:10.1016/j.bbabio.2009.09.005

Turner, A. J. and Coyle, A., 'What does it mean to be a donor offspring? The identity experiences of adults conceived by donor insemination and the implications for counselling and therapy' (2000) 15(9) *Human Reproduction* 2041–51

Tutton, R., 'Personalizing medicine: futures present and past' (2012) 75(10) *Social Science and Medicine* 1721–8
  Genomics and the Reimagining of Personalized Medicine (Farnham: Ashgate, 2014)

Tutton, Richard and Prainsack, Barbara, 'Enterprising or altruistic selves? Making up research subjects in genetics research' (2011) 33(7) *Sociology of Health and Illness* 1081–95

Twenge, Jean M. and Campbell, Keith W., *The Narcissism Epidemic. Living in the Age of Entitlement* (New York, NY: Free Press, 2009)

Tymstra, T., 'At least we tried everything: about binary thinking, anticipated decision regret, and the imperative character of medical technology' (2007) 28(3) *Journal of Psychosomatic Obstetrics and Gynecology* 131

UK Biobank, 'Participants' (2016) www.ukbiobank.ac.uk/participants/, accessed 6 November 2017

'Umbilical cord blood banking Richard Branson's way' (2007) 369(9560) *The Lancet* 437

United Nations Office on Drugs and Crime, *Assessment Toolkit: Trafficking in Persons for the Purpose of Organ Removal* (New York, NY: United Nations, 2015)
  Issue Paper: Abuse of a Position of Vulnerability and other 'Means' within the Definition of Trafficking in Persons (New York, NY: United Nations, 2013)

Ursin, Lars Ø., 'Biobank research and the welfare state project: the HUNT story' (2010) 20(4) *Critical Public Health* 453–63

Valcarcel-Nazco, C., Perestelo-Perez, L, Molinuevo, J. L. et al., 'Cost-effectiveness of the use of biomarkers in cerebrospinal fluid for Alzheimer's disease' (2014) 42(3) *Journal of Alzheimer's Disease* 777–88

Van Assche, Kristof, Gutwirth, Serge and Sterckx, Sigrid, 'Protecting dignitary interests of biobank research participants: lessons from *Havasupai Tribe* v. *Arizona Board of Regents*' (2013) 5(1) *Law, Innovation and Technology* 54–84

van Beers, Britta, *Persoon en Lichaam in het Recht: Menselijke Waardigheid en Zelfbeschikking in het Tijdperk van de Medische Biotechnologie* (The Hague: Boom Juridische Uitgevers, 2009)

'Is Europe "giving in to baby markets?" Reproductive tourism in Europe and the gradual erosion of existing legal limits to reproductive markets' (2014) 23(1) *Medical Law Review* 103–134

'The changing nature of law's natural person: the impact of emerging technologies on the legal concept of the person' (2017) 18(3) *German Law Journal* 559–94

van Beers, Britta, Corrias, Luigi and Werner, Wouter G. (eds.), *Humanity across International Law and Biolaw* (Cambridge: Cambridge University Press, 2014)

Van der Wees, P. J., Nijhuis-Van der Sanden, M. W. G., Ayanian, J. Z. et al., 'Integrating the use of patient–reported outcomes for both clinical practice and performance measurement: views of experts from 3 countries' (2014) 92 (4) *The Milbank Quarterly* 754–75

Vayena, E. and Tasioulas J., 'We the scientists: a human right to citizen science' (2015) 28 *Philosophy and Technology* 479–85. doi:10.1007/s13347-015-0204-0

Veatch, Robert M., 'Why liberals should accept financial incentives for organ procurement' (2003) 13(1) *Kennedy Institute of Ethics Journal* 19–36

Venter, J. C., *A Life Decoded: My Genome, My Life* (New York, NY: Viking/ Penguin, 2007)

Verbeek, P.-P., *Moralizing Technology: Understanding and Designing the Morality of Things* (Chicago, IL: University of Chicago Press, 2011)

Vezyridis, Paraskevas and Timmons, Stephen, 'Dissenting from care. data: an analysis of opt-out forms' (2016) 42(12) *Journal of Medical Ethics* 792–6

'Understanding the care.data conundrum: new information flows for economic growth' (2017) *Big Data and Society*. doi:10.1177/2053951716688490

Volk, Michael L., 'Organ quality as a complicating factor in proposed systems of inducements for organ donation' (2014) 77(3) *Law and Contemporary Problems* 337–45

Wadmann, S., Johansen, S., Lind, A. et al., 'Analytical perspectives on performance-based management: an outline of theoretical assumptions in the existing literature' (2013) 8(4) *Health Economics, Policy and Law* 5–27

Wahlberg, A. and Streitfellner, T., 'Stem cell tourism, desperation and the governing of new therapies' in A. Leibing and V. Tournay (eds.), *Technologies de l'espoir. Les débats publics autour de l'innovation médicale* (Montreal: Université de Montréal, 2009)

Wakefield, J., 'Google Deepmind: Should patients trust the company with their data?' (23 September 2016) *BBC News*, www.bbc.com/news/technology-37439221

Waldby, Catherine, 'Umbilical cord blood: from social gift to venture capital' (2006) 1(1) *Biosocieties* 55–70

Wallace, Douglas C., Singh, Gurparkash, Lott, Marie T. et al., 'Mitochondrial DNA mutation associated with Leber's hereditary optic myopathy' (1988) 242 (4884) *Science* 1427

298

BIBLIOGRAPHY

Walzer, Michael, *Spheres of Justice: A Defense of Pluralism and Equality* (New York, NY: Basic Books, 1983)

Wancata, Andrew, 'No value for a pound of flesh: extending market-inalienability of the human body' (2003) 18(2) *Journal of Law and Health* 199–228

Wang, Min-Kang, Chen, Da-Yuan, Liu, Ji-Long et al., 'In vitro fertilisation of mouse oocytes reconstructed by transfer of metaphase II chromosomes results in live births' (2001) 9(10) *Zygote* 9–14

Wellcome Trust/IPSOS Mori, *The One-Way Mirror: Public Attitudes to Commercial Access to Health Data* (2016) www.ipsos.com/sites/default/files/publication/5200-03/sri-wellcome-trust-commercial-access-to-health-data.pdf, accessed 6 November 2017

Wevers, Kate, 'Prenatal torts and pre-implantation genetic diagnosis' (2010) 24(1) *Harvard Journal of Law & Technology* 257–80

Widdows, Heather, *The Connected Self. The Ethics and Governance of the Genetic Individual* (Cambridge: Cambridge University Press, 2013)

Widdows, H. and Cordell, S. 'Why communities and their goods matter: illustrated with the example of biobanks' (2011) 4(1) *Public Health Ethics* 14–25

Wigmore, Stephen J., Lumsdaine, Jen A. and Forsythe, John L. R., 'Ethical market in organs: defending the Indefensible' (2003) 325(7368) *British Medical Journal* 835–6

Wijlaars, Linda, '"Goldilocks" gene response to TB suggests best treatment' (6 February 2012) *Bionews*

Wilkinson, Stephen, 'Commodification arguments for the legal prohibition of organ sale' (2000) 8(2) *Health Care Analysis* 189–201

    Bodies for Sale: Ethics and Exploitation in the Human Body Trade (New York, NY: Routledge, 2003)

    'The exploitation argument against commercial surrogacy' (2003) 17 *Bioethics* 169–87

Wilkinson, Stephen and Garrard, Eve, 'Bodily integrity and the sale of human organs' (1996) 22(6) *Journal of Medical Ethics* 334–9

Wolf, G., *Gary Wolf: The quantified self | TED Talk | TED.com.* (2010) Available at: www.ted.com/talks/gary_wolf_the_quantified_self (accessed 2 February 2018).

Woods, Simon, 'Big Data governance: solidarity and the patient voice' in Brent Mittelstadt and Luciano Floridi (eds.,), *The Ethics of Biomedical Big Data* (Springer International, 2016), pp. 221–38

Woolley, J. Patrick, McGowan, Michelle L., Teare, Harriet J. A. et al., 'Citizen science or scientific citizenship? Disentangling the uses of public engagement rhetoric in national research initiatives' (2016) 17 *BMC Medical Ethics* 33

Working Group on Incentives for Living Donation, 'Incentives for organ donation: proposed standards for an internationally acceptable system' (2012) 12(2) *American Journal of Transplantation* 306–12

World Alzheimer Report: The Global Impact of Dementia: An Analysis of Prevalence, Incidence, Cost and Trends (London: Alzheimer's Disease International, 2015).

Wright, Caroline F., Hall, Alison and Zimmern, Ron L., 'Regulating direct-to-consumer genetic testing: what is the fuss about?' (2011) 13(4) *Genetic Medicine* 295–300

Wyverkens, E., Provoost, V., Ravelingien, A. et al., 'The meaning of the sperm donor for heterosexual couples: confirming the position of the father' (2017) 56(1) *Family Process* 203–16

Yakupoglu, Yarkin K., Ozden, Ender, Dilek, Melda et al., 'Transplantation tourism: high risk for the recipients' (2010) 24(6) *Clinical Transplantation* 835–8

Yamada, Mitsutoshi, Emmanuele, Valentina, Sanchez-Quintero, Maria J. et al., 'Genetic drift can compromise mitochondrial replacement by nuclear transfer in human oocytes' (2016) 18(6) *Cell Stem Cell* 749–54. doi:10.1016/j.stem.2016.04.001

Zargooshi, Javaad, 'Quality of life of Iranian kidney "donors"' (2001) 166(5) *Journal of Urology* 1790–9

Zetterberg, H., Wilson D., Andreasson U. et al., 'Plasma tau levels in Alzheimer's disease' (2013) 5 *Alzheimers Research and Therapy* 9

Zhang, John, Liu, Hiu, Luo, Shiyu et al., 'Live birth derived from oocyte spindle transfer to prevent mitochondrial disease' (2017) 34(4) *Reproductive Biomedicine Online* 361–8. doi:10.1016/j.rbmo.2017.01.013

Zhang, John, Zhuang, Guanglun, Zeng, Yong et al., 'Pregnancy derived from human nuclear transfer' (2003) 80 *Fertility and Sterility* 56. doi:10.1016/S0015-0282(03)01953-8

Zhang, John, Zhuang, Guanglun, Zeng, Yong, 'Pregnancy derived from human zygote pronuclear transfer in a patient who had arrested embryos after IVF' (2016) 33(4) *Reproductive Biomedicine Online* 529–33. doi:10.1016/j.rbmo.2016.07.008

Zhou, Q., Wang, M., Yuan, Y. et al., 'Complete meiosis from embryonic stem cell-derived germ cells in vitro' (2016) 18(3) *Cell Stem Cell* 330–40

Žižek, S., *Organs without Bodies: on Deleuze and Consequences* (London/New York, NY: Routledge, 2004/2012)

Zwart, Hub, *Technocratie en Onbehagen: de Plaats van de Ethiek in Het Werk van Michel Foucault* (Nijmegen: Sun, 1995)

'Next: book review' (2007) 3(1) *Genomics, Society and Policy* 48–51

'Francis Collins, *The Language of Life*: book review' (2011) 6(3) *Genomics, Society and Policy* 67–76

'Genomics and identity: the bioinformatisation of human life' (2009) 12 *Medicine, Health Care and Philosophy* 125–36

'Woyzeck and the birth of the human research subject: genetic disposition and the nature-nurture debate through the looking-glass of fiction' (2013) 6(3) *Bioethica Forum* 97–105

'The genome as the biological unconscious – and the unconscious as the psychic "genome": a psychoanalytical rereading of molecular genetics' (2013) 9(2) *Cosmos and History: the Journal of Natural and Social Philosophy* 198–222

'The obliteration of life: depersonalisation and disembodiment in the tera-byte age' (2016) 35(1) *New Genetics and Society* 69–89. doi:10.1080/14636778.2016.1143770

'"Extimate" technologies and techno-cultural discontent: a Lacanian analysis of pervasive gadgets' (2017) 22(1) *Techné: Research in Philosophy and Technology* 24–54. doi:10.5840/techne20174560

Legislation

Council of Europe

Additional Protocol to the Convention on Human Rights and Biomedicine, concerning Genetic Testing for Health Purposes (2008) (CETS No. 203)

European Union

Regulation (EU) 2016/679 of the European Parliament and of the Council of 27 April 2016 on the protection of natural persons with regard to the processing of personal data and on the free movement of such data, and repealing Directive 95/46/EC (General Data Protection Regulation), *Official Journal* L 119/1, 4 May 2016

United Kingdom

Care Act 2014, www.legislation.gov.uk/ukpga/2014/23/contents, accessed 6 November 2017

Data Protection Act 1998, www.legislation.gov.uk/ukpga/1998/29/contents, accessed 6 November 2017

Data Protection Bill [HL], https://publications.parliament.uk/pa/bills/lbill/2017–2019/0066/18066.pdf, accessed 6 November 2017

Digital Economy Act 2017, www.legislation.gov.uk/ukpga/2017/30/contents/enacted, accessed 6 November 2017

Health and Social Care Act 2012, www.legislation.gov.uk/ukpga/2012/7/
  contents, accessed 6 November 2017
National Health Service Act 2006, www.legislation.gov.uk/ukpga/2006/
  41/contents, accessed 6 November 2017

United Nations

Universal Declaration of Human Rights, UDHR (1948) www.un.org/en/
  universal-declaration-human-rights, accessed 29 January 2018

United States

42 CFR 493.129(1)
Clinical Laboratories Amendments Act of 2014
Drug Efficacy Amendment ('Kefauver Harris Amendment') PL 87–781
  (10 October 1962)
Federal Food, Drug and Cosmetics Act (FD and C)
Orphan Drug Act of 1983. Pub L. No. 97–414, 96 Stat. 2049

INDEX

Books in the Series

Anne-Maree Farrell
The Politics of Blood: Ethics, Innovation and the Regulation of Risk

Stephen Smith
End-of-Life Decisions in Medical Care: Principles and Policies for Regulating the Dying Process

Michael Parker
Ethical Problems and Genetics Practice

William W. Lowrance
Privacy, Confidentiality, and Health Research

Kerry Lynn Macintosh
Human Cloning: Four Fallacies and Their Legal Consequence

Heather Widdows
The Connected Self: The Ethics and Governance of the Genetic Individual

Amel Alghrani, Rebecca Bennett and Suzanne Ost
Bioethics, Medicine and the Criminal Law Volume I: The Criminal Law and Bioethical Conflict: Walking the Tightrope

Danielle Griffiths and Andrew Sanders
Bioethics, Medicine and the Criminal Law Volume II: Medicine, Crime and Society

Margaret Brazier and Suzanne Ost
Bioethics, Medicine and the Criminal Law Volume III: Medicine and Bioethics in the Theatre of the Criminal Process

Sigrid Sterckx, Kasper Raus and Freddy Mortier
Continuous Sedation at the End of Life: Ethical, Clinical and Legal Perspectives

A. M. Viens, John Coggon and Anthony S. Kessel
Criminal Law, Philosophy and Public Health Practice

Ruth Chadwick, Mairi Levitt and Darren Shickle
The Right to Know and the Right Not to Know: Genetic Privacy and Responsibility

Eleanor D. Kinney
The Affordable Care Act and Medicare in Comparative Context

Katri Lõhmus
Caring Autonomy: European Human Rights Law and the Challenge of Individualism

Catherine Stanton and Hannah Quirk
Criminalising Contagion: Legal and Ethical Challenges of Disease Transmission and the Criminal Law

Sharona Hoffman
Electronic Health Records and Medical Big Data: Law and Policy

Barbara Prainsack and Alena Buyx
Solidarity in Biomedicine and Beyond

Camillia Kong
Mental Capacity in Relationship

Oliver Quick
Regulating Patient Safety: The End of Professional Dominance?

Thana C. de Campos
The Global Health Crisis: Ethical Responsibilities

Jonathan Ives, Michael Dunn and Alan Cribb
Empirical Bioethics: Theoretical and Practical Perspectives

Alan Merry and Warren Brookbanks
Merry and McCall Smith's Errors, Medicine and the Law (second edition)

Donna Dickenson
Property in the Body: Feminist Perspectives (second edition)

Rosie Harding
Duties to Care: Dementia, Relationality and Law

Ruud ter Meulen
Solidarity and Justice in Health and Social Care

David Albert Jones, Chris Gastmans and Calum MacKellar
Euthanasia and Assisted Suicide: Lessons from Belgium

Muireann Quigley
Self-Ownership, Property Rights, and the Human Body

Françoise Baylis and Alice Dreger
Bioethics in Action

John Keown
Euthanasia, Ethics and Public Policy: An Argument Against Legislation (second edition)

Amel Alghrani
Regulating Assisted Reproductive Technologies: New Horizons

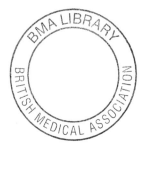